HOME NURSING CARE
FOR THE ELDERLY

Editor
Mildred O. Hogstel, R.N., C., Ph.D
Professor of Nursing
Harris College of Nursing
Texas Christian University
Fort Worth, Texas

Brady Communications Company, Inc.
A Prentice-Hall Publishing Company
Bowie, MD 20715

Publishing Director: David Culverwell
Acquisitions Editor: Ann Moy
Production Editor/Text Design: Patricia King Macht
Art Director/Cover Design: Don Sellers, AMI
Assistant Art Director: Bernard Vervin
Manufacturing Director: John Komsa

Typesetting: Mid-Atlantic Photocomposition, Baltimore, MD
Printing: R. R. Donnelley & Sons Company, Harrisonburg, VA
Typefaces: Novarese Bold, display; Novarese book, text.

Home Nursing Care for the Elderly

Library of Congress Cataloging in Publication Data
Home nursing care for the elderly
Includes bibliographies and index.
1. Geriatric nursing.   2. Home nursing.   3. Aged—Home care.
4. Home care services.   I. Hogstel, Mildred O.
[DNLM: 1. Geriatric Nursing.   2. Health Services for
the Aged.   3. Home Care Services.   WY 152 H765]
RC954.H58   1985   610.73'65   84-25760

ISBN 0-89303-498-3

Prentice-Hall of Australia, Pty., Ltd., *Sydney*
Prentice-Hall Canada, Inc., Scarborough, *Ontario*
Prentice-Hall Hispanoamericana, S.A., *Mexico*
Prentice-Hall of India Private Limited, *New Delhi*
Prentice-Hall International (UK) Limited, *London*
Prentice-Hall of Japan, Inc., *Tokyo*
Prentice-Hall of Southeast Asia Pte. Ltd., *Singapore*
Editora Prentice-Hall Do Brasil LTDA., *Rio de Janeiro*
Whitehall Books, Limited, Petone, *New Zealand*

Printed in the United States of America

85 86 87 88 89 90 91 92 93 94 95   1 2 3 4 5 6 7 8 9 10

Cover logo is an artist's rendering of a wide-barked oak tree, symbolizing a long and full life.

To nurses and family members everywhere
who give knowledgeable, skillful, and
loving care to older people in the home.

CONTENTS

Preface

Contributors

Acknowledgments

v

SECTION III: MANAGEMENT OF HEALTH PROBLEMS AT HOME

SECTION IV: THE FUTURE OF HOME HEALTH CARE

The need for home nursing care is increasing tremendously as the emphasis on care of chronic diseases expands because of a growing older population. Costs for institutional care, both hospital and nursing home, continue to increase also, thus making home health care more attractive to clients and families. Most older people want to continue to stay in the home for as long as possible when illness and/or disability occurs.

Not only is most home health care ultimately less expensive than institutional care, it is far more acceptable to most older people and their families. Institutional care is necessary during acute illness and certain phases of chronic illness, but much of the care needed during the recovery and rehabilitative period can be provided in the home.

The primary purpose of this book is to provide assistance to the practicing nurse who gives care to older clients and their families in the home. The nurse in the home setting is in a unique position to provide skillful and comprehensive health care, including the prevention of possible health problems through teaching, the assessment of potential problems before they become major ones, and the prevention of complications before they become severe when disease is present.

This book is also written for nurses who teach and supervise others who give direct nursing care to older people in the home. It is intended for nurses in all types of home health care agencies, visiting nurse associations or services, proprietary agencies, home services provided by hospitals or long term care facilities, and city and county health agencies which provide home care.

Nursing students in community health nursing courses will find a realistic overview of home health care as well as specific information on nursing care for the most common health problems which are found among the elderly in the home. Students in medical-surgical nursing courses will find adaptations for home care for specific diseases of the elderly.

Section I discusses the external and internal support systems available for home health care in the community. Chapter 1 presents the development and expansion of home health care and the types and organizations of home health care agencies. The multiple resources available in the community which help to provide additional services for older persons who need assistance in the home are discussed in Chapter 2. The important role of the family as the primary support system for most older people who need an increasing amount of assistance of some type is presented in Chapter 3. Chapter 4 provides an overview of hospice care which is increasing as a support system for terminally ill older clients and their families. Legislative, socio-cultural and financial factors affecting these support systems are also included.

Section II emphasizes the important role of the nurse in home health care, especially as a supervisor of home health care and as the leader of the interdisciplinary health care team. Chapter 5 discusses the unique qualities needed by the nurse in home health care and presents the specific functions and role of the nurse who works in this area. The importance of assessing and adapting the home environment to meet the older clients' and families' needs are included in a very practical and realistic way in Chapter 6.

Each of the seven chapters in Section III presents the essential nursing care of specific chronic health problems commonly found among the elderly because many older people live with one or more chronic illnesses for years. Chronic health problems, perhaps more so than many acute conditions, require the cooperation, support, and assistance of the client and the family because these conditions often last a life time. The client and family should be involved in the development of the care plan, if possible, so that the personal, physical and financial resources of the client and family can be utilized in the most effective way possible.

The problems presented are arthritis and osteoporosis, cardiovascular disease, cancer, mental health problems, diabetes and thyroid disease, pulmonary problems, and sensory deficits. Each of the major conditions/problems is discussed together with the related nursing care applicable for the older adult in the home.

Sample master care plans follow each chapter in Section III. Plans are organized to include one or more of the priority nursing diagnoses for the condition and specific observations to make during the assessment phase of the nursing process.

Based on the assessment, the planning phase includes short term and long term patient/client goals. Intervention includes specific realistic nursing orders, including suggestions for patient teaching, as well as a list of related community resources and/or other support systems available for the older adult client in the home. Evaluation includes statements of expected outcomes in an attempt to evaluate to what degree the nursing orders will be effective and the patient goals met.

These master care plans are not meant to be comprehensive. But they will provide the practicing nurse and/or nursing student with a quick reference and review of the major problems to expect, together with the related nursing care needed, when planning to assess and/or care for specific older clients in the home. More detailed implications for nursing care are included within the text of each chapter.

The book concludes with Section IV which proposes some future trends and developing needs in the rapidly expanding and changing field of home health care.

Home health care for the elderly is expanding rapidly. It is my hope that nurses in home health care agencies of all types will carefully assess that expansion, and that they will continue to use their professional and personal knowledge, judgment, and skills in providing high quality care for the elderly in the home.

LAZELLE EMMINIZER BENEFIELD, R.N., M.S.N., Assistant Professor, Department of Nursing, Old Dominion University, Norfolk, Virginia and President, L. Benefield Associates, Home Health Care Consultants, Virginia Beach, Virginia

PATRICIA BOHANNON, R.N., Ph.D., Associate Professor, Graduate Program in Oncology, The University of Texas School of Nursing, Houston, Texas

LINDA KOONCE BROWN, R.N., M.S., Assistant Professor, Harris College of Nursing, Texas Christian University, Fort Worth, Texas

MARTA ASKEW BROWNING, R.N., M.S., Director of Professional Services, Visiting Nurse Association of San Diego County, Inc., San Diego, California

MARY FLO BRUCE, R.N., M.P.H., M.S., Director of Nursing, Cook County College, Gainesville, Texas

ALICE LE VEILLE GAUL, R.N., M.S., Assistant Professor, Harris College of Nursing, Texas Christian University, Fort Worth, Texas

MONETTE GRAVES, R.N., M.S., Emeritus Associate Professor, Harris College of Nursing, Texas Christian University, Fort Worth, Texas

MILDRED HOGSTEL, R.N., C., Ph.D., Professor of Nursing, Harris College of Nursing, Texas Christian University, Fort Worth, Texas

KAREN KAPKE, R.N., C., Ph.D., Associate Professor, University of Wisconsin—Milwaukee School of Nursing and Director, Center for Adult Development, University of Milwaukee—Wisconsin and Deputy Director, Milwaukee Long Term Care Gerontology Center

RODNEY L. LOWMAN, Ph.D., Assistant Professor, Department of Psychology, North Texas State University, Denton, Texas

DAVIDA MICHAELS, R.N., M.S.N., Clinical Specialist, Visiting Nurse Association, Springfield, Massachusetts

LINDA RICHARDSON, R.N., Ph.D., Assistant Professor, Harris College of Nursing, Texas Christian University, Fort Worth, Texas

CAROL A. STEPHENSON, R.N., Ed.D., Assistant Professor, Harris College of Nursing, Texas Christian University, Fort Worth, Texas

SUZANNE DIXSON THOMAS, R.N., C., Ph.D., Assistant Professor, College of Nursing, University of Tennessee, Center for Health Sciences, Memphis, Tennessee

VIRGINIA MAJOR THOMAS, R.N., M.A., Hospice Clinical Specialist, Home Health Services of Dallas, Inc., Dallas, Texas

SUSAN DOUGHERTY WILLIAMS, R.N., M.S., Assistant Professor, Harris College of Nursing, Texas Christian University, Fort Worth, Texas

ACKNOWLEDGMENTS

Much appreciation is expressed to the contributing authors, most of whom are involved in home health care in one way or another. Thank you for sharing your thoughts, ideas, and nursing experiences with the readers. Appreciation also goes to the following for their specific contributions:

—To **Mary Suther**, President of American Affiliated Visiting Nurse Associations/ Services and to **Pam West**, Home Health Services and Staffing Association, for information they provided about their respective organizations contained in Chapter 1.

—To **Janet Henne**, Executive Director, and **Lucille Bub** and **Barbara Verklereen**, clinical coordinators of the Visiting Nurse Association of San Diego, California whose professional example and clinical expertise have provided the framework for the content of Chapter 6.

—To **Andrew Haskett**, Director of Learning Resources Center, Harris College of Nursing, Texas Christian University, for his drawings in Chapter 6.

I also wish to thank typists **Barbara Hancock, Susan Moore, Karen Rudisill, Donna Taylor,** and **LaVonna (Becky) Wilson** for their valuable contributions.

Finally I want to thank my 88-year-old father, **Ole G. Hogstel**, for his patience and continuing support. He often sits quietly beside me while I write or edit.

SECTION I
HOME HEALTH SERVICES
AND SUPPORT SYSTEMS

CHAPTER 1

AN OVERVIEW OF HOME HEALTH CARE

Linda Koonce Brown
and Marta Askew Browning

Need for Home Health Care of the Elderly Grows

In the next decade and beyond, the need for quality home health care of the aged will escalate. The number of older adults in the United States is growing at a staggering rate. Consider these facts:

- The average life expectancy in the U.S. has increased by more than 25 years since 1900. (*Developments in Aging*, 1980, pp. vii–xii)
- In 1970, 20 million people, or 9.8% of the population of the U.S., were 65 years or older. By 1980 these figures rose to 25 million, or 11.3% of the population.
- By the year 2000, more than 35 million people, or 13.1%, will be 65 years or older. By 2050, these numbers will rise to 67 million, or 21.7%. (*Statistical Bulletin*, 1984, p. 17).

Not only will there be more people 65 and older, fewer younger people will be around to take care of them. While the older population of the U.S. has grown almost sevenfold, the population as a whole only tripled, according to *Developments in Aging*, 1980, p. xiii. For example, in the decade of the seventies, the rate of growth for the population under 65 was only 6.3%, compared to 23.5% for the 65-and-over group.

Of course, just because someone is 65 years old, he or she is not automatically in ill health and in need of home nursing care. But one cannot dispute the fact that older Americans are at increased risk for multiple chronic health problems. Some 80% of older Americans have one or more chronic diseases, and half the elderly population have limitations because of these conditions. They can have arthritis, reduced vision, hearing loss, or hypertension (*Healthy People*, 1979, p. 77).

Besides these physical infirmities, psychological factors can create problems for the older adult as well. Among the most common are depression, perhaps from the death of spouse, family or friends; low and fixed-income; fear of financial constraints or difficulty adjusting to retirement.

Most of these problems mentioned will be managed in the home setting with support services from health professionals. Most older people live in their own homes. Rauckhorst, Stokes and Mezey (1980, p. 319) reported that only 5% of people over 65 are institutionalized. Some 13% live with their children, but 82% live at home.

This is where the home health care professionals come in. They can assess the home environment and patient and family behavior, then work for appropriate nursing interventions so that the older adult can remain independent in his or her own home.

To appreciate today's home health care industry, it is important to look at how it emerged, its current condition and where it may be headed.

The Evolution of Home Health Care

At the beginning of this century, health care was provided for older adults in their homes, usually by members of the immediate family and/or by other relatives. Family members were often given emotional support and technical guidance by private duty nurses, nurses from a local Visiting Nurse Association and family physicians. Often, the only people who went to the hospital were those without family or those whose conditions had progressed to a stage beyond the expertise of family or the nursing support system.

Health Care: From Home to Institution

From the 1950s to the 1970s, the trend shifted away from home care. The pendulum began to shift toward institutionalization because of some of these factors:

- Construction of major medical centers and local community hospitals.
- Rapid expansion of medical knowledge and development of new technology.
- Increased mobility of the population, separating family members from traditional support systems.
- Economic pressures which forced women, the traditional caregivers, into the work force.
- The woman's movement, which prompted some women to redefine traditional roles.
- Fragmentation of family units which decreased a sense of responsibility and moral obligation of the family to care for its own.
- Expectation of increasing affluence enabling each generation to rely on its own financial resources.
- Excitement and glamour associated with the hospital which lured health care providers to this new center of practice.

In addition, the course of health care was affected radically by another trend: nurses relinquished their influential roles as the major providers of at-home services to become more dependent on the physician in the institutional setting. As the century progressed, the proportion of nurses remaining actively engaged in community-based or home care practice grew progressively smaller.

This shift is evident in data from a national survey of registered nurses conducted by the American Nurses' Association. An estimated 978,234 registered nurses were employed in 1977. Only 7.9% were practicing in community health settings. The overwhelming majority of nurses, 69.5%, were associated with institutions; 61.4% in hospitals; and 8.1% in nursing homes (Moses, 1979, p. 1752).

The centralization of health care—with the physician as chief and the hospital at the center of the delivery system—defined the character of the health care system and the role of the consumer who used the system. Following are some of the most significant trends.

Financial Incentives Promoted Acute Care

Funding for acute care disease-focused services with the physician as the primary provider increased steadily over the decade. Although verbal support was given to the concepts of prevention and health maintenance, funding for this area was poor.

The Medical System Assumed Responsibility for Health Care

The explosion of medical knowledge and the focus of the delivery system on cure of disease gradually led the public to believe that most health problems could be "fixed". If one did not feel well, he or she simply went to the physician. The physician was expected to write a prescription for a medication which, when taken, would bring a swift cure. As cures were discovered for acute illnesses, such as pneumonia, deaths from communicable diseases decreased and longevity increased. However, chronic disease rates began to rise for conditions associated with poor health habits and altered life styles. Inadequate nutrition, cigarette smoking, physical inactivity, and stress took their toll and were eventually reflected in the rising rates for heart disease, cancer, obesity and emotional disorders.

Focus on Episodic Illness

Health care personnel increasingly derived satisfaction from meeting and resolving acute and/or crisis health needs and began admitting patients for diagnosis and treatment. The acute need having been met, the case was considered resolved. As a result, health care professionals failed to develop adequate strategies for dealing with other needs on the health care continuum, such as:
- prevention of illness
- creation of effective services for the elderly and disabled requiring long term care

- provision of comfort and support to the dying and their families
- involvement of the patient and family in health care decision making.

Development of programs and services to meet these needs were financially unrewarding to the health care professionals and, compared to surgery and modern technology, were not very exciting.

Health Practitioners Preferred Institutions

The home was ignored as a locus of health care delivery, not because it was an inappropriate site, but because providers familiar with the institutional system of care simply were not conditioned to consider the home as a setting for health services.

Home care was overlooked as a field of practice by the universities and teaching hospitals which provided clinical practicums for professional students almost exclusively in familiar in-patient acute care settings. Thus, upon graduation, these new practitioners continued to practice their profession with the in-patient institution as the chief center of practice.

Costs Shifted from Consumers to Insurance

Technology and the training to use technology, along with the cost of operating institutions, caused the financing of health care to exceed the average consumer's pocketbook. Insurance began to shield Americans from the financial impact of unexpected illness. Over the decades, insurance benefits expanded and employers, who had identified health insurance as a major employee benefit, began to subsidize the cost of insurance. The federal government became involved and, in the 1960s, created the Medicare and Medicaid programs which provided an insurance cushion for the elderly, disabled and indigent with acute health care needs. Today, health care is financed in this country primarily by third-party health insurance. The principle provider of such insurance is the federal government, which provides funding through the Medicare and Medicaid programs. In addition, the federal government, through its health insurance programs, provides the major source of financing for home health services, a field the private insurance sector has been reluctant to enter thus far.

Costs Escalated for Health Care

The cost of hospital care, combined with the high costs of medical technology, inflation, and capital expansion of facilities, has brought the Medicare/Medicaid programs to the threshold of collapse. For example, since the introduction of Medicare in 1965, government spending for hospital care has increased eightfold. In 1980, 72% of Medicare payments were for care received in hospitals. The steep and steady increase in hospital costs (approximately 15% per year in 1981 and 1982 respectively) is a major reason why the Medicare program faces bankruptcy between 1986–89 (Dole, 1983). In contrast, estimates of the total amount of money spent for home care in 1981 was $3.1 billion. This amount is a sizable sum, but it comprises only about 1% of the total national expenditure for health care and approximately one-eighth the amount spent for care in a nursing home (Pepper, 1983).

The escalation of costs has caused the delivery of health care to return once again to the home. The system appears to have come full cycle.

Return of Health Care to the Home

The federal government has been forced to seek alternate methods of providing health care to recipients of Medicare and Medicaid benefits. Great interest in home care has evolved in the state and federal legislatures. Numerous demonstration projects are underway and proposed legislation will, if enacted, provide funding for additional ventures which will give data on true costs of home care compared to the financing of institutional services.

These home care demonstration projects test:

- the impact of expanded Medicare/Medicaid benefits on utilization of home care services
- the relationship between home care and the satisfaction of clients
- the cost of treating at home people who are at greatest risk of institutionalization (GAO, 1982, 32–42).

The Effect of Client Consumerism

Economic constraints are forcing professional caregivers, provider organizations, and consumers of service to re-examine their own roles in promoting health and well-being. Changes include:

- participation in physical conditioning
- stress management
- evaluation of the role of nutrition in promoting health and preventing disease
- initiation of no-smoking regulations in public areas
- self-help groups
- publication of self-help assessment and diagnosis manuals
- advocacy for reduction of environmental pollution.

These programs portend an upheaval in the current system of institution-based acute care. Health care in America is in a state of transition with both new and old modes of delivery and multiple provider groups (including the individual consumer) vying for dominance and control of the marketplace.

John Naisbitt (1982, pp. 40–41) in his book *Megatrends,* expressed the opinion that Americans are starting to place technology in a less-exalted role and want "high touch" interactions with other people. This shift in attitude is already becoming apparent in subtle changes occurring in the health care delivery system. Patients and their families are expressing a desire to participate in decisions related to health care.

Patients and their families want the right to:

- know health care alternatives
- choose treatment and/or type of practitioner
- refuse treatment
- give informed consent
- initiate living wills
- receive health care and support services which will enable the patient to remain at home for as long as possible.

The public's desire to return health care to the home and community has resulted in such legislation as the Medicare hospice benefit (described in Chapter 4) Desire for expanded government support for home health care has become a serious political issue. The elderly, a potent political force, have clearly expressed a desire to be maintained and helped at home in non-institutional settings. U.S. Rep. Claude Pepper (D., Fla.), a loyal advocate for the older adult, summarized the need for care as follows (Pepper, 1983):

> "There is compelling evidence that over 3 million older Americans who are in desperate need of home health services are going without the care they need. We allow those people to suffer in neglect until the only choice they have is placement in a nursing home. As a social policy, this is nonsense. Our priorities are misaligned. As a nation, we spend in excess of $25 billion a year to pay for the care of the infirm aged in long-term care facilities and only about $3 billion to maintain them in their own homes. We must do better. We should do our best to take care of our older Americans in their homes and only when this proves to be impossible, only as a last resort, should they be placed in an institution."

Finally, the General Accounting Office (GAO) recognized the desire of government to expand and revise Medicare coverage in its report titled "The Elderly Should Benefit from Expanded Home Health Care but Increasing these Services Will Not Insure Cost Reductions."

The GAO noted the need for the older adult to have care provided in a personal and familiar environment that allows freedom of choice in scheduling daily activities, unrestricted visits by family and friends, and personal control over types of health care services utilized. This study also reported that evidence exists supporting the premise that home care may lengthen the lives of the elderly and most certainly provides a greater sense of independence, satisfaction and well-being (GAO, 1983, p. 45). The major dilemma remains one of financing:

"It has been suggested that the most challenging issue for expanded home care is not whether non-institutional alternatives are less expensive but whether it is feasible, with the resources available, to provide every individual who needs services with a full range of options" (GAO, 1982, p. 39).

Actions taken by the federal government in the funding of home health services over the next few years will be critical for the survival of the home health care industry. Until decisions are made and the direction of the federal government can be determined, the private sector third-party insurance providers are unlikely to expand coverage for home care services for the older adult.

Agencies Providing Home Health Care

Home health care is provided by a variety of community agencies and organizations in the United States. These agencies are classified in various ways. The following categories are based primarily on the Health Care Financing Administration Cost Form (1983–1984):

- Official (governmental) health agencies
- Voluntary non-profit agencies, including Visiting Nurse Associations/Services
- Combination official and voluntary agencies
- Private non-profit agencies
- Proprietary agencies
- Hospital-based programs
- Extended care facilities

Governmental Health Agencies

Official agencies are organizations whose existence is mandated by law and whose primary funding comes from tax revenues. Examples of official agencies include city, county, combined city-county, and state health departments. The populations served by health departments are generally the residents of geographical subdivisions. For example, a city health department provides its health services to people who reside within the geographical limits of the city. State health departments may provide direct services in small or rural communities which do not have their own established local health departments.

The purpose of most health departments is the prevention of illness and promotion of health. In implementing this philosophy, health department programs provide such services as communicable disease control, environmental sanitation, maintenance of birth and death records, laboratory services, public health nursing programs, community analysis, and health education activities.

When home health care is included as one service of an official health department, the nursing division provides the direct services. The public health nurse provides home health care in addition to other types of health care services. Stewart (1979, p. 30) stated that although about half of the Medicare certified home health agencies in 1977 were official agencies, many of these health departments were small and offered limited services. She further stated that official agencies should be considered an important source of home health care.

Voluntary Non-Profit Agencies

Voluntary agencies are not mandated by law or funded by taxes as are government agencies. They are non-profit agencies financed by private funds and exempt from federal income tax. Private funding sources for voluntary health care agencies may include grants, foundations, donations, United Way contributions, insurance reimbursement and client payment. Voluntary home health agencies may also receive indirect tax revenues through the payment of fees from sources such as Medicare and Medicaid.

Jarvis (1981, p. 54) reported that voluntary agencies frequently are founded by groups or individuals who recognize needs for services. These perceived needs may focus on specific population groups or diseases. A voluntary agency is then formed to meet the identified needs through service, education and research. Examples of voluntary agencies that provide home health care include Visiting Nurse Associations/Services and religious or church-related agencies.

Visiting Nurse Associations/Services

Established about 1885 (Stewart, 1979, p. 31), Visiting Nurse Associations (VNA) or Visiting Nurse Services (VNS) are the classic example(s) of home health care agencies with a voluntary structure. The size of the agency and services tend to vary across the United States, from small agencies (with one registered nurse and two or three services), to large, well-established agencies offering the full range of home health care services and employing several hundred health professionals. There are over 500 Visiting Nurse Associations/Services in the United States. They are more common in the Northeast than in the South or Midwest.

Combination Official and Voluntary Agencies

Stewart (1979, p. 33) defined a combination agency as a home health agency created by the merger of an official and voluntary agency. The services of both previous agencies are made available to clients, and funding is usually received from the same sources as before the merger. Advantages of a combination agency are reduced health care costs, less duplication of services, reduced overhead, and lowered capital outlay (Stewart, 1979, p. 33). The nurse in a combination agency may function in a variety of nursing roles similar to the nurse in an official agency (Wiles, 1984, p. 783).

Private Non-Profit Agencies

Private non-profit home health care agencies are privately-owned and exempt from federal income tax. Ownership of this type of agency is held by either an individual or a corporation, with the ultimate authority being the owner. Funding for the private non-profit agency is from client payment, private insurance, and Medicare and Medicaid (if certified) (Stewart, 1979, pp. 34–36). The same basic home health care services are offered, depending upon the size of the agency.

Proprietary Agencies

Another type of agency that provides home health care is the private profit-making (proprietary) agency. These agencies are owned by individuals, partnerships or corporations. Some proprietary agencies are certified to receive Medicare and Medicaid funds, while others are not so certified. Direct payment from clients, third-party reimbursement from insurance programs, Worker's Compensation, and automobile insurance are additional sources of funding (Home Health Care, Upjohn, 1980).

Services offered by proprietary agencies are generally the same as those found in official and voluntary agencies. Services are similar if the private agency is Medicare–and Medicaid–certified. Proprietary agencies often provide extensive in-home services for which the federal health insurance programs will not reimburse. These services, such as nursing or homemaker services, are usually financed by direct client payment and/or private health insurance.

Proprietary agencies have been increasing in number in the United States in recent years. Since the requirement for certificate of need to establish a new health care facility from a Health Systems Agency has been eliminated in some states, proprietary agencies have proliferated. Prior to 1980, proprietary agencies could not be Medicare-certified and reimbursed unless they obtained state licensure. The federal government discontinued the licensing requirement in the Omnibus Reconciliation Act of 1980 that took effect July 1, 1981 (Chiarello, 1983, p. 1C).

Hospital-Based Programs

According to Lundberg (1982, p. 81), a number of factors have contributed to the sizable increase in home health services sponsored by hospitals. Some of these factors are improvements in third-party and Medicare payments, the increasing geriatric population, and emphasis on discharge planning. Changes in home care services have allowed more severely ill clients to be cared for in the home. There has also been an increased awareness of home health care as a viable alternative for clients who wish to remain independent and avoid institutionalization.

Another factor influencing the entrance of hospitals into the home health care field has been the implementation of the Social Security Amendment of 1983. This law provides for a prospective reimbursement system for Medicare based on 467 diagnostic related group (DRG) categories. The large federal deficit, potential bankruptcy of the Medicare system, and the high cost of hospital treatment provided the impetus for this legislation. The law began its three year phase-in period in October, 1983. It applies to Medicare only and not to other third-party insurance payers. The key feature of the legislation is that Medicare payment for hospital costs will be determined and fixed in advance according to the patient's diagnosis, rather than based on the length of stay or services utilized. This fixed fee will be considered full payment and hospitals may not charge the patient more than the deductible and the cost of services not covered by Medicare.

The health care delivery system, as we know it, will change permanently as a result of this legislation (Shaffer, 1983, pp. 388-396). For example, to conserve revenues, patients will be discharged from hospitals earlier to reduce costs of service. Many of these patients will require complex, technological care in the home.

Hospitals themselves, like home health agencies, may be official, voluntary, or proprietary. Structurally, the home health unit may be an independent department or a component of another department. Authority for the home health component ultimately rests with the owner or executive board, depending upon the type of agency. An administrator is generally appointed to direct the home health agency's activities (Stewart, 1979, pp. 36–40).

One advantage of a hospital-based home health agency is its close tie to the hospital—with the wide variety of health professionals such as nutritionists and therapists who deliver the in-patient care and who are also available as resources for home care. Most of the home health agency clients are those who have been patients of the hospital, discharged early and in need of extensive care. Continuity of care in addition to discharge planning and re-admission processes are expedited due to the proximity of the health professionals, the client, and client records.

Extended Care Facility Based Program

Some nursing homes have been adding home health care services to their organizational structure in much the same way and with similar advantages as those discussed for hospital-based home health care services. In this way, clients can be cared for in their homes as long as possible and then be admitted to the nursing home when they need more extensive nursing care. Coordination of care is facilitated for those clients who need alternating maintenance and constant care.

Services Offered by Home Health Care Agencies

Regardless of the type of agency or ownership, most home health agencies provide one or more of the same types of services. Agency staff members must be familiar with the services available in their specific agency to provide their clients and themselves with the services and expertise of the interdisciplinary health care team. Some of the major services offered by home health agencies are:

- skilled nursing care
- physical therapy
- speech pathology services
- occupational therapy
- medical social services
- homemaker-home health aide services
- nutrition services
- medical equipment and supplies.

Skilled Nursing Care

Stewart (1979, p. 47) stated that nursing services provide the "foundation of home health care," because "nursing was the first health service to be provided and remains the one most frequently utilized." Stewart (1979, pp. 46–56) described the role of the home health care nurse as follows:

- providing direct care
- providing indirect care
- acting as case manager
- functioning as a clinical nurse specialist and/or nurse practitioner.

Direct Care

Direct care refers to bedside nursing care, including all phases of the nursing process. The home health care nurse assesses the physiological, emotional and social status of the client and family. Based on the nurse's assessment and information from other health care providers, the nurse formulates nursing diagnoses and establishes the plan of care with the client and family. Implementation includes a full range of nursing care activities such as administration of medications, treatments and procedures. Teaching the client and family self-care techniques and consulting with the physician regarding the client's status are other important aspects of implementation. Interventions to prevent illness and promote health are implemented with skilled nursing care activities (Wiles, 1984, p. 984).

The evaluation phase of the nursing process includes the ongoing assessment of the client's progress toward the resolution of problems, accompanied by modifications in the nursing plan of care.

Indirect Care

Wiles (1984, p. 786) defined indirect care as care that is administered without having direct contact with the client. The nurse serving in the role of consultant or supervisor is delivering indirect care to clients. The home health care nurse may consult with various health care professionals for the benefit of the client. The nurse may work with members of the home health care team in team conferences and with hospital personnel who provide the client's inpatient care. As a supervisor, the home health care staff nurse supervises the care given to the client by paraprofessionals such as the homemaker/home health aide.

In the case manager role, the home health nurse provides for coordination and continuity of the client's care. The nurse does this by facilitating communication between all members of the health care team. The clinical nurse specialist or nurse practitioner functions by providing direct care, consulting with the health care team on managing client problems, and providing inservice education programs to agency staff (Stewart, 1979, p. 55). The specific role of the nurse is discussed in detail in Chapter 5.

Physical Therapy

Although the nurse is responsible for assuring that proper posture and body alignment, normal range-of-motion exercises, and other similar types of physical activities are continued, the physician may order restorative physical therapy to regain, maintain or improve muscle tone and joint movement. The physical therapist, like the home health care nurse, provides direct and indirect care in the home health setting. In providing direct care, the physical therapist evaluates neuromuscular status and implements corrective treatment measures as ordered by the physician (Wiles, 1984, pp. 790–791). Examples of direct care include such procedures as heat packs, gait evaluation and training, ultrasound, therapeutic exercise and massage ("Conditions of Participation," 4-1980, 205.1 A, B, C).

Indirect services provided by the physical therapist include consultation with staff and other health professionals, case management activities, supervision of para-professionals such as physical therapy assistants, and recommendations on equipment and home adaptations.

Speech Pathology Services

Speech pathology services are defined as " . . . those services necessary for the diagnoses and treatment of speech and language disorders which result in communication disabilities" ("Conditions of Participation," 10-81, 205.3A). Restorative therapy may first be implemented until the client's response is insignificant or has reached a plateau. If the patient's response is insignificant, a maintenance program may be implemented and the family instructed in this program ("Conditions of Participation," 10-81, 205.3C). Like the home health care nurse and physical therapist, the speech therapist provides direct and indirect care to the client. The provision of direct care includes evaluation of the client's speech and language abilities. Corrective measures are instituted by the therapist directly and taught to the client and/or family (Wiles, 1984, p. 791). Indirect care includes consultation with and education of other home health care personnel, case management activities and supervision of paraprofessional staff (Stewart, 1979, p. 78).

Occupational Therapy

Occupational therapy is defined as "medically prescribed treatment concerned with improving or restoring functions which have been impaired by illness or injury, or where function has been permanently lost or reduced by illness or injury, to improve the individual's ability to perform those tasks required for independent functioning" ("Conditions of Participation," 11-78, 205.2A). Direct care includes testing muscles and joints to evaluate the client's functional abilities together with assessment of the home for barriers and safety. Treatment plans are designed to restore upper extremity muscle strength and mobility, teach compen-satory mechanisms to aid in independence, and modify the home to enhance the client's activities of daily living. Indirect care consists of consultations with staff regarding compensatory mechanisms and home adaptations for client care (Wiles, 1984, p. 791).

Medical Social Services

Medical social services are those social services that enable clients and families to cope effectively with social and emotional factors affecting their functioning. These services are particularly important when the social and emotional factors affect the client's response to treatment and adjustment to illness. Medical social services are provided by a social worker with a master's degree in social work (Wiles, 1984, p. 791). Direct care begins with assessing the client, family and home situation. The interventions carried out may include counseling, referral to community resources, and advocacy to assist clients in obtaining needed services.

The social worker performs important indirect care by counseling with other staff members regarding family dynamics and difficult or inappropriate behavior by the client/family. Agency personnel may be assisted to understand the client's behav-ior and appropriate responses to that behavior (Stewart, 1979, pp. 79–82).

Homemaker/Home Health Aide Services

When the plan of care for the elderly person is to maintain that person in the home, the most appropriate intervention may be the services of a homemaker/home health aide. This classification of personnel is known by several titles. However, Brickner (1978, pp. 217–220) described the function in three areas: domestic chores, personal care, and paraprofessional health care.

Domestic chores include activities such as washing dishes, preparing meals, sweeping and dusting, running errands, shopping for needed items, doing the client's laundry, ironing and reading to the client. Examples of personal care functions include bathing, mouth care, assisting the client in toileting needs, dressing and walking. Paraprofessional health care services include such activities as observing vital signs, assisting with prescribed skin care regimens, and observ-ing and reporting the client's general condition to the registered nurse (Brickner, 1978, pp. 218–219).

Home health aide services are defined by Medicare as those functions involving the personal care of a patient. These services are included in the physician's plan of care. The specific personal care requirements of the patient are determined by the registered nurse and are supervised by the nurse. In some instances a physical, speech or occupational therapist may supervise the home health aide.

Stewart (1979, p. 59) noted that the homemaker often serves as a role model in teaching and demonstrating personal care to the client. Both Brickner (1978, pp.

220–222) and Stewart (1979, pp. 60–62) stressed the importance of adequate training and supervision of the homemaker/home health aide. They are a part of the health care team and function in a plan of care that is designated by the physician, registered nurse, and/or case manager.

Nutrition Services

Nutrition services in the home health care agency are provided by the nutritionist directly to the client or indirectly through consultation with agency health care professionals. The nutritionist assesses the client's nutritional needs and plans specific interventions, with the physician prescribing therapeutic diet regimens. Dietary teaching and counseling are done with the client and family, and any other person who may be participating in meal planning and preparation for the client. The nutritionist serves as a consultant and educator to home health agency staff when direct services to the client are not feasible. The nutritionist can assist the staff—and in particular the homemaker/home health aide who may be purchasing, planning and preparing meals—in implementing dietary interventions while considering the client's social, cultural and economic status (Stewart, 1979, pp. 84–85). Although client visits by a nutritionist are not Medicare reimbursable, this service is an important one for clients and is offered by some home health agencies.

Medical Equipment and Supplies

Home health agencies provide medical equipment and certain nondurable supplies necessary for client care. Medical equipment constitutes appliances which can be used repeatedly and includes items such as hospital beds, trapeze bars, wheelchairs and crutches. These items may be owned or rented by the agency and placed in the client's home to facilitate treatment ("Conditions of Participation," 3-82, 206 B). Nondurable supplies are those expendable items needed for the home health agency personnel to carry out the plan of care to treat or diagnose a client's illness or injury. Examples of medical supplies include catheters, syringes, irrigating solutions, dressing materials, and oxygen ("Conditions of Participation," 10-81, 206.3A).

Funding for Home Health Care

Funding for home health care comes from a variety of sources. Services for clients may be paid with client and/or family funds, community funds, private or group insurance, Worker's Compensation, Medicare, and/or Medicaid. Although all aspects of health care are expensive, home health care is less expensive than hospital care. The costs for home health care and nursing home care are about the same; (Stewart, 1979, p. 14) however, the benefit of having the client remain in his or her home or the home of a relative increases the advantages of home health care. Because many of the regulations for funding are subject to redefinition or change, the person working in a home health agency will need to be aware of the most current regulations.

Medicare

Medicare is federal health insurance for persons who are 65 years of age or older or disabled. Created by Title XVIII of the Social Security Act, Medicare first became effective on July 1, 1966. Medicare insurance has two separate programs: one part is hospital insurance and one part is medical insurance. Briefly, the hospital insurance component covers in-patient care in a hospital, post-hospital care in a skilled nursing facility, and home health care. The medical insurance covers physician's services, outpatient hospital services, home health services, and other health care services such as X-rays, laboratory work, and rental or purchase of medical equipment (*Medicare and Private Health Insurance* N.D., pp. 6–9).

Medicare pays all costs for an unlimited number of medically needed home health visits. Services covered include part-time skilled nursing care, physical therapy, and speech therapy. If any of the above three services are needed, Medicare can also provide for occupational therapy, home health aide services, medical equipment and supplies, and services of a medical social worker. Disallowed costs include full-time nursing service, visits by a nutritionist, medications, home-delivered meals, and homemaker services that are custodial in nature (*Guide*, 1982, pp. 1–6). Medicare will not reimburse for prevention and health promotion activities. However, the health professional implements these measures in conjunction with visits for reimbursable skilled care (Wiles, 1984, p. 794).

Effective July 1, 1981, Medicare implemented changes that made the financing of home health care less restrictive. Flory (1981, p. 16) summarized the conditions to be satisfied for Medicare *hospital* insurance to provide home health services:

1. The care provided by the home health agency must be skilled care.
2. The care provided must include skilled nursing care, physical therapy, or speech therapy.*
3. The client must meet the definition of homebound.
4. A physician must prescribe the need for home care and establish a plan of treatment within two weeks of hospital or nursing home discharge.
5. The agency providing the home health care must be certified by Medicare to receive reimbursement.

To have home health care services reimbursed under Medicare *medical* insurance, these conditions must be met:

1. A physician must determine the need for skilled nursing and therapy services, (physical or speech)*.
2. The physician must prescribe a plan of treatment for the client.
3. The client must meet the definition of homebound.
4. The home health agency must be certified to receive Medicare reimbursement (Flory, 1981).

---

* Flory (1981, p. 16) also included occupational therapy as a basis for entitlement. However, effective 12/1/81 occupational therapy was eliminated as a basis for entitlement.

Additional requirements for reimbursement are that the nursing or therapy services must be:

- intermittent;
- reasonable and necessary to the treatment of an illness or injury; and
- of such complexity that qualified nurses or therapists deliver or supervise the care ("Conditions of Participation," 5/81, 204.1; 4/80, 205.1; 11/78, 205.2; 10/81, 205.3).

It is also important to note that maintenance or custodial types of care are not reimbursed. Medicare reimburses for services when the client's medical condition is unstable. Once the client has reached the maximum level of functioning and no more improvement can be expected, Medicare coverage ceases. "The key words to remember for Medicare home health coverage are skilled, homebound, intermittent, and unstable" (Wiles, 1984, p. 796). Once all the conditions are satisfied, Medicare will pay 100% of the allowed costs (there is no deductible) for an *unlimited* number of visits (Flory, 1981, p. 16).

Medicaid

Medicaid is funded through Title XIX of the Social Security Act and was implemented at the same time as Medicare. Medicaid is a federal program administered by the states. The federal government provides matching funds to states for development of the state's own health program. The target groups towards whom Medicaid is directed are families with dependent children (AFDC) and the disabled, blind or elderly; and those who lack the funds necessary to pay for care and are receiving Supplemental Security Income (SSI). Medicaid is provided for AFDC and SSI recipients and for the medically indigent (Stewart, 1979, p. 111).

Home health care is one health service provided by Medicaid. Each state must provide nursing services, home health aid service, and medical equipment and supplies. The physician must establish a written plan of care and review it every 60 days. Additional services are determined by each state (Stewart, 1979, pp. 111–12).

Private Insurance

An increasing number of private insurance companies are beginning to offer home health care benefits. The benefits vary from policy to policy and are generally found in the basic policy benefits, major medical benefits, and/or Medicare supplemental policies. Services covered may include any of the full range that home health agencies offer: nursing, therapy services, and medical supplies. There may be limits on the number of visits provided, and the client may be required to pay a portion of the cost of care (Stewart, 1979, pp. 119–20).

Direct Pay

Home health agencies are also able to receive payments directly from clients for services rendered. Direct pay may be necessitated when: the client has no insurance benefit that provides home health care; when benefits expire; when the client must make co-payments with insurance; or when needed services are disallowed by the insurance plan in question. Funds such as United Way may subsidize part or all of some non-covered costs in agencies that receive such funds when clients have no other source of payment.

Licensure, Certification and Accreditation of Home Health Agencies

Home health care agencies are subject to several sets of external standards. The most important of these are the various requirements for state licensure, specific criteria which must be met for Medicare and Medicaid certification, and standards for national accreditation by various organizations such as the national home health care associations and the National League for Nursing.

Gallagher (1981, p. 213) pointed out that there is no consistent method of quality control for home health care. Many states do not have licensure laws. Agencies do not have to be Medicare-certified if they choose not to participate in Medicare, and accreditation is a voluntary process. "This issue should be of concern to community health nurses because there may be a number of agencies for whom there is no means of quality control" (Gallagher, 1981, p. 213).

Licensure

Each state has the option of requiring state licensure for home health agencies. The licensure requirements vary from state to state but may resemble standards for Medicare regulations. If the state has a licensure law, the home health agency's license is issued by the state health department or licensure board. If a state licensure law exists, all home health agencies are required to be state licensed before they can receive Medicare reimbursement. Less than half of the states have licensure requirements, although this trend may increase with the proliferation of home health agencies (Gallagher, 1981, p. 211).

Certification

A second method of providing for quality control is that of Medicare certification. In order to receive Medicare funds, the agency must be Medicare certified (Gallagher, 1981, p. 212). Agencies are evaluated on conditions such as:

- compliance with federal, state and local laws;
- organization of services;
- acceptance of patients, plan of treatment, and medical supervision;
- services delivered;
- maintenance of clinical records;
- agency evaluation (*Federal Register*, July 16, 1973, pp. 18978–18983).

Accreditation

The accreditation procedure is a voluntary process for quality assurance that is jointly sponsored by the National League for Nursing and the American Public Health Association ("The National League," ND., pp. 1–2). The purposes of accreditation are to assess an agency's quality as compared to nationally-accepted standards and to stimulate improvement in home health agencies (NLN Council, 1982, pp. 1–2).

In order to be accredited, an agency conducts a self study report based on the stated standards. Following the self study, a team visits the agency to conduct an on-site visit, after which an accreditation decision is made. The standards on which accreditation are based relate to the agency's community assessment, organization and administration, programs established in response to community needs, agency staff, evaluation processes, and future plans (*Criteria and Standards*, 1980, pp. 1–42).

An accredited agency submits interim reports every three years and repeats the accreditation process in five years. Some 105 home health agencies and community nursing services were accredited as of October, 1982 ("Home Health Agencies," 1983, p. 48).

Organizations of Home Health Care Agencies

Home health care agencies may belong to a variety of national organizations and/ or associations. Appendix A lists the name, address, major functions, and membership requirements for the major national organizations.

National Association for Home Care (NAHC)

The largest of these organizations is the National Association for Home Care, formed in 1982. It provides five classes of membership. Voting members are designated as follows:

- *Provider Members*—Organizations which, as their primary purpose, provide direct health and/or social services to the sick and disabled in their homes.
- *Affiliate Members*—State organizations of home care provider organizations.
In addition, non-voting categories of membership are:
- *Associate Members*—Other organizations interested in home care services.
- *Individual Members*—Persons who are interested in home care but are not eligible for provider or affiliate membership.
- *Honorary Members*—Persons who have distinguished themselves in furthering the purposes of the Association.

The principal purpose of this growing national organization is to provide an organized and unified voice for the home care industry through:

- compilation and dissemination of industry data;

- promotion and interpretation of home care services to those groups, public and private, affecting the financing and delivery of home care services;
- political visibility and action directed toward creating legislation and regulations favorable to the home care industry;
- promotion of high standards of patient care for home care services;
- initiation, promotion and presentation of educational programs;
- initiation, promotion and underwriting of research in home care;
- collaboration with organizations at state, national, and local levels representing home care interests.

This increasingly vocal organization represents more than 1,000 provider-members, including official, voluntary, proprietary, institution-sponsored, and private not-for-profit home health agencies (Bylaws 1982, pp. 1, 2, 9). Issues and activities of this organization are presented in the monthly publication, *Caring*, the National Association for Home Care Magazine.

American Federation of Home Health Agencies, Inc.

The American Federation of Home Health Agencies (AFHHA) is an organization composed of Medicare-certified home health agencies throughout the nation. The board of directors consists of experienced home health agency directors. The AFHHA attempts to influence public policy regarding home health agencies by lobbying for member agencies before Congress, fiscal intermediaries, and the Health Care Financing Administration. This organization has successfully lobbied and testified about numerous health and home health care issues. The organization's newsletter *Home Health Agency Gazette*, reports from Washington on legislative issues. Meetings and educational programs are planned and implemented to keep members updated on home health care issues. The organization also offers its members an insurance package that includes health, life, employee benefits, professional liability and other types of insurance (American Federation of Home Health Agencies, Inc., 1984).

National HomeCaring Council

Organized in 1962 as the National Council for Homemaker Services, the organization adopted its new name—the National HomeCaring Council—in 1981. The mission of this organization is "to promote, develop and ensure provision of responsible homemaker/home health aide and related services of high quality for all families and individuals in need of such service" (National HomeCaring Council, 1982, p. 2).

The Council sets, and promotes adoption of, basic standards for homemaker/home health aide services, provides education for those working with homemaker/home health aide services, provides public information about the services and works for legislation and public policy changes favorable to the expansion of homemaker/home health aide services.

The Council conducts research on methods of service delivery, promotes long-range planning for the use of these paraprofessionals for in-home services and works with organizations on the local, state, national and international level to advance the aims of its programs (National HomeCaring Council, 1982, p. 2).

National League for Nursing (NLN)

The principal purpose of the NLN Council of Community Health Services is to promote NLN's commitment to nursing and quality health care by assisting community health agencies in planning, developing and evaluating their service programs. Voting membership in the NLN Council is available to agencies providing community health services. The NLN Council of Community Health Services provides leadership in establishing standards for accreditation of community health services, provides continuing education workshops and seminars, promotes research, and disseminates information on techniques and approaches in the delivery of community health services. This organization also collaborates with other national groups concerned with quality health care. It interprets community health services to the public, collaborates with other NLN membership groups and develops and publishes materials related to community health nursing and community health services (NLN Council, 1982, p. 1).

Home Health Services and Staffing Association (HHSSA)

HHSSA is a trade organization whose purpose is to advance the views of the home health care industry before Congress, federal regulatory bodies, and state legislatures. The organization is comprised of approximately 1,000 home health agencies from 44 states. This organization represents free-standing (not facility based), investor–owned, proprietary home agencies. Many of the larger home health care chains belong to HHSSA. Being primarily an advocacy organization, it does not focus on research or education activities.

American Affiliated/Visiting Nurse Associations/Services (AAVNA/S)

The American Affiliated Visiting Nurse Associations/Services was organized in 1983 to promote voluntary, non-profit Visiting Nurse Associations/Services as the provider of choice in the delivery of home health care. AAVNA/S is an economic alliance of Visiting Nurse Associations/Services that assists the agencies in networking with each other. Sharing of expertise and such concerns as quality assurance methods and protocols promotes efficient functioning in affiliate agencies. Affiliation with AAVNA/S is open to all VNA/Ss across the country.

Summary

Health care in America has come full cycle in the 20th century: from home-based care, to the high-tech institutional setting and back to an emphasis on home health care. The primary factors in the shift in emphasis to the institution include the construction of major medical centers, expansion of technology, increased population mobility, economic pressures, and centralization of health care with the physician as the leader.

The shift has switched back to home health care because of factors such as: the high cost of institutional care; the trend toward prevention of illness; the increasing number of vocal and politically active elderly and handicapped persons; government financing of health care; and evidence of the cost effectiveness of home health care. This change is receiving increased emphasis in the United States as the number of older adults continues to increase into the 21st century.

Home health care today is offered by a variety of agencies: official, voluntary non-profit, combination, non-profit, proprietary, hospital-based, and extended-care facilities. The major services offered by these agencies include: skilled nursing care; physical therapy, speech pathology services and occupational therapy; nutritional services; medical social services; and homemaker/home health aide services.

Funding for services provided by home health agencies comes from sources such as Medicare, Medicaid and private insurance. Clients may pay directly for services, or United Way funds may subsidize care for indigent clients. The three major sources of quality control that affect home health agencies include state licensure, certification and accreditation. However, home health agencies may not be affected by any of these standards if the state in which they function has no such licensure laws or if the agency elects not to participate in Medicare/Medicaid reimbursement and chooses not to pursue accreditation. The promotion of high quality standards of home care is the primary thrust of national organizations representing various components of the home health care delivery system.

REFERENCES

American Federation of Home Health Agencies, Inc., 429 N. Street, S.W., Suite S-605, Washington, D.C., 20024, 1984

Brickner PW: *Home Health Care for the Aged: How to Help Other People Stay in Their Own Homes and Out of Institutions.* Appleton-Century-Crofts, New York, 1978, pp. 159–64, 217–22

Bylaws of National Association for Home Care. (NAHC) Article II, pp 1, 2, 9, as adopted June 28, 1982

Chiarello B: "There's no place like home—for health care" *Fort Worth Star-Telegram,* Sunday, February 20, 1983, pp. 1C, 7C

"Conditions of participation in home health agencies: Federal health insurance for the aged." *U.S. Department of Health, Education, and Welfare.* Reg. 203–206, August 27, 1968

Criteria and Standards Manual for NLN/APHA Accreditation of Home Health Agencies and Community Nursing Services. National League for Nursing, New York, Publication Number 21-1306, 1980

Development in Aging: 1980 Part I, Special Committee on Aging, United States Senate, Washington: U.S. Government Printing Office, Washington, D.C., 1981, pp. vii–xiii

Dole R: Chairman of the Senate Finance Committee, Keynote Address given at the Spring Legislative Conference of the National Association for Home Care, Washington, D.C., March 14, 1983

Federal Register. Vol 38, No. 135, Washington, D.C., Monday, July 16, 1973, pp. 18,978–18,983

Flory G: "Medicare changes ease home health care financing." *Pennsylvania Medicine*, Vol 84, No. 9, pp 16–17, September 1981

General Accounting Office "Report to the chairman of the Committee on Labor and Human Resources, United States Senate: The elderly should benefit from expanded home health care but increasing these services will not insure cost reductions," Gaithersburg, Md. GAO/IPE-83-1, December 7, 1982

Gallagher B M: "Nursing role in home health care," in Jarvis LL: *Community Health Nursing: Keeping the Public Healthy.* F. A. Davis Company, Philadelphia, 1981, pp. 199–218

Guide to Health Insurance for People With Medicare. National Association of Insurance Commissioners and the Health Care Financing Administration of the U.S. Department of Health and Human Services, Washington, D.C.: U.S. Government Printing Office, HCFA - 02110, pp 1–6, April 1982

Health Care Financing Administration: Cost Report Form, 1983–1984

Healthy People: The Surgeon General's Report on Health Promotion and Disease Prevention. U.S. Department of Health, Education, and Welfare DHEW (PHS), Publication No. 79-55071, 1979, pp. 71–80

"Home care providers join forces as first NAHC meeting convenes," *Am J Nurs*, Vol 82, No. 12, December 1982, pp. 1817–1905

"Home health agencies and community nursing services accredited by NLN/APHA" *Nurs Health Care*, Vol 4, No 1, January 1983, pp. 48–49

Home Health Care. Upjohn Health Care Services, Inc., U.S.A., Pamphlet No HM-6551, 1980

Jarvis, L L: "Health care delivery system", In *Community Health Nursing: Keeping the Public Healthy.* F.A. Davis Company, Philadelphia, 1981, p. 54

Lundberg C J: "Home care legislation," *Hospitals*, Vol 56, No 21, November 1, 1982, pp 81–84

Medicare and Private Health Insurance: A Training Text. Health Care Financing Administration, U.S. Department of Health and Human Services, HCFA 82-01 1101, pp 6–9, N.D.

Moses E, Roth A: "Nurse power," *Am J Nurs*, Vol 79, No 10, October 1979, pp 1745–56

"NLN Council of Community Health Services", *Rules of Procedure.* National League for Nursing, 1982, p. 1

Naisbett J: *Megatrends.* Warner Books, New York, pp 39–53, 1982

"National HomeCaring Council celebrates twenty years of service to the nation," *National HomeCaring Council News,* Special Issue, Vol 20, No 3, 1982, pp 1–4

Pepper C: Chairman of House Subcommittee on Health and Long Term Care, Briefing paper: home health care, to Aging Committee Members, March 11, 1983

Pepper C: Chairman of House Subcommittee on Health and Long Term Care, "Pepper calls hearing to explore home care issues", *News—Select Committee on Aging*, U.S. House of Representatives, Washington, D.C., March 14, 1983

Rauckhorst L M, Stokes S, Mezey M D: "Community and home assessment," *J Gerontol Nurs*, Vol 6, No 6, June 1980, pp. 319–27

Shaffer F A: "DRG's: History and Overview," *Nurs Health Care*, Vol 4, No 7, September 1983, pp. 388–96

Statistical Bulletin, Metropolitan Life Insurance Company, New York, Vol 65 No 1, Jan–Mar 1984, p. 17

Stewart, J E: *Home Health Care.* The C. V. Mosby Co., St. Louis, 1979, pp. 25–45, 46–67, 96–124

The National League for Nursing/American Public Health Association Program for Accreditation of Home Health Agencies and Community Nursing Services. National League For Nursing, New York, Publication no 21-1505, N.D., pp. 1–2

Wiles E: "Home Health Care," Stanhope M and Lancaster J: *Community Health Nursing: Process and Practice for Promoting Health.* The C.V. Mosby Company, St. Louis, 1984.

BIBLIOGRAPHY

Branch L G, Jette A M: "A prospective study of long-term care institutionalization among the aged." *Am J Pub Health*, Vol 72, No 12, December 1982, pp 1373–79

Butler R N: *A Generation at Risk*, Hogg Foundation for Mental Health, The University of Texas, Austin, Texas, 1984

Clemen S A, Eigsti D G, McGuire S L: *Comprehensive Family and Community Health Nursing.* McGraw-Hill Book Company, New York, 1981

"Home care today," *Am J Nurs*, Vol 84, No 3, March 1984, pp 340–342

Jenkins E H: "Homemakers: The core of home health care," *Geriat Nurs*, Vol 5, No 1, January/February 1984, pp 28–30

Livengood W, Smith C, Hallstead, S: "The Impact of DRGs on home health care," *Home Health Care Nurse*, Vol 1, No 1, September/October 1983, pp 29–31, 34

Medeiros C, Barreto-Vega G: "Projecting need for home health services: Analysis of need and demand," *Home Health Review*, Vol 4, No 3, December 1981, pp 32–42

Skellie F A, Mobley G M, Coan R E: "Cost-effectiveness of community-based long-term care: Current findings of Georgia's alternative health services project," *Am J Pub Health*, Vol 72, No 4, April 1982, pp. 353–58

Weinstein S M: "Specialty teams in home care," *Am J Nurs*, Vol 84, No 3, March 1984, pp 343–345

CHAPTER 2

COMMUNITY SUPPORT SYSTEMS FOR HOME HEALTH CARE

Karen A. Kapke

The health status of older people is related to their socioeconomic status, family and living arrangements (Havighurst, 1977, Shanas, 1965; Weil, 1977). Chronic illnesses of older adults are often long-term and require many life style adaptations. The financial and emotional cost of care involved in multiple chronic illnesses is high. The self-care skills needed to manage the chronic illnesses commonly experienced by older adults are often demanding and complex (Goldfarb, 1964). The leading causes of disability and death among the elderly are cancer, heart disease, stroke, diabetes, arthritis, accidents, cirrhosis, pneumonia and suicide (Henricks & Hendricks, 1981). Many older people experience two or three chronic illnesses simultaneously, often compounded by depression or a general state of poor health and nutrition (Estes, 1977, pp. 99–110; Lawton, 1974).

Older people use the health care system more frequently than younger people (*Facts About Older Americans - 1979*, 1980):

> In 1977, older people had about a one in six chance of being hospitalized during a year, higher than for persons under 65 (1 in 10). Among those hospitalized during the year, the proportion with more than one stay was greater for older persons than for younger ones (26% vs. 15%) and the average length of stay was about four days longer (11.1 vs. 7.0 days).
>
> On the average, older people paid more physician visits than did those under 65 (6.5 vs. 4.6 visits) in 1977, and a higher proportion had visited a doctor within the last six months (70% vs. 57%).

In 1977, the nation spent about 29% of its $143 billion dollar expenditure for personal health care on older persons. The per-capita health care cost for an older adult was about two-and-one-half times higher than for younger adults. On the average, the health care of an older adult cost $1745 compared to the $661 spent for younger adults (*Facts About Older Americans - 1979,* 1980).

The demographic and health care utilization characteristics of the older adult population, therefore, support the need for increased services aimed at assisting older people to remain as independent as possible in their own homes. Services are needed not only for the management and self care adaptations for the chronic illnesses experienced by older adults, but services are also needed that will enable people to remain living independently in the community.

In order to accomplish the goal of independence in the home setting, the purposes of home health care should be to provide: (1) family-centered care; (2) comprehensive services supporting independence and self care, and (3) skilled nursing and other professional care that emphasizes prevention, health education, self care, therapeutic interventions, screening and coordination with other health resources (Brody, 1974; Hammerman, 1974; *Home Health—The Need for a National Policy to Better Provide for the Elderly,* 1977; Stewart, 1979).

While considerable progress has been made by communities in providing such services for older adults, significant gaps in services still exist. The nursing profession plays a key role in enhancing the availability of community-based service options for older adults. The nurse has a role to play in planning, implementing, coordinating and evaluating such community-based supportive care systems.

The Spectrum of Support Services for Older Adults

The overall goal of community-based support services for older adults is to allow the person the opportunity to remain living in the community at the highest level of independence possible. Functional independence includes the ability to perform usual activities of daily living, such as dressing, bathing, eating, toileting and ambulating (Lawton, 1971).

The ability to perform other tasks of daily living are important. The older person's ability to remain living independently in the community may depend upon the accomplishment of such tasks as managing personal finances, shopping or getting groceries, using a telephone, performing light or heavy housekeeping tasks, cooking, doing laundry, or engaging in social and recreational activities. Community-based supportive care systems are designed to assist older adults with those tasks necessary for independent community living.

Support services are not intended to replace those areas of functioning in which the person or family is already independent. Neither are they intended to replace the services provided to the older adult by the natural networks of relatives, neighbors or friends. Community supportive care systems are intended to provide services that the older adult or family is not able to perform or obtain. The services are intended to assist older adults to be less isolated and more independent in activities of daily living (Milloy, 1964).

Ideally, supportive care systems for home health would be comprehensive and reflect a long-term care continuum:

> The major goal of a long-term care system is to develop a "continuum of care"—that is, a wide range of services and facilities to provide any level of care needed by a consumer and to have other levels of care available as they may be needed (American Health Planning Association, 1982, p. 8).

This continuum of care includes a full range of health and social services coordinated to accomplish rehabilitative, maintenance, preventive and protective services. This service spectrum also needs to encompass a range of services that focus on the mental and social health needs of the older adult, as well as on the physical health needs.

The home health nurse is often in a key position to assist the older adult to utilize effectively the services across this continuum of care. The homebound older adult may need access to a variety of services provided by multiple agencies. It is helpful for the nurse to become familiar with services available in a particular community. The nurse also needs to be aware of gaps in the continuum of supportive care. The nurse may be able to work with formal or informal care systems to create services where gaps exist.

Various authors have proposed lists of services to be included in the continuum of supportive care services (Brody & Mascrocchi, 1980, p. 1197; Butler & Lewis, 1982, p. 260; Remnet, 1981, p. 445; Stewart, 1979, p. 68). In general, services span in-home, access, protective, supportive, health/medical, recreational, housing and home maintenance services.

Figure 2-1 illustrates those community services most typically targeted to the older adult in the home. This spectrum of services is designed to permit older adults to remain living independently in the community as long as possible. The continuum of care includes such services as: housing alternatives, home repair and maintenance, homemaker services, shopping assistance, friendly visitor, telephone reassurance, pastoral counseling, home-delivered meals, public health department services, mental health services, legal and advocacy services, and adult day care. Transportation and information and referral are access services discussed later in the chapter. These community services supplement those normally provided by home health care agencies.

Housing Alternatives and Home Maintenance

The majority of older adults live in single-family homes for 20 years or longer (Atchley, 1980, p. 321). About half of all older adults in urban areas and about 70% of older adults in rural areas live in a husband-and-wife family unit (Atchley, 1980, p. 321). Many of the 95% of older adults who are living in independent households need some supportive services to maintain that household, however.

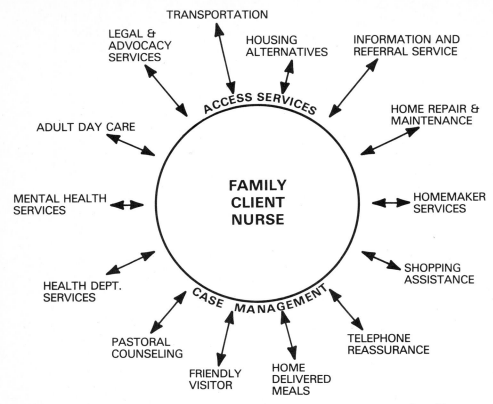

Figure 2.1 The spectrum of community-based supportive care systems for older adults in the home.

Functionally disabled older adults may require increased assistance with home maintenance activities over a long period of time. Other persons may need assistance with household tasks or home repair services temporarily and for a short period of time. In either case, the services provided by community agencies for older adults may include heavy housecleaning, home repair and maintenance (e.g., painting and plumbing services), or yard work (e.g., mowing and snow shoveling). Such services are provided by a variety of agencies, including volunteer groups, churches, senior centers, work exchange programs, youth employment services, county offices on aging, or private companies.

In addition, several programs assist low-income older adults with basic household expenses. For example, older adults may utilize federally subsidized financial assistance services to purchase home heating fuel. They may also pay for their utilities on an annual budget plan. Older adults with low incomes may also benefit from lower cost telephone services, such as limited use or party-line services. Certain tax credits, such as the homestead tax credit, may also apply to low-income older adults who rent or own their home.

Congregate housing and share-a-home programs also help to meet the housing and home maintenance needs of older adults. Congregate housing provides the older adult with an independent living environment in which repairs and upkeep are provided by the landlord. Options include private rental units; condominiums; life-care programs (in which the older person pays an endowment for an apartment and a monthly maintenance fee in exchange for the assurance of nursing home care at the same fee if it is ever needed); federally subsidized low-rent housing complexes; community-based residential facilities or group homes where meals and housekeeping services are provided; or share-a-home programs (in which older adults purchase or rent a home together and share in the tasks and costs of home maintenance).

Home maintenance and repair services are essential for those older adults who are unable to perform these tasks due to functional impairment, low income, or lack of skills. The location of the housing, the resources within the neighborhood, the safety of the neighborhood, or the presence of physical barriers such as stairways are also factors that influence the ability of older adults to live independently in the community. All of these factors should be considered by the home health nurse when assessing the supportive care needs of the older adult client.

Homemaker Services

Another important support service for older adults is homemaker or chore services. Depending upon the functional limitations of the person, a wide range of homemaker services may be needed by older adults. Services should be matched to the person's abilities, with care being taken not to provide more services than needed. For many older adults, housework may be therapeutic. Housework can provide physical exercise, meaningful activity, and a sense of control over one's own environment.

Homemaker services range from assistance with occasional heavy housecleaning (e.g., cleaning the oven, moving furniture, washing windows, washing and waxing floors) to weekly or daily chore services (e.g., dusting, vacuuming, laundry, dishwashing, cleaning the bathroom). Homemaker services are provided by a wide variety of agencies in the community such as volunteers in church programs, county aging units, county welfare agencies or departments of social services, proprietary or non-profit home care agencies, or private businesses.

Homemaker services are often provided in conjunction with home health aide or personal care services. In this way, the homemaker/home health aide would assist the older adult with such activities as bathing and dressing, as well as with basic household chores such as cleaning, cooking, and laundry.

Homemaker, housing and home maintenance services are essential for many homebound older adults. These are services that prevent the need for institutionalization and enable the person to remain living independently in the community. A variety of other supportive services may be available in the community for the home health client.

Shopping Assistance

Home delivery of groceries is a service provided by some merchants. This service is another valuable, although sometimes more expensive, alternative for the older adult unable to go out and buy groceries. The use of catalogue shopping services through major department stores is also a useful shopping strategy for home health clients. Another in-home service provided in some areas is barber or beautician services. In addition, some pharmacies deliver medications and medical supplies to the home. The pharmacist can also answer client's questions about medications and give advice about the use of over-the-counter medications.

Friendly Visitor

A variety of programs are available in communities to provide older adults with social support. For example, friendly visitor services are offered by voluntary health and social service agencies or by church groups. Friendly visitor programs are usually staffed by volunteers. Older adults often serve as the volunteers, thus providing a valuable service for the home-bound older adult and a meaningful activity for the functionally independent older adult volunteer. Friendly visitors often provide a variety of services, such as assistance with correspondence, companionship for visits to the physician, shopping and errand service, recreational activities, and most important, friendship and concern.

Telephone Reassurance

A related program is telephone reassurance. This service gives the older adult a source of daily contact with the outside world and provides reassurance that if the person becomes ill or injured, assistance will be provided within 24 hours. Harbert and Ginsberg explain the function of telephone reassurance programs:

> [A]n unanswered telephone is an alert to the volunteer to have another person visit the residence to determine why the client was.unable to answer the phone (1979, p. 219).

Most programs that check daily on the well-being of the older adult either use a phone call or an emergency signalling device that is worn by the person or that is contained in the apartment to detect lack of movement by the person within the environment (for example, LifeLine and Care Line). These programs are sponsored by various community agencies, including hospitals, nursing homes, and fire departments.

Pastoral Counseling

Another area of significant support for the older adult is pastoral counseling provided in the home. Many churches or synagogues also provide home visiting by parishioners to homebound members. Such services provide a valuable connection to the religious community and serve as a way to meet the spiritual needs of the older adult.

Home—Delivered Meals

Another service that may prevent institutionalization for older adults is the home-delivered meals or Meals-on-Wheels program. These programs may provide one or two meals daily from five to seven days a week. Some programs provide therapeutic diets; others only serve a general diet. Creative approaches by some communities to the development of home-delivered meals programs has extended this resource to greater numbers of older adults. For example, a friend, relative or a volunteer can obtain a meal from a congregate nutrition site and deliver it to the homebound older adult. In other programs, older adults living in remote rural areas are provided with one or more weeks supply of complete frozen dinners. This method of home delivery of meals is less expensive than the delivery of a daily hot meal, and it still provides the person with a way to easily heat a meal and obtain a well-balanced diet.

Butler and Lewis (1982, pp. 266–267) described several other programs that assist older adults to obtain adequate nutrition. Food stamps, for example, increase the purchase power of low-income older adults. They enable older adults to purchase a greater quality and quantity of nutritious foods at a cheaper cost. From time to time, surplus commodities such as cheese and butter, are distributed to low income adults.

Public Health Department Services

Besides the funding sources previously mentioned, city and county health departments prove to be a great resource for the homebound older adult.

Health departments typically provide home visit, clinic and health education services, some targeted to older adults. The health department may also be an important source of information and referral for those in need of supportive home care.

Yet another service provided by many health departments is the health clinic. Public health nurses in these clinics may provide screening measures to detect common chronic illnesses, health assessment, individual health counseling, immunization and group health education programs. Sites for family health clinics may vary by community. In some cases, health departments have developed clinics in congregate housing projects for the elderly or as part of a senior center's programs so that the services are accessible to older adults.

Mental Health Services

Many older adults need mental health services. Wantz and Gay (1981, pp. 106–109) noted that the trend in mental health services has gone from institutional treatment toward home and community-based care.

The incidence of mental health problems is higher among older adults than among the general population. The Task Panel on the Elderly of the President's Commission on Mental Health reported in 1978 that an estimated 15 to 25% of older persons have significant mental health problems ("Elderly Remain", G.A.O., 1982, p. 8).

Mental health services for older adults are not well-developed in many communities, however. Their mental health needs can be complex, including such problems as alcoholism, suicide, depression, Alzheimer's Dementia, neuroses or psychoses. Their needs can be complicated by problems such as poverty, loss of family and friends, isolation, societal stereotyping, or abuse. Mental health services provided by communities may or may not be targeted specifically to the elderly. Ideally, services would include crisis intervention, outpatient therapy, family or group therapy, support groups, and inpatient care. In some communities, home visits are made by mental health professionals for crisis, therapy or follow-up services.

One important component of the community mental health system for older adults is protective services. Atchley describes protective services as those:

> used by the community when it becomes clear from the behavior of older people that they are mentally incapable of caring for themselves and their interests (1980, p. 315).

Protective services are needed by an estimated 20% of older people (Atchley, 1980, p. 315). One challenge of protective services is to gain the cooperation of agencies and the family for referral and follow-up care. The protective services caseworker, working in conjunction with the home health nurse and the family, can help assist the older adult to remain living independently in the community. It is especially important for the home health nurse to assist the older adult to obtain mental health services immediately when a change in the memory, cognition or judgment of the client is noted. In many instances, in the older adult, confusion is a symptom of an underlying physical health problem. When the health problem is treated, the confusion is reversed. Many other mental health problems of older adults, such as depression and alcohol abuse, are known to be readily treatable in an older adult if the appropriate services are available and acceptable to the client.

Legal and Advocacy Services

A variety of legal services have been developed for older adults.

> Older adults are beginning to be viewed as a distinct client group with its own set of problems, such as taxes, wills, pensions, Medicare, Medicaid, Social Security, nursing homes, and involuntary commitment (Harbert & Ginsberg, 1979, p. 222).

In some communities, paralegals employed by social service agencies or law firms provide assistance to older adults in areas related to housing, finances, rights or insurance. Retired attorneys serve as volunteers in some communities and provide legal counsel to older adults.

Monea defined advocacy as "defending and promoting the needs of a client" (1981, p. 614). In conjunction with case management, the advocacy services in many communities help the older adult to negotiate and utilize the many community services designed to meet needs ranging from home maintenance to mental health.

In many instances, the home health nurse may function as a client advocate working with other professionals and community agencies on behalf of the client and the family. In some communities, organized advocacy services are available to older adults. These services may be provided by a variety of sources: ombudsman programs, councils of senior citizen organizations, resident councils or tenant unions of housing complexes, or caseworkers in social service agencies.

Adult Day Care

One last area of supportive care for home health clients is adult day care. The purpose of adult day care is to provide health promotion, maintenance and rehabilitation services by a team of health and social service professionals (Pegels, 1981, p. 61). Generally, the client attends the day care program for two to five days per week. Meals and transportation are often provided as part of the day care program. Socialization and recreational activities are an important part of the services of the day care center. A variety of direct services such as personal care, counseling or health education are also included in adult day care programs. Depending upon the particular thrust of the day care program, specific rehabilitation services may also be provided.

There are many variations of day care programs designed to meet different needs of the older adult client. Some programs are primarily social in nature, providing an outlet for supervised recreational activities, respite for the family, and some personal care services provided within a sheltered environment. Other programs are targeted to special populations, such as adults with mental health problems or groups for Alzheimer's Dementia. Other programs are intended to serve as an intensive rehabilitation program and are often referred to as day-hospital programs.

Other Voluntary Agencies and Organizations

There are a wide variety of specialized organizations in most communities funded in whole or in part by private contributions. (Wilson & Neuhauser, 1982, pp. 239–240). Nurses need to have a working knowledge of these agencies and their basic services. Often, the use of a phone book listing or a community services directory will serve as a good place to begin finding agencies in a particular community.

Some organizations providing services for older adults include: the American Cancer Society, the American Heart Association, the American Diabetes Association, the Arthritis Foundation, the Alzheimer's Disease and Related Disorders Association, the National Society for the Prevention of Blindness, the National

Kidney Foundation, the American Lung Association, and the National Association for Mental Health. These national organizations have local chapters and affiliates in most communities.

A major function of these organizations is community education. They publish excellent teaching tools for the public and the professional. Many have a variety of pamphlets and films available at minimal or no cost. Another service many of the voluntary agencies provide is a speakers' bureau for community education programs. These organizations often fund research and provide scholarships or fellowships for nurses to pursue further education in specialized areas of practice.

Local chapters of these organizations may also provide a wide range of direct services, such as a loan closet of supplies and equipment for home care clients, screening programs, counseling services for individuals and families, support groups for families or clients experiencing a specific major chronic illness, or transportation for visits to the physician.

In addition to these organizations, other programs relevant to the home health care needs of older adults may exist. Programs are targeted for: the hearing impaired, people with colostomies or ileostomies, women who have had mastectomies, individuals who have recently been widowed, or older adults with alcohol or drug abuse problems. Many of these programs are provided by voluntary self-help associations, such as Alcoholics Anonymous, United Ostomy Association, Reach to Recovery, and others. An awareness of the local resources available as support services for home health care will enable the nurse to better meet the needs of clients through effective referrals.

The Coordination of Support Services

Supportive services can be coordinated in a variety of ways. Case management, single agency coordination, or county-wide or state-wide long–term care systems abound. In each case, a wide range of support services are coordinated to enable older adults to remain living independently in their own homes.

The effectiveness of this spectrum of services depends upon: (1) the comprehensiveness of the range of services available to the homebound older adult; (2) the adaptability of the service system in responding to socioeconomic and cultural differences among clients; (3) the mechanisms provided for coordinating and financing the service components; and (4) the strategies used for serving those most in need.

Figure 2–1 depicts the spectrum of community support services for the elderly in the home. It also illustrates the relationship between the client, family and the nurse, who is at the hub of the service spectrum. It also shows how the link between the client and the services is achieved through access and case management services.

Discharge Planning and Case Management

One model used to coordinate community support services for older adults is discharge planning and case management. The nurse in home health often assumes responsibility for case management.

Discharge planning is the process whereby the client's needs are assessed and resources identified. Clemen, Eigsti, and McGuire point out that: "The discharge planning needs of many clients are complex and long-term. Planning for discharge should start the day a client begins using a health care resource (1981, p. 236)."

Many hospitals now have discharge planners and an ongoing multidisciplinary team discharge planning process. Through the discharge planning process, the client's needs are identified and community resources are matched to those needs. Referral to community resources is a critical step in implementing the discharge plan. It is important for the nurse involved in discharge planning to be aware of the range of community-based supportive care systems available for the older adult client. In the discharge planning process, care must be taken not to duplicate services already used by the client or provided by the family or informal support networks of the client. It is also important to recognize that the family and the client have the right to select among service alternatives and accept or reject referral suggestions.

Some barriers to effective referral in the discharge planning process include: (1) the attitudes of the professionals that can discourage or frustrate clients; and (2) cost or accessibility of the community resources (Clemen, Eigsti, & McGuire, 1981, p. 250).

The referral process is best accomplished by a team approach that brings a thorough knowledge of the client's needs, community resources, and potential barriers for the client in gaining access to or in using resources. For example, a Jewish client may refuse to use home-delivered meals unless the meals are prepared in a Kosher kitchen. Minimally, the referral team needs to include the client, the family, the informal support networks of the client, the physician, the nurse, and the social worker. Depending upon the needs of the client, there may also be a need for other professionals to be involved with the discharge planning process, such as therapists, the clergy, or legal advocates.

In planning for discharge and in providing referral and case management, the home health nurse may need to consider the following questions as a guide to discharge and case management decisions:

1. How much of the case management and the provision of services should be provided by the nurse or other service providers, versus by the client or the family directly?
2. Does the assessment and the discharge planning process encompass concern for the mental, social, physical and environmental needs of the client?

3. Does the mix of supportive services to be provided compensate for the activities of daily living that the client is not able to do without compromising the client's ability to regain the strength to perform these activities?
4. Does the client have access to a sufficiently broad range of services to maintain the safety and quality of the environment as well as the health and well-being of the client?
5. Are the services the best possible match for the social and cultural characteristics of the client?
6. Will the client have access to a team of multi-service providers who will respect the client's rights for self-determination?

Single Agency Coordination

One model targeted to older adults is the single agency approach. This approach seeks to provide a broad spectrum of services within the context of one organizational structure, thereby enhancing the coordination of the services as the client moves through the various components of the continuum of care (Fisk, 1982). In this model, a hospital, for example, would develop a continuum of care and would manage the case for the clients as they moved through the care system.

This model has been extended into countywide or statewide programs for the coordination and financing of community-based long–term care systems (e.g., Quinn, Segal, Raisz, & Johnson, 1982; Seidl, Applebaum, Austin, & Mahoney, 1981; Hageboeck, 1982). As such programs develop, nurses should be involved in drafting the enabling legislation, in implementing the programs, in evaluating the programs, in articulating the role of nursing in community-based long-term care, and in developing innovative models for the delivery and financing of home health nursing care for older adults.

The Aging Network

A most important set of resources for communities involved in planning, implementing and coordinating supportive care systems for older adults are the aging network services funded by the Older Americans Act. Each state unit on aging serves as the funding channel for a variety of services (Leach & Martin, 1981, pp. 453–455). The services provided to communities through Older Americans Act funding include in-home, transportation and nutrition services. In addition, area agencies fund many of the supportive care services that have been described in this chapter. The Area Agency on Aging network serves a critical role in the assessment of the long-term care needs of older adults in each community. Based on their assessments, the aging network then assumes a leadership role in most communities by planning and implementing services that assist older adults in remaining independent in the community.

Access Services

Access services are a critical link in the provision of community-based support services for older adults in need of home health services. Access services include transportation as well as information and referral services. Such services give the older adult access to information, resources and services in the community.

Many communities provide a centralized information and referral service. With a telephone call, the older adult can get information about any of the services in the community targeted to the health and social service needs of the elderly. In some communities, there may also be a specialized information and referral service just for older adults. The information and referral numbers are not only useful to the client but also to the family and nurse.

Transportation is often a problem for the elderly in the home. Atchley distinguished three groups of older adults who have transportation needs:

(1) those who could use existing public transportation but could not afford it;
(2) those who for one reason or another need to be picked up and returned directly to their homes; and
(3) those who live in areas where there is no public transportation (1980, p. 319).

In some communities there is specialized transportation for handicapped adults. In addition, reduced fares may be available for older adults able to use traditional forms of transportation such as buses and taxis. A van or bus may be available through the Y.M.C.A., a senior center, or a congregate housing site. Some communities have a system called Dial-A-Ride, in which older people call to arrange transportation. Some grocery stores bring older adults to the store one day a week. In some communities, the local transit authority may provide free access to a bus one or more times a year for nonprofit groups serving older adults. Some senior centers, for example, use the municipal bus service to provide groups of older adults with recreational trips.

In addition to the access services provided through publicly financed programs, there may also be a variety of services funded through the private sector. In some communities, organizations such as the American Red Cross, the American Cancer Society, or the Arthritis Foundation provide transportation or referral services.

A very important resource in many communities is a program provided through churches for older adults. Church-sponsored programs include friendly visitor services; shopping services, companion services for trips to the doctor; outreach and referral services; directories of community agencies, and others. In some communities, clusters of churches and synagogues working together have developed a powerful network of outreach and access services for homebound older adults.

The nurse working with home health clients needs to know types of transportation services available and their limitations. Some communities, especially in rural areas, lack services. Often, there is a requirement of a one- to two-week reservation. This lead time can work against an older adult who needs to see a physician within a week. Some older adults find any form of public transportation frightening. They may be agoraphobic or paranoid, or afraid of falling, getting lost, or being assaulted. Therefore, the nurse may need to do more than inform the client about available services. The client may need help identifying the fears and setting up strategies to cope.

CASE PRESENTATION: MRS. MAY

Mrs.May, a 90-year-old white female, lived in a large federally subsidized apartment complex for the elderly. She lived there for eight years and had many friends in the building. Her daughter-in-law lived about 20 miles away, and three children lived in other states. Her telephone was a primary source of communication. She enjoyed watching television and occasionally did sewing and mending.

In general, Mrs. May described her health as good for her age, despite her very frail physical health state. She said her strength was her mental outlook and her positive self-concept. She had been hospitalized about 30 times, most occurring during the past 20 years. She took Inderal for her blood pressure and Donnatol to prevent the recurrence of an ulcer.

Mrs. May was most recently hospitalized with pneumonia. She was found in her apartment by a friend. She was very short of breath and incoherent. When she was hospitalized for the episode of acute pneumonia, a gerontological nursing clinical specialist visited her at the hospital. The nurse, who gave weekly clinics at her apartment building, was able to provide the hospital staff with background information about Mrs. May's condition prior to hospitalization. This was very important because she was experiencing an hypoxia-induced aphasia, and she was unable to communicate effectively with the staff.

Discharge planning began as soon as Mrs. May started responding to medical and nursing interventions. After a few weeks of hospitalization, she was ready to go home. Discharge planning meetings were held with Mrs. May, her daughter-in-law, the nurse from the apartment complex, the physician, the social worker, and the hospital discharge planner. The physician wanted to admit Mrs. May to a nursing home for an extended convalescence, but the nurse and Mrs. May were able to convince him that adequate resources were available to her at her apartment.

Services were obtained from the Visiting Nurse Association, including home health aide services. One of her neighbors was recruited to cook her a hot meal a day and eat with her. This met some of her needs for socialization. Mrs. May was able to prepare the other two meals herself. The pharmacist delivered medications. Her daughter-in-law or friends brought her groceries.

The nurse from the apartment complex continued to monitor Mrs. May's progress and the effectiveness of the supportive care systems. After a few weeks, Mrs. May's strength improved significantly. Her cardiac and respiratory status were stable, and she had gained back the weight lost in the hospital. She was ambulating around the apartment complex and taking short trips with her daughter-in-law. The Visiting Nurse Association services were discontinued, and Mrs. May resumed preparing her own meals.

Over the next year, Mrs. May had several other health problems. With ongoing nursing interventions from the gerontological nursing clinical specialist and occasional home visits by the physician, Mrs. May's problems were treated successfully, and she was able to remain living independently in her own apartment. The nurse continued to help Mrs. May as her health needs changed. Through effective case management, the nurse was able to monitor the effectiveness of the community support systems.

Summary

Community-based supportive care systems are designed to help the older adult remain living independently in the community. Most older adults live in their own homes and need services either on a long-term or a short-term basis. Supportive care services are intended to supplement those activities that the older adult is able to accomplish independently or with the assistance of family or friends.

A full spectrum of services are needed in the community to assist older adults to remain living independently. The services often needed by older adults include: housing and home repair services; shopping assistance; friendly visitor; telephone reassurance; pastoral counseling; home-delivered meals; public health department services, including health clinic and home visits by public health nurses; mental health services spanning crisis intervention, outpatient, inpatient, and protective services; legal and advocacy services; and adult day care services.

These services are provided in many communities by: government agencies, voluntary groups, churches, centers on aging, and other health and social service agencies.

The nurse needs to be familiar with the range of services provided in a community targeted to the home care needs of older adults. It is also important for the nurse to understand how to coordinate community-based supportive care systems. The nurse often assumes an important role in discharge planning and case management. The nurse may also work with an agency that uses a single-agency coordination approach for supportive care services. Access services, such as information, referral and transportation, provide the vital link between the client and the service network.

The case presentation of Mrs. May illustrates the role of the nurse in information and referral, discharge planning, and coordination of community-based care for a healthy vulnerable older adult in the community. A wide range of services enabled this client to remain living independently in the community.

REFERENCES

American Health Planning Association: *A Guide for Planning Long Term Care Health Services for the Elderly.* American Health Planning Association, Washington, D.C., 1982.

Atchley, R: *The Social Forces in Later Life* (3rd ed.). Wadsworth Publishing Co., Belmont, California, 1980

Brody S: "Evolving health delivery systems and older people." *Am J Pub Health*, Vol 64, No 3, 1974, pp 245–48

Brody S, Mascrocchi C: "Data for long-term care planning by health systems agencies." *Am J Pub Health.* Vol 70, No 11, 1980, p. 1197

Butler R, Lewis M: *Aging and Mental Health* (3rd ed.) C.V. Mosby Co., St. Louis, 1982.

Clemen S, Eigsti D, McGuire S: *Comprehensive Family and Community Health Nursing.* McGraw-Hill, New York, 1981

Elderly Remain in Need of Mental Health Services (G.A.O. Publication No. HRD-82-112). General Accounting Office, Washington, D.C., 1982

Estes E: "Health experience in the elderly." In Busse E, Pfeiffer E (eds.): *Behavior and Adaptation in Late Life* (2nd ed.). Little, Brown & Co., Boston, Mass 1977

Facts About Older Americans—1979 (DHEW Publication No. OHDS 80-20006). Administration on Aging, Washington, D.C., 1980

Fisk A: "Comprehensive health care for the elderly." *J Am Med Assoc*, Vol 249, No 2, 1983, pp 230–36

Goldfarb A: "Responsibilities to our aged." *Am J. Nurs*, Vol 64, No 11, 1964, pp 78–82

Hageboeck H: *A Training Manual on the Components of a Community Based Long Term Care System for the Elderly.* University of Iowa, Iowa City, Iowa, 1982

Hammerman J: "Health services: Their success and failure in reaching older adults." *Am J Pub Health*, Vol 54, No 3, 1974, pp 253–56

Habert A, Ginsberg L: *Human Services for Older Adults: Concepts and Skills.* Wadsworth, Belmont, California, 1979

Havighurst R: "Perspectives on health care for the elderly." *J Geront Nurs*, Vol 3, No 2, 1977, pp 21–24

Hendricks J, Hendricks C: *Aging in Mass Society: Myths and Realities* (2nd ed.) Winthrop, Cambridge, Massachusetts, 1981

Home Health—The Need for a National Policy to Better Provide for the Elderly. U.S. General Accounting Office, Washington, D.C., 1977

Lawton M: "The functional assessment of elderly people." *J Am Geriat Society*, Vol 19, No 6, 1971, pp 465–81

Lawton M: "Social ecology and the health of older people." *Am J Pub Health*, Vol 64, No 3, March 1974, pp. 257–60

Leach, R, Martin C: "Governmental Resources for the Elderly," in Hogstel MO (ed): *Nursing Care of the Older Adult.* John Wiley and Sons, Inc., New York, 1981, pp 453–55

Milloy M: "Casework with the older person and his family." *Social Casework*, Vol 45, No 8, 1964, pp 45–56

Monea H: "The geropsychiatric public health nurse: A model for comprehensive mental health care." In Ebersole P, Hess P (eds.): *Toward Health Aging: Human Needs and Nursing Response.* C.V. Mosby, St. Louis, 1981

Pegels C: *Health Care and the Elderly.* Aspen Systems Corp., Rockville, Maryland, 1981.

Quinn, J, Segal J, Raisz J, Johnson C: *Coordinating Community Services for the Elderly.* Springer Publishing Co., New York, 1982

Remnet V: The home assessment, in Burnside I: *Nursing and the Aged* (2nd ed.), McGraw-Hill, New York, 1981

Seidl F, Applebaum R, Austin C, Mahoney K: *Delivering In-Home Services to the Aged and Disabled: The Wisconsin Experiment.* University of Wisconsin, Madison, Wisconsin, 1981.

Shanas E: "Family help patterns and social class in three countries." In Neugarter B (ed.): *Middle Age and Aging: A Reader in Social Psychology*. The University of Chicago Press, Chicago, 1968

Shanas E: "Health care and health services for the aged." *The Geronto*, Vol 5, No 3, September 1965, pp 240, 276

Stewart J: *Home Health Care*. C.V. Mosby, St. Louis, 1979

Wantz M, Gay J: *The Aging Process: A Health Perspective*. Winthrop, Cambridge, Massachusetts, 1981

Weil, P: "Dominant patterns of older persons' health status and health services use." *J Geront Nurs*, Vol 3, No 2, 1977, pp 25–32

Wilson F, Neuhauser D: *Health Services in the United States* (2nd ed.), Ballinger, Cambridge, Massachusetts: 1982

BIBLIOGRAPHY

Abel N: "Daytime care lets elderly people stay home at night." *Modern Health Care*, Vol 6, No 1, 1976, pp 23–28

Brody E: "Long-term-care for the elderly: Optimums, options, and opportunities." *J Am Geriat Society*, Vol. 19, No 6, 1971, pp 482–94

Chamberlain R: "Geriatric day care—filling the service gap between home and nursing home." *Health Values: Achieving High Level Wellness*, Vol 5, No 2, 1981, pp 67–69

Dunlop B: "Expanded home-based care for the impaired elderly: Solution or pipe dream?" *Am J Pub Health*, Vol 70, No 5, 1980, pp 514–19

Ehrlich P: *Mutual Help for Community Elderly: Mutual Help Model, Volumes 1 & 2* Southern Illinois University, Carbondale, Illinois

Federal Council on the Aging. *The Need for Long Term Care: Information and Issues* (USDHHS Publication No. OHDS 81-20704). Office of Human Development Services, Washington, D.C., 1981

Freeman R, Heinrich J: *Community Health Nursing Practice* (2nd ed.), W.B. Saunders, Philadelphia, 1981

Hennessey M, Gorenberg B: "The significance and impact of the home care of an older adult." *Nurs Clin North Am*, Vol 15, No 2, 1980, pp 349–60

Hickey T: *Health and Aging*. Brooks/Cole, Monterey, California, 1980

Holmes M: *Program Development Handbook for State and Area Agencies on Homemaker and Home Health Services for the Elderly* (USDHEW Publication No. OHDS 78-20019). Administration on Aging, 1980

Home Health Care Programs: A Selected Bibliography (USDHEW Publication No. HRA 79-60). Division of Nursing, Health Resources Administration, 1979

Kahana E, Coe R: "Alternatives in long-term care," in Sherwood S (ed): *Long-Term Care: A Handbook for Researchers, Planners, and Providers*. Spectrum, New York, 1975

McKeehan K (ed): *Continuing Care: A Multidisciplinary Approach to Discharge Planning*. C.V. Mosby Co., St. Louis, 1981

Murray R, Huelskoetter M, O'Driscoll D: *The Nursing Process in Later Maturity*. Prentice-Hall, Inc., Englewood Cliffs, New Jersey, 1980

O'Brien C: "Adult day health care and the bottom line." *Geriat Nurs*, Vol 2, No 4, 1981, pp 283–86

Oktay J, Sheppard F: "Home health care for the elderly." *Health and Social Work*, Vol 3, No 3, 1978, pp 36–47

Somers A: "A Long-term care for the elderly and disabled: A new health priority." *N Eng J Med*, Vol 307, No 4, 1982, pp 251–52

Somers A, Moore F: "Homemaker services—essential option for the elderly." *Public Health Reports*, Vol 91, No 4, 1976, pp 354–59

Spencer M: "Nursing role in gerontology." In Jarvis L (ed): *Community Health Nursing: Keeping the Public Healthy*. F.A. Davis Co., Philadelphia, 1981

Steinberg R, Carter G: *Case Management and the Elderly*. Lexington Books, Lexington, Massachusetts, 1983

Wan T, Weissert W, Livieratos B: "Geriatric day care and homemaker services: An experimental study." *J. Geront*, Vol 35, No 2, 1980, pp 256–74

Ward R: *The Aging Experience: An Introduction to Social Gerontology*. J.B. Lippincott Co., New York, 1979

Warhola C: *Planning for Home Health Services: A Resource Handbook* (USDHHS Publication No. HRA 80-14017). Health Resources Administration, 1980

Wells T: *Aging and Health Promotion*. Aspen Systems Corporation, Rockville, Maryland, 1982

CHAPTER 3

THE ROLE OF THE FAMILY IN HOME HEALTH CARE

Susan Dougherty Williams

The family continues to be a valuable resource in preventing the institutionalization of an older family member. The combination of home health care agencies, other support systems in the community, and the family will provide care and support to older persons and allow them to maintain more independence by staying at home alone or with family members. The increase of elderly in the home will require more home health nurses to provide care and to teach the family techniques of care.

When the family has agreed to ask the ill older person to live in their home, there are changes this situation will bring to their lives. The family takes on the role of caregiver, teacher, counselor and supporter. Many families do not have the knowledge, resources or skills to provide older family members with optimum care and support. It is often necessary for the family to contact a home health agency or other community support groups which can provide home health care and teaching for the client and the family. The family can act as a support to the older adult only when they have the needed knowledge, understanding and skills. The family should learn how to enjoy the older person at home.

Changes in Family Roles

The home health nurse has to have a good understanding of family structure and the ways family roles change when an older adult moves into the family's home. Each family member will be affected differently by an older person being in the home. Adults have established lives away from parents, and when one or more parent is introduced back into their lives in a closer relationship, the relationship may go through a major change. In the parent-child relationship, the parent nurtures and cares for the child. Roles often change when the child becomes the caregiver and supporter for the older person.

Family roles may change when the older person relates to the younger children in the family. The children see their own parents being "parented" and find it hard to understand why their parents can be told what to do. With multiple generations living under one roof, there will be differences of opinion on how to discipline and on what is acceptable behavior for the children. What is considered appropriate behavior, based on the values and beliefs of the older person, may be different from the younger parent. For example, the two generations may disagree on allowances and dating patterns of the grandchildren.

The young person can gain a better understanding of the aged and the problems they face when they see these problems in the older person living with them. However, the older adult can also become an adviser and confidant of the child and give the child a wider sense of family.

Changes may also occur in the husband-wife relationship. The wife's major role may have been the care of her husband and children. When she adds another responsibility—care of the older person—conflict may develop. The wife may have to give up her career for a period of time. Role fatigue often occurs for caregivers when they are confined at home, and their activities outside the home are diminished (Goldstein, 1981). Fatigue leads to hostility, anger, guilt and depression. It would be wise to encourage everyone in the family to make time for themselves apart from the new family responsibilities.

Changes of life style and adjustments in relationships will also be part of the changes a family will experience as they introduce the older person into their family circle. Role conflict, generational differences, and loss of some freedom are other problems the family may experience. A family can gain much, however, by the experience the older person brings to the family.

In interventions with the client, the home health nurse should assess the strengths and coping skills of the family. Without these strengths, the family cannot be an active support group for the older person. The home health nurse also can help the family and older person during their discussions about the pros and cons of staying at home when skilled care is needed.

Changes for the Elderly Person

Moving into a family member's home will cause role changes for the older family member. Moving into a family member's home is an example of a "maturational" crisis for the older person. Maturational crises occur across the life spectrum when a person perceives a stressful event as a threat to his equilibrium. His usual coping mechanisms are not sufficient to handle the situation (Williams, 1974, p. 43). Independence is often hard to relinquish. This problem is especially true if the older person owned his or her own home for a long period of time. When older people live in someone else's home, they have to consider others before making some decisions. It takes time for older people to realize that they will have to accept assistance from the child and adjust to the new relationships their physical or mental limitations have caused.

Sense of identity can also be altered. An older person who has always been Mrs. Brown who lives at 1200 Elm Street is now the mother of Sally Smith and lives with her at 2400 Macon Drive. Mrs. Brown begins to become identified with her daughter rather than maintaining her own independent identity.

The freedom the older person has had in the past will also be altered by physical and mental conditions. A change in physical or mental status may be the main reason the older person is moving in with the family. It is very difficult and frustrating for older people to accept the fact that they can no longer care for themselves and that they have to be dependent on someone else. It is well to remember that the best action by the nurse is to have the family plan *with* the older person and not *for* him or her. This action gives older clients a greater sense of independence and control over their lives.

Potential Family Problems

With the introduction of any new member into an established home, problems can occur. If all members of the family do not agree that the older person should move in with the family, there will be immediate problems. If the husband, wife, children or other family members are reluctant to have the older person move into the home, the problem should be discussed. Reasons why individual family members do not want the older person in the home should be explored and discussed. Questions that often arise are: "Am I going to have to give up my room?" "How will I have time to care for my husband and the children too?" "Will we be able to take care of her?" Does this mean we can't take any more of our short weekend trips?" If agreement cannot be reached, the family should explore other options.

Questions that the family and older person must consider and discuss before the older person moves into the home are:

- Do all family members agree to have the relative move in with the family?
- What kind of nursing care will be needed, and who will provide that care?
- What community resources are available to assist the client and the family?
- Is the home structurally safe for an older person?
- What adaptations will be required in steps, rails and bathrooms?
- What changes can be expected to occur in the family?
- What changes can be expected to occur in the older person?
- What are the potential problems?

By being aware of some of the potential problems that might develop, families and the older person can avoid or diminish these conflicts by discussing how they will handle them. The home health nurse should be aware of potential problems that could develop and assist the family early to plan for these. Potential problems which may occur are described below.

Space

If someone in the family has given up a room for the older person, conflict may develop because each person in the family does not have his or her own private space at home. A specific area of the house or a scheduled time to use a certain room should be allotted to each member for some private time. Family caregivers who work at stress-producing jobs particularly need some place to unwind. Stress levels will increase, for example, when the caregiver is exposed to the noisy voices of children while receiving requests for physical assistance from an older parent as soon as the caregiver arrives. The nurse could help the family understand this type of problem and suggest that the caregiver have 15 to 20 minutes of quiet time alone initially before getting involved with family requests and tasks.

Possessions

Older people may want to move some of their personal possessions into the family home. A favorite chair, a grandfather clock, or another piece of furniture the older person has had for many years will ease the transition from one home to another. Other family members may not like the possessions or have room for them, however, so the family should first decide what possessions will be moved into the home and what adjustments will need to be made.

Entertaining

There will be times when the older person or younger family member will not want to include each other while entertaining friends. All family members should be asked ahead of time if they can have this night "just for my friends." Other family members could stay in their room or plan to be out for the evening. Older family members are encouraged to maintain their own friends and/or seek new friends their own age, thus not solely relying on their adult children for entertainment.

Responsibilities and Chores

Older family members should feel that they are part of the family and, therefore, should be included in the responsibilities of the household, if able. The parent should not be made to feel like a guest but like a responsible family member. Children often find it difficult to understand that if the parent is "waiting" on grandmother, why can't she "wait on me?" Chores and responsibilities should be explained and assigned to *all* family members so that everyone does his or her part.

If physically able, the older person could assume the responsibility of taking out the garbage, working in the yard, doing minor repairs around the house, washing dishes, or dusting furniture. Perhaps older family members could start a small garden in the back yard, thus giving them a worthwhile activity, much-needed exercise, and fresh vegetables. An older person in a wheelchair can even dry dishes or fold clean linen.

Expenses

Added expenses for food, home maintenance and utilities often occur with the addition of another person in the home. The thermostat may have to be set higher in the winter because older family members get cold easily. The purchase of drugs or medical supplies may be a major expense. The question arises as to whether the family should pay all of the additional costs or whether the other children who live far away should pay their share of expenses. Discussions should be held ahead of time on the problems of finances and how the family will meet these costs. One solution is to arrange for the out-of-town children to send a fixed amount of money each month to help the family that is caring for the older person in their home. The adult children should resolve this possible problem very early in order to prevent hidden hostility, anger and broken family relationships later. Open and frank family discussions about money are essential.

Vacations

A debate often occurs in the family concerning vacation plans. A frequent comment is: "We want to go here for our vacation, but I don't think Grandmother could keep up with us and who would stay with her at home?" What does the family do? The family should determine how mobile and physically able the older person is to take a trip and whether he or she wants to go. The family should decide whether or not the older family member should be included on the vacation. If the older family member is not able to take a trip or prefers not to go, perhaps an out-of-town family member could stay with the older person while the family is away. This plan gives the older family member something special and allows the rest of the family to take their vacation alone. If the older family member is quite dependent, arrangements could be made for care in a nursing home for the length of time the family is on vacation.

Childrearing

An older family member can often be heard saying something like this: "If I would have done that when I was his age, I would be sent to my room." It is often hard for different generations to accept behavior that differs from what they believe. Older people need to understand that they can offer advice, but that the rearing of the children rests with the parents.

Coping with Family Problems

When family problems develop, the home health nurse can assist the family in resolving them. Some stress is normal and essential for life and growth. Stress can provide the stimulus needed to adapt to the changing conditions caused by the addition of an elderly family member. Selye (1975, p. xi) found that any emotion or activity causes stress. Family problems described previously cause stress. If enough stresses are added, a crisis occurs. Caplan (1964, p. 18) identified the four characteristic phases of a crisis as: 1) the initial phase when tensions rise; 2) a second stage when tensions increase because the crisis has not been resolved; 3) a third stage when increased tension stimulates new problem solving; and 4) an acute stage when the situation is extremely difficult to tolerate.

If the family and the home health nurse are aware of how crises develop, intervention may prevent the crisis from occurring. What interventions can facilitate a solution? The nurse can:

- assist the client to confront the crisis;
- help the client confront the crisis in manageable doses;
- assist the client to discover the facts surrounding the perceived crisis;
- give the family honest assurances;
- encourage the family not to blame others;
- encourage the family to accept help;
- aid the family with everyday tasks and situations.

Solving problems takes time. The home health nurse and the family should guard against expecting change too rapidly. Supportive guidance and positive reinforcement need to be continued on a long-term basis.

Assessment of Potential Client Problems

A tool to help the nurse assess the problems the family will have in managing chronic illness at home has been suggested by Straus (1975). Using this framework, the nurse can help the family explore problems that might arise while caring for a chronically ill older person in the home. This model also will help the nurse, family and older person develop a plan of care. The framework includes:

- the prevention of medical crises and their problems once they occur;
- control of symptoms;
- carrying out the prescribed regimens;
- prevention of or living with social isolation;
- adjustment to the course of the disease;
- normalizing interactions with others and other life styles;
- finding the money necessary to pay for treatment and care.

Assessment of Nursing Care Needed and Capabilities of Family Caregivers

The home health nurse will assess the needs of the client, determine what skilled nursing care is needed, and help the family decide how much of the care they will be able to provide. The family needs to know if care will be needed on a 24-hour basis. They also need to decide who will be the primary caregivers. If the family believes that they will be unable to meet all of the older person's needs, the nurse should help them explore various resources in the community. (Many of these resources are discussed in Chapters 1 and 2.) The nurse can also teach and counsel them about how to provide as much of the care as they can.

Nursing Care of The Older Person and The Family In The Home

After the family has examined all possible factors and invited the older person to live with them, they will need to learn how to perform the required nursing care and where to seek their own support groups to relieve the stress of long-term care in the home.

The family has the responsibility for both mental and physical support of the older person at home. Unless a nurse is employed on a 24-hour-basis, much teaching will need to be done with the older client and the family on how to maintain the maximum health potential of the older person. Care is not just given when the home health nurse visits, but care is an ongoing process. Seven major areas that require teaching of the family and the older person in the home are:

- drug administration and storage
- treatments
- nutrition
- mobility
- activities of daily living
- hygiene
- elimination

Drug Administration and Storage

Administration of drugs presents one of the major problems for the older client in the home. The nurse should instruct the family and older client about the purpose of each drug and how it is to be administered. The family should have a clear understanding of how many tablets or capsules are to be taken and when. The nurse should use client education cards that can be left with the family for later reference. These cards state the name of the drug, what it looks like, the effect on the body, possible side effects, dose and method of administration. This information should be stated in language easily comprehended by family and client.

To help assure that the medication is taken as ordered, there are various types of manufactured drug dispenser containers with separate compartments for each day of the week. Other types of containers have compartments for different times of the day. The family places medicines into the time compartments each day. Another method is to use an egg carton or ice cube tray and mark the days or times on the carton or tray. There are other devices such as a medication clock that can be set to ring every two, four, eight or 12 hours. The clock rings each time to remind the person to take his or her medication.

The client or family needs to record that the medication has been taken. It is very easy to become busy and not remember if they gave the medicine. Also, the older person may forget when or if the medicine was taken. A chart can be made that states the name of the medication and the different times it is administered. When the client takes the medicine or the caregiver gives it, they put a mark on a certain date. See Table 3.1 for a simple example of a Medicine Flow Sheet. This sheet can be taped to the inside of the kitchen cabinet (where the medicines are kept), or on the refrigerator door as an obvious reminder to record each medicine when it is given.

Medication should be stored properly. If it is not stored according to the instructions on the container, the medication could be of no use. Clients and family members should also be taught to monitor expiration dates on medicines. As with any medication, the caregiver must be careful where the medication is stored because of other family members in the home, particularly children. Caps should be placed back on bottles and closed. Requests for a screw-type cap can be made to the pharmacist, so the older person can open the bottle easier. But such a cap means that it is also easier for a child to get into the bottle. Bottles should be stored up and out of reach of children and the confused or disoriented older person. All medications should be kept in one place to avoid mixing them up with the medications of other family members.

Clients and family members should be taught about the dangers of the misuse of over-the-counter drugs, taught not to take old drugs or drugs prescribed for another person and taught that they should not place several drugs in one medicine bottle.

Treatments

A home health nurse is often asked to visit the home to give treatments necessary in the care of the older person. These procedures may need to be performed several times a day. Treatments could include monitoring vital signs and blood pressure, as well as range-of-motion exercises, dressing changes, catheter care, or the administration of medications. The nurse should instruct the family how to do these treatments as needed. In teaching the family or older client, the nurse should: 1) tell the family and older person the purpose of treatment; 2) instruct the family and client why the treatment is being done and when they need it; 3) gather all necessary equipment for the procedure; 4) demonstrate how to do the treatments; 5) have the family or client demonstrate the treatment while the nurse is present; 6) leave step-by-step written instructions; 7) list signs and symptoms of possible complications with this treatment and 8) leave a number to call in case of questions or problems.

The older person needs to understand the importance of the treatment and the benefits gained from the procedure. The caregiver should demonstrate the treatment while the nurse is present, so questions can be clarified or a technique perfected. If several treatments are being done, equipment for each procedure can be kept in different clear plastic shoe boxes so the equipment will not get mixed up.

Recordkeeping is essential. The nurse needs to know what treatment was given and when to help monitor the older person's progress. The nurse can then

TABLE 3.1
Medicine Flow Chart

NAME _____

MEDICATION	MONDAY		TUESDAY		WEDNESDAY		THURSDAY		FRIDAY		SATURDAY		SUNDAY	
	Time	Dates	Time	Dates	Time	Dates	Time	Dates	Time	Dates	Time	Dates	Time	Dates

TABLE 3.2
Record of Daily Treatments

Date	Time	Treatment	Remarks

determine if the care is being given at the appropriate times. A recording system can be used to indicate the specific treatment and the hours it is to be done. The caregiver then records the results under the date and time the care was given. An example may be found in Table 3.2.

Nutrition

Maintaining the nutritional level of the home health client is often very challenging. Factors that influence meal planning are food likes and dislikes of the person, diet restrictions, medications, chewing ability, and eating habits. The nurse will need to perform a thorough assessment of the person's diet restrictions, likes, dislikes, and eating habits before planning a proper diet. After the assessment, the nurse or a nutritionist works with the older person and the caregiver to plan nutritious meals that the person will eat and that will not cause extra preparation. Instructions or resources may need to be given to the caregiver regarding preparation of some of the special diet food requirements.

Smaller, more frequent meals may have to be given to the older person rather than one or two large meals a day. The older person should join the family for meals, if possible. This allows the person important socialization. If the older person is unable to eat at the family dinner table, family members could take turns eating with the person in his or her room.

Mobility

Keeping the older person as mobile as possible is a goal for all home health care personnel. Older clients need to perform normal range-of-motion exercises every day to keep their joints and muscles in good tone. Short term goals can be set for the older client who tends to be inactive, such as having the client get up and walk to the table every morning to have breakfast with the family.

The home environment needs to be assessed for safety factors and easy accessibility to needed areas (see chapter 6). Aids, such as canes, walkers or railings, can be used by the older person as a support, and this allows the person more mobility. Being up and moving around increases older adults' circulation and keeps them from becoming socially isolated in their own bedroom.

Activities of Daily Living

The nurse should help plan a schedule and determine methods to help the client in the normal activities of daily living. Collecting a family health history in the early phases of contact will facilitate this planning. The nurse will need to assess the client's needs and determine how much, if any, help the client will need in bathing, dressing, mouth care, toileting and ambulating.

If possible, different types of assistance may be given by various members of the family. For example, although the adult daughter may help her disabled father with his bath, her husband may help him go to the bathroom; a grandson may help him to shave, if needed; and a granddaughter may help him finish dressing by putting on his shoes and sweater. This plan has several advantages. It provides a sharing of the tasks among family members, thus decreasing the problem of fatigue for any one person. It helps all family members understand the needs of the older person and provides time for a relationship between the older family member and each member of the family. Problems can occur, for example, if an adolescent grandson or granddaughter is forced to assist with these tasks. Careful planning with the entire family, therefore, is essential.

Hygiene

The need for essential hygiene—bathing, shaving, mouth care—is important. The needs and wishes of the older family member should be followed as far as possible. For example, a daughter-in-law may believe that her father-in-law should have a complete bath every day because that is her custom. However, he may not want or need a daily bath. Perhaps he has not taken a daily bath routinely during his entire lifetime. The nurse can help the caregiver understand that a complete daily bath is not always necessary and, in fact, may cause the older person's skin to become dry and irritated. The father-in-law will probably want to wash his hands and face, shave, comb his hair, and dress. If he seems to be comfortable with this routine, it will cause fewer concerns for all. If there is an odor because of uncleanliness, however, the caregiver may need to provide the materials for the bath and hope that, with encouragement, the client will go ahead and bathe. If there are no major pressures or hostilities shown, usually the older person will take the bath.

If the client is in bed most of the time, the family will need to be taught how to bathe the client, give special skin care, and maintain oral hygiene. The family caregiver should be taught to use a soap with oil or cold cream in it, emollient lotions, and very little or no powder because it tends to dry out the older person's skin. A complete bath is not necessary every day, even for clients confined to bed, unless they particularly enjoy the stimulation and communication which accompanies the bath. However, the family must be taught specific techniques about how to prevent the formation of pressure sores. Some lay persons seem to believe that pressure sores are inevitable in the person who has to remain in bed most of the time. Therefore, they need to be taught about the importance of cleanliness, dryness, massage, positioning and appropriate types of mattresses and pads that decrease pressure to the skin.

Oral hygiene, including total mouth and teeth care, should be demonstrated by the nurse or home health aide. Family members need encouragement and support to assist with or perform effective mouth care for the older adult so that complications will not occur.

Elimination

Elimination can be a special problem, both for the older family member and the caregivers. Even if the older person is able to go to the bathroom alone, he or she may not recognize abnormalities or remember when elimination, especially bowel elimination, last occurred. For this reason, at least one family member should note when the older person went to the bathroom and ask about the type of elimination that occurred as soon as possible because the older person may forget later. A simple record of bowel elimination can be kept on a chart similar to the one shown in Figure 3.2. Or, a simple abbreviation or check on a monthly calender in the client's room may be used.

Caregivers should be taught to be alert for the signs of constipation in the older family member (for example, decreased appetite, drowsiness, confusion, irritability, headache, and frequent toileting). If diet, exercise, and/or bulk laxatives are not effective in maintaining adequate bowel elimination patterns, the nurse may need to obtain a physician's order for an enema and teach the primary caregiver the most effective and safe method to perform the procedure. If the client is unable to go to the bathroom, a bedside commode can be purchased, rented or perhaps borrowed. A bed pan, fracture pan, old flat bath basin, or other flat utensil of some kind can be used on a straight back chair by the bed if necessary.

If the client has a retention catheter in the bladder, the caregiver will need to be taught the technique for and importance of catheter care and perineal care. Some caregivers may be interested in learning how to do a catheterization if necessary. Incontinence of the client in the home is always a problem. The family can be taught about bowel and bladder training if appropriate. The family needs to be sure that an appropriate container is readily available for use by the older person. Sometimes they do not have time to get out of bed and go to the bathroom.

Sociocultural and Spiritual Beliefs

Home health nurses are concerned with the physical condition of the older client, but they should also consider the heritage and beliefs of the older client and family while planning nursing care. If sociocultural and spiritual beliefs are explored, this process provides information that will help the nurse understand the older person and the family.

Old ways and beliefs need to be recognized and incorporated into home health care. Cultural beliefs determine how one defines health and illness and how the older person accepts nursing care. Nurses need to be aware of how different cultures view the aged. Culture may structure, facilitate or hinder individual and group adjustment to the physical and psychological constraints of aging (Holzberg, 1982 p. 249). These cultural beliefs will influence how well the family accepts the older person who moves in with them and provides for them.

Jewish

Jewish people are concerned with the quality of life, so they seek and utilize medical care and treatment to preserve and enhance the quality of life. The family is very important, particularly when illness occurs, and members are very supportive of one another. The older family member is visited and provided with care and support in the home, if possible, where his or her needs can be met and kosher dietary practices can be maintained. Family members would work with the home health nurse to help provide quality and supportive care for the older family member in the home.

Chinese

The Chinese believe that health is a physical and spiritual harmony (Campbell, 1973, pp. 245–40). The individual must adjust oneself in the environment. The body is viewed as a gift, given by the parents and forebearers that should be well cared for and maintained. The older person is expected to be respected and cared for by their children (Rose, 1978, p. 54–63). Home health care of the elderly would be very acceptable to this family who is culturally expected to care for their aging parents. The philosophy of maintaining the body would help the nurse get cooperation from the older person in treatment at home.

Blacks

The American black comes from many different settings. Often health is viewed as something that one can do nothing about. "It's going to happen anyway so why bother?" is a phrase commonly expressed (Stokes, 1977, p. 51–66).

The family has had a more matriarchal family structure in the past where the older female was the head of the family. She retained the respect and loving care of all family members into old age. The home health nurse needs to be aware of the matriarchal system in planning care. In many homes, care is given by many different generations who live under one roof (Carrington, 1978, p. 34–52).

Self help and folk practices are not uncommon in many of the older black persons' homes. Older black clients are usually eager to be independent and to try to help themselves. More self-care activities could be planned with these older clients.

Hispanics

Many Hispanics believe that health and illness are "God's Will." Illness is something they do not have any control over and is punishment for something (Herrera, 1977, pp. 65–85). Prevention of illness is associated with prayer, maintaining religious symbols in the home, and adornment with religious medals. The family is very supportive of the older person who is usually cared for by the children. The home health nurse will have to consider that older Hispanics may feel that they are being punished for something they did, and when the punishment is over, they will get better. Folk medicine may also be used to ward off the punishment.

Native American

Native Americans perceive health as a harmony with nature and the ability to survive different circumstances. Direct questioning is not considered proper, and the health care provider is expected to deduce the problems more by intuition than by direct questioning. An older person's self-esteem is based on the ability to help others by giving advice to younger family members and being regarded as a source of wisdom (Primeaux, 1977, p. 55). The home health nurse will find data collection hard to do by direct questioning and, therefore, not appropriate. Asking advice of the older person on what care should be given and how it could be done would increase the self-esteem of the older person. Listening is one of the best communication techniques with the older Native American.

Spiritual Beliefs

Moberg (1977, pp. 47–49) found that involvement in religious activities outside the home decreased in later life, but religious attitudes and feelings increased. For the home health client who becomes less physically and socially mobile, religion becomes more of a personal home activity. Many older persons turn to religious television programs for sermons, study and comfort. Other older people will read their Bible and find personal support from this activity.

Many churches are promoting an active outreach program for elderly shut-ins. Home visitation teams make calls, bring tapes of Sunday sermons, and update the person on the activities of the church. Communion is brought to members at home. Many congregations are recognizing an increase of older persons in their homes who want to continue their religious activities but cannot attend worship services in the church. Outreach programs will continue to expand from churches to the elderly in their homes.

The home health nurse needs to consider the spiritual needs and beliefs of the older person when planning care. Religion is often a major support system along with the family.

Support Groups for the Family

After the older person has been in the home for some time, the family adjusts. Family members have learned how to perform treatments and nursing care, plan nutritional diets, and adjust their lives to the situation. The stress and strain of changes and constant responsibilities may begin to cause them concern. Support groups are developing to assist families who compose this "sandwich generation" (Silverman, Brachce, and Zielinski, 1981).

The middle or "sandwich" generation is pulled in three directions: 1) raising their own children, 2) leading their own lives, and 3) helping their aging parents (Silverman, 1981, p. 43). When the older person is in the family home, family members try to balance themselves between their family, their own interests, and caring for their parents or other older relatives. Families are often afraid to voice some of the frustrations that the additional care for this older person is causing them. Support groups for the family are a way for family members to examine their feelings and find other people who have similar concerns.

"As Parents Grow Older"

One example of an educational support group is the "As Parents Grow Older" (APGO) program (Silverman, 1981). In 1978 the Administration on Aging, under the Department of Health Education and Welfare, awarded a grant to the Institute of Gerontology at the University of Michigan to develop, implement and evaluate the APGO model. As a result of this grant, support groups for families have been formed to discuss the topics presented in the program. These topics include: 1) increasing understanding of the psychological aspects of aging; 2) chronic illness and behavioral changes with age; 3) sensory deprivation and communication; 4) decision making and alternative living situations; 5) availability of community resources; and 6) dealing with situations and feelings (Smith, 1982, p. 16).

Members of these groups have discovered that other families face similar problems and experiences. They can also talk with other people who share similar situations and help them see things in perspective. By increasing the knowledge of families about aging, many better understand the behavior of their parents. Similar groups have been developed in different areas around the country under other grants and funding. The nurse should contact the local unit of the American Red Cross or mental health association, the Area Agency on Aging, or local universities for information about the "As Parents Grow Older" program or other similar support systems for persons with aging family members.

Senior Centers

Senior Centers in some communities have a time when family members can meet together and discuss mutual problems. It has been helpful within this setting because of the resource people who can facilitate this group. They know resources for the older person and can help families find the appropriate agency.

Mental Health Centers

Mental health centers provide more individualized support for family members. Often, caregivers need to discuss their situation with someone else and discover better coping skills to manage the situation. A mental health counselor is an objective, neutral person who can help people explore their situation and determine how they might possibly develop better coping skills or solutions.

Area Agency on Aging

Local agencies on aging are responsible for local planning, administration, evaluation and ongoing technical assistance to agencies serving older people in a certain area. This organization is one that families could contact to determine if there are other families with similar problems and what agency or groups could best help them. Since they are responsible for planning, it is feasible that the agency could help start a family support group in the area.

Churches

Some churches have developed informal support groups for older members and families by giving the phone number of one family to another. This process works like a "buddy system." When caregivers feel stressed, they call another family and talk with one of the members, or another family who has had a bad day will call the first family. Individual counseling to support the family is done by many ministers or counselors working closely with the church.

Respite Care

Respite care is another method of care that helps support the family by giving them some time alone away from an older family member. As noted earlier, all families or individuals need some time away from each other. Caregivers need to withdraw from a demanding situation periodically to renew their energy. Temporary care can be arranged from agencies, neighbors and/or other family members.

Nursing Homes

Some nursing homes will consider a short-term stay for an older person needing skilled nursing care. A variety of different arrangements can be made. Often, if older family members have been hospitalized and need continuing nursing care but not in an acute care setting, they will temporarily be sent to the nursing home for care. When they are stronger and less care is necessary, they are discharged to go home with the family. The family is relieved of the intensive nursing care often needed for the just-released hospital patient.

Other Support Systems

Neighbors often come in for an afternoon or a couple of hours a day so that the caregiver has some time to run errands or have a few minutes alone. If neighbors and friends rotate this responsibility, it does not pressure anyone and allows the caregiver some free time.

Family members who live out of town can be called upon if the family wants to go on a short vacation or has some activity planned for which they need a few days away from home. Other family members could make this stay part of a vacation or be of assistance temporarily.

Elder Abuse and Neglect

Some families overwhelmed by the burdens and lack of support may abuse and/or neglect the elderly person. On a home visit, a daughter became upset and admitted "pushing her mother" because "she is always there." Another daughter explained that when tension between her and her mother became intolerable, she gave her mother additional sedatives to make her go to bed and stay asleep (Johnson, 1979, p. 11).

Lau and Kosberg (1979, p. 18) interviewed 404 elderly clients at a chronic illness center and found one in 10 was a victim of abuse or neglect by a family member. Neglect and abuse of the elderly is not new. The problems that lead a son or daughter to abuse or neglect a parent may be financial or physical. They may be due to role reversal, social isolation, fatigue, crowding or difficult family relationships. The incorporation into the nuclear family of an additional person who is seen as dependent, roleless and uncontributing, creates additional stress within the family, and in some cases, leads to neglect and abuse of the elderly in the same way that it leads to abuse of a child (Johnson, 1979, p. 14).

Anderson (1981, p. 77) suggested that elderly abuse or neglect may take one of four forms: 1) physical abuse, 2) physical neglect, 3) emotional abuse, or 4) emotional neglect. Physical abuse is hitting or beating the elderly person. Improper use of drugs or giving multiple drugs is also a form of physical abuse. Unintentional abuse usually is caused by the daughter who is the major caregiver. The abuse is not usually premeditated, but is crisis-precipitated. There are cases of intentional abuse where battering of parents was done "to make them mind." Physical neglect usually occurs when the family does not provide sufficient care and/or food. Strain from caring for the older person over a long period of time will cause the caregiver to neglect the older person. Emotional abuse occurs from the negative attitude many people in society have regarding the elderly. Belittling, stereotyping, isolating, and berating the elderly are all methods of emotional abuse. Emotional neglect results often when elderly persons no longer can control or manipulate the environment around them (Anderson, 1981, p. 83). This neglect results in helplessness, depression, withdrawal and loss of territory.

The home health nurse needs to be alert for signs and symptoms of elderly abuse or neglect and be aware of situations that provoke it, so that appropriate interventions can be taken. Philips (1983, p. 167) has developed a tool to help nurses identify abusive situations. By using such tools, and by working with the client and family in assessing potential problems, some of the abusive and neglectful situations could be resolved. The home health nurse can help bring to the attention of lawmakers the significance of elder abuse.

Summary

With an increase in the number of older people living at home, more families will be faced with care of the older family member. This trend will change and enrich families. The family will continue to be a major support system for the older person. When an older person is living in the home with adult children, added stresses will cause family support groups to grow.

Home health care allows the person to remain in the home, to continue to practice individual cultural and spiritual beliefs, and to retain his or her values while receiving home nursing services. There are many other support systems the home health nurse will continue to assess and recommend to help keep the family together and meet the total needs of the older client and family. Various forms of elder abuse may occur when families who are caring for chronically ill older adults in the home do not have needed assistance or support.

REFERENCES

Anderson C: "Abuse and neglect among the elderly." *J Geront Nurs*, Vol 7, No 2, February 1981, pp 77–85
Campbell T, Chang B: "Health care of the Chinese in America." *Nurs Outlook*, Vol 21, No 4 April 1973 pp 245–49
Caplan G: *An Approach to Community Mental Health*. Grune and Stratton, New York, 1961, p 18
Carrington B: "The Afro-American, " in Clark A L (ed): *Culture Childbearing Health Professional*. F. A. Davis, Philadelphia, 1978, pp 34–52

Goldstein V, Regnery G, Willin E: "Caretaker Role Fatigue." *Nurs Outlook*, Vol 29, No 1, January 1981, pp 23–29

Herrera T, Wagner M: "Behavioral Approaches to Delivering Health Services in a Chicano Community," in Reinhardt A, Quinn S M (eds): *Current Practices in Family Centered Community Nursing*. C. V. Mosby Co., St. Louis, 1977, pp 67–85

Holzberg C: "Ethnicity and aging." *The Gerontol*, Vol 22, No 3, 1982, pp 249–57

Johnson D: "Abuse and Neglect." *J Gerontol Nurs*, Vol 5, No 4 July/August 1979, pp 11–13

Lau E, Kosberg J: Editorial. *JAMA*, Vol 241, No 10 1979, p 18

Moberg D O: "Religion and the aging family." *Family Coordinator*, Vol 21, 1972, pp 47–49

Philips L: "Elder abuse—what Is It? Who says so?" *Geriat Nurs*, Vol 4, No 3, May/June 1983, pp 167–170

Primeaux M: "American Indian health care practices—A cross-cultural perspective." *Nurs Clin North Am*, Vol 12, No 1, 1977, p 55

Rose P: "The Chinese American," in Clark A L (ed), *Culture Childbearing Health Professionals*. F. A. Davis Company, Philadelphia, 1978, pp 54–73

Selye H: *The Stress of Life*. McGraw-Hill, New York, 1975, p xi

Silverman A, Brache C, Zielinski C: *As Parents Grow Older*. Institute of Gerontology, University of Michigan, Ann Arbor, Michigan, 1981

Smith B K, LeLong J, Adelberg B: *Aging Parents and Dilemmas of Their Children*. Hogg Foundation for Mental Health, University of Texas, Austin, Texas, 1981

Stokes L: "Delivering Health Services in a Black Community," in Reinhardt A, Quinn M D (eds) *Current Practice in Family-centered Community Nursing*. C. V. Mosby Co., St. Louis, Mo., 1977, pp 51–66

Straus A L: *Chronic Illness and the Quality of Life*. C. V. Mosby Company, St. Louis, 1975

Visiting Nurse Association, *VNA Adult Day Care Centers*. Visiting Nurse Association, Dallas, Texas, 1981

Williams F: "Intervention in Maturational Crises," in Hall J, Weaver B. *Nursing of Families in Crises*. J. B. Lippincott Co., Philadelphia, 1974, pp 43–50

BIBLIOGRAPHY

Abril I: "Mexican American folk beliefs that affect health care." *Arizona Nurse*, Vol 28, 1975, p 14

Archbold P: "Impact of parent caring on middle aged offspring." *J Gerontol Nurs*, Vol 6, No 2, 1982, pp 78–85

Banzinger C H: "Intergenerational family households: Recent trends and implications for the future." *The Gerontol*, Vol 19, No 5, 1979, pp 471–80

Beam I M: "Helping families survive." *Am J Nurs*, Vol 84, No 2, February 1984, pp 229–32

Brody E: "Women in the middle and family help to older people." *The Gerontol*, Vol 21, No 5, 1981, pp 471–80

Brody S J, Poulshock S W, Masicocchi C F: "The family caring unit: A major consideration in the long-term support system." *The Gerontol*, Vol 18, No 6, 1978, pp 556–61

Burnside I M: *Nursing and the Aged* (2nd ed.). McGraw-Hill Publishing Co., New York, 1981

Cheung L: "The Chinese elderly and family structure: Implications for health care." *Public Health Reports*, Vol 95, No 5, 1980, pp 491–95

Cohen P: "A group approach for working with families of the elderly." *The Gerontol*, Vol 23, No 3, 1983, pp 248–49

Ebersole P, Hess P: *Toward Healthy Aging.* C. V. Mosby Co., St. Louis, 1981

Epstein C: *Learning to Care for the Aged.* Reston, Reston, Virginia, 1977

Grobe M E, Ilstrup D, Ahmann D: "Skills needed by family members to maintain care of an advanced cancer patient." *Cancer Nursing*, Vol 4, No 5, 1981, pp 371–75

Haber D: "Promoting mutual help groups among older persons." *The Gerontol*, Vol 23, No 3, 1983, pp 251–52

Hickey T, Douglass R: "Neglect and abuse of older family members." *The Gerontol*, Vol 21, No 2, 1981, pp 171–76

Hildebrandt E: "Respite care in the home." *Am J Nurs*, Vol 83, No 10, October 1983, pp 1428–31

Hogstel M O: "Skin care of the aged." *J Geront Nurs*, Vol 9, No 8, August 1983, pp 430–37

Johnson C: "Dyadic family relations and social support." *The Gerontol Vol 22, No 4, 1983, pp 377–83*

Kay M: "The Mexican American" in Clark A (ed.): *Culture Childbearing Health Professionals.* F. A. Davis Co., Philadelphia, Pennsylvania, 1978

Kauffman J, Ames B: "Care of aging family members." *J Home Eco*, Spring 1983, pp 215–46

Mace N L, Rabins P V: *The 36-Hour Day.* The Johns Hopkins University Press, Baltimore and London, 1981

Mindel C H: "Multigenerational family households: Recent trends and implications for the future." *The Gerontol*, Vol 19, No 5, 1979, pp 456–63

Mindel C, Wright R: "Satisfaction in multigenerational households." *J Geront*, Vol 37, No 4, 1982, pp 483–89

Nydegger C: "Family ties of the aged in cross cultural perspective." *The Gerontol*, Vol 23, No 1, 1983, pp 26–31

Olsen J: "Helping families cope." *J Gerontol Nurs*, Vol 6, No 3, 1980, pp 152–54

Oppeneer J E, Vervoren T M: *Gerontological Pharmacology*, The C. V. Mosby Company, St. Louis, 1983

Reinhardt A M, Quinn D (eds.): *Current Practice on Family-centered Community Nursing.* C. V. Mosby Co., St. Louis, 1977

Smith K F, Bengston V L: "Positive consequences of institutionalization: Solidarity between elderly parents and their middle aged children." *The Gerontol*, Vol 19, No 5, 1979, pp 438–48

Staller E P: "Sources of support for the elderly during illness." *Health and Social Work*, Vol 7, No 2, 1982, pp 111–12

Sullivan T: "The subculture of the aging and its implications for health and nursing care of the elderly," in Reinhardt A, Quinn M D (eds.): *Current Practices in Gerontological Nursing.* C. V. Mosby Co., St. Louis, 1979

Texas Department of Human Resources. *Directory of Services Offered.* Region 05

Wan T T, Weissert W, Livieratios B: "Geriatric day care and homemaker services: An experimental study." *J Geront*, Vol 35, No 2, 1980, pp 256–74

Weeks J, Cuellar J: "The role of family members in the helping networks of older people." *The Geront*, Vol 21, No 4 1981, pp 388–94

Yurick A G, Robb S S, Spier B E, Ebert N J: *The Aged Person and the Nursing Process*. Appleton-Century-Crofts, New York, 1980

CHAPTER 4

HOSPICE CARE

Virginia Major Thomas

In spite of considerable newspaper and television publicity, many people are still unfamiliar with the term *hospice*. Some think of it in terms of a building or a place. This interpretation probably results from the fact that the most famous 20th century hospice—and the first to familiarize the term hospice in this century—is a unique and interesting building—St. Christopher's Hospice, Sydenham, London, founded by Dr. Cecily Saunders.

The word hospice, however, has a much more comprehensive meaning. Hospice refers to a program of care for terminally ill persons and their families. This care is provided by an interdisciplinary team of professionals and volunteers educated in hospice philosophy and methods. The care is provided on a part-time, intermittent basis with 24-hour, 7-days-a-week availability. In times of great crisis, continuous care is possible. This care can be given anywhere, perhaps best in the home but also in a nursing home, a hospital, or a special hospice in-patient facility. Place is less important than the care given and the philosophy underlying that care.

History and Development of Hospice

More than 150 years ago no hospice program existed in the United States, and there was little need for one. Most people died at home, attended by large, extended families, neighbors and friends who provided support and treatment. The person's physician and minister, if available, also assisted.

The post-World War II emergence of the modern health care system has created the need for hospice programs. The amazing technology has made the cure of formerly incurable conditions possible. Therefore, more and more, modern hospitals have become the setting of care for acute illnesses and injuries. The hospitals' focus is the cure of these acute conditions.

In such settings, incurable illnesses and their victims appear out of place except when curative therapy is still being attempted. Persons with terminal illnesses have found that in modern hospitals, either their care comes second to that of persons with curable conditions, or they have been avoided by professionals, abandoned as failures in a cure-oriented system.

This frequently tragic situation led to the rise of the hospice movement in this century. Hospices as refuges for lonely, weary, sick or dying travelers on life's road have a long history. Although they antedate the Crusades, they became more numerous in medieval times with the rise of the saints' cults and subsequent pilgrimages to saints' shrines. They provided simple hospitality and safe resting places for pilgrims and crusaders and offered care to the sick or dying. One example is the Hospital of St. Thomas the Martyr Upon Eastbridge in Canterbury, England. This building served pilgrims to the shrine of Thomas à Becket, who was murdered in Canterbury Cathedral in 1170. Today it is a museum. Another example is L'Hospice de Beaune in Beaune, France, still functioning as a hospital.

More recent predecessors of the 20th century hospices are the Hospice of the Sisters of Charity in Dublin, founded in the late 19th century by Sister Mary Aikenhead; the hospitals of the Hawthorne Dominican sisters in the United States; the Anglican St. Luke's in London; and St. Joseph's Hospital for the Dying, now St. Joseph's Hospice, in Hocking, London, established by the English Sisters of Charity in the first decade of the 20th century. Both of the latter are still in operation.

Dr. Cecily Saunders worked at both. It was at St. Joseph's that she worked on controlling pain in the terminally ill before she founded the most famous of this century's hospices, St. Christopher's, in 1967. Inspired by a cancer-plagued refugee of the Warsaw ghetto whom she cared for in London in 1948, Dr. Saunders envisioned for the dying a combination of hospital and home. She saw combined in one setting medical care and personal, individual attention that reflected loving regard for each individual as a person of inestimable value (Saunders, 1969). St. Christopher's, along with St. Joseph's and St. Luke's, has inspired imitators in many countries. From St. Christopher's, Dr. Sylvia Lack came in 1973 to Connecticut to be medical director of Hospice, Inc., now The Connecticut Hospice, Inc. This Connecticut hospice and the Hospice of Marin in California have assisted with educational programs in many hospices that have sprung up throughout the United States in the last decade.

These hospices have taken a wide variety of forms. Some consist of a hospice team within a hospital, where the hospice patients are scattered on different floors, the so-called "scattered bed" approach. Other hospice teams are functioning within hospitals but with all hospice patients in one wing or on one floor. Some teams are autonomous, that is, unconnected with any other hospital, and have a combination of "free-standing" hospice in-patient facility and home care teams. Some are hospices operating as teams or programs out of home care agencies, with contractual agreements with acute care hospitals or extended care facilities for the use of their beds if that becomes necessary for pain control or family relief. There has been a great deal of variety in the organization of hospices, but many professionals, non-professionals, patients and families feel that the best place for care is the client/family home. There is no place like home, and it is with home care that this chapter chiefly deals. However, hospice care is greatly affected by the setting; the home care described here may vary in many details from the hospice care given on an acute care hospital wing.

Principles of Hospice Care
Death Is A Part of Life

What is involved in hospice care? One fundamental conviction underlying hospice care cannot be too strongly stressed: *death is regarded as a natural part of life whether it results from disease or not.* In a technology-dominated health care system oriented primarily toward cure, and in a society that exalts life, productivity and progress, this insistence on the naturalness of death is a desperately needed antidote, a contact with reality.

Recognition and acceptance of this means a wonderful freedom from the heavy burden of attempting to conquer death when that is not possible. Heavy responsibilities remain: psychosocial care, symptom relief, and constant alertness to uncomfortable or dangerous physical symptoms and problems which may be unrelated to the terminal illness—the development of gall stones in a client with cancer, for example. There is never room for diagnostic laziness. Still, hospice caregivers are not involved in the frustration of fighting the inevitable.

Care is Client- and Family-Directed

Another fundamental conviction underlying hospice care is that a different criterion of success must be used from that prevailing in today's health care. As Dr. Cecily Saunders put it, success is measured not in "how our treatment is working, but how the patient is, what he is doing . . . what he is being in the face of physical deterioration" (Stoddard, 1978, p. 73). Relief of pain, nausea and vomiting may be achieved completely, but the client may be anxious, fearful, terror-filled. Hospice caregivers may be able to alleviate much of the client's concern, yet not all of it. Another way of putting this conviction is to say that hospice is not just client–centered but, to a large degree, client-*directed;* better yet, client and family directed. The dying of a client almost always involves family or others important to the client.

Much is made, correctly so, of the interdisciplinary team. Less often is it understood that the client/family is the unit of care in hospice and is an active member/unit of that team. The following example shows how this works:

A hospice nurse was expressing her frustration in the presence of the nursing director of the home health agency where her hospice team was based. Her frustration stemmed from the fact that neither client nor family would cooperate with her suggestions for pain control. The client had a great deal of pain, and both the client and the client's daughter said they wanted the pain reduced if not eliminated. But after several periods of instruction and explanations by the nurse, the home health assistant, and the social worker, the client and her daughter were still not following procedures that would probably have reduced her pain. Although she realized that the client might have subconscious or unacknowledged reasons for needing to have pain, the nurse still felt frustration. The nursing director listened, then quietly suggested that, like other noncompliant clients of the home health agency, this client be discharged from service for refusal to follow the care plan. "Is there anything more we can do for them?" she asked. Discharge for noncompliance is a familiar procedure in home health agencies.

As the hospice nurse immediately realized, discharge for noncompliance is an impossible procedure in hospice. Although pain and other symptom control were part of the care plan the client and her family had actively participated in making, she couldn't be discharged from hospice care until she and her family refused hospice care and indicated they wanted no more to do with the hospice team. Her manner of dying belonged to her; it was her decision to make; and the way her family shared her death was for them to decide. If, although fully understanding that pain control was possible and fully understanding how to do this, she still chose to have severe pain, the choice was hers, and the hospice team members went along with it. And there was something more they could do for her: team members could at least be with her and sit with her in her pain.

It is at such a time as this, when feeling frustrated and helpless, that hospice caregivers most want to run away. Paradoxically, this is the time when they are most needed by client and family. This was not an easy choice for the team to accept, and those involved in her care needed much support from other team members. Characteristic of hospice care, the choices of the client and family were respected. To the end, the mystery remained: the team never knew or understood why she and her family made the choice they did. Similarly, less traumatic choices are respected, such as whether or not to use a hospital bed and whether or not to use the services of a volunteer.

Client/Family Is The Unit of Care

As indicated above, the client, family, or close friends (if no family is available) are considered the unit of care in hospice. The interweaving of these lives, often over long periods of time, makes the dying of one member of enormous significance to the others. The consent of both client and family are required for hospice care. They must know—at some level—that hospice care is palliative, not curative. The family or friends contribute to the plan of care for the client and are usually involved in the physical care of the client after being taught care measures and techniques by the nurse and the home health assistant. Family and friends are, at the same time, the recipients of care and support themselves during the stressful time of dying and afterwards. They have their own needs separate from those of the client.

It is an interesting fact that the physical care of the dying family member by the family very often fulfills the need of the family to "do something," alleviates the frustrating feelings of helplessness among family members, and after the death of the client, serves to relieve the guilt of family members for not having done something earlier. If family members have assisted with physical care during the dying period, they recognize that they *have* helped the deceased. Hospice care also attempts to respect the beliefs and values of the client and family by not trying to judge, change or influence them. Hospice care reflects the conviction that there is no one "right" way to die; dying is a part of each individual's total way of living. Some are comforted by prayers, some by music, and some by silent companionship.

Cultural variations must be noted and respected. In some cultures, loud lamentation and profuse crying are considered appropriate expressions of impending loss or of grief after death. The sister of one client was not in the room at the moment of death. When she returned and found her sister dead, she started a deafening wailing and keening and even lifted the body in her arms. The behavior of the sister might have stunned the nurse if the nurse had not witnessed similar displays of grief in other families from the same cultural background. On the other hand, numerous family members gathered at another client's deathbed and uttered not one sound during the final death struggle. When one teenager uttered a stifled sob a few moments after the client's breathing ceased, at least four family members immediately frowned at her reprovingly, and she quickly composed herself into stiff silence.

Client/Family Conflicts

Although hospice care is delivered to both client and family or friends, the client and the family or friends may need different care. Conflicting desires and interests may surface and find expression. The client, for example, may be ready and anxious to settle affairs and write a will, while the family is not yet ready to face the finality these acts imply. Very often, hospice team members find the family very concerned because the patient "won't eat" when the patient is long past the point in life where food is desired, relished, or even needed. It is very difficult for most families to disengage themselves from the lifelong habit of nurturing with food.

Sometimes client-family conflicts are greater than those illustrated by these examples. The hospice team members must often find a balance between client desires and family desires. They must do counseling and provide much psychological or emotional support. They must also be realistic and recognize that certain lifelong patterns of intrafamilial relationships cannot be changed and should not be changed.

One couple, whom a hospice team cared for, had a 14-year marriage which included endless nagging and insults by the wife; drunkenness, infidelity and forgery by the husband; divorce and remarriage. They had mutual hostility and distrust. The wife frankly referred to her sick husband as "that poor old thing" and stated she would leave him except that she felt sorry for him and besides, if they were married when he died she would get his social security which was more than hers. When radiation therapy improved his superior vena cava syndrome, she became extremely angry and irritable. When he had good periods, she was angry; when he seemed to be declining, her spirits picked up and she talked frankly in front of him about his imminent death. Aside from encouraging them—separately—to ventilate their feelings, there was little that could be done to change these family dynamics. He died without being reconciled to her and as he died, her pre-existing ulcer became dramatically better.

Thus hospice team members come to realize that not every death will occur with peace, with dignity, and with resolutions of tasks and problems. They come to realize that hospice helpers must be careful not to impose their own conceptions on others about how a patient should die or how a family should act or react. Hospice team members should try not to bring their own beliefs to client/family care. However, that is easier said than done.

The Interdisciplinary Team

The hospice interdisciplinary team, of which the client/family is a crucial part, devises the plan of care for the patient and delivers the care. This team is the heart of the hospice program. The number of members of the professional disciplines may vary on the team but there must always be, in addition to the client/family unit, nurses, physicians, social workers, counselors (pastoral and/or others), home health assistants, volunteers, and sometimes physical therapists, occupational therapists, nutritionists and speech language pathologists. Of these disciplines, the National Hospice Reimbursement Act requires the hospice program to provide nursing care, physician direction, medical social services, and counseling. The other professional disciplines may be contracted for with other agencies or sources.

The need for multiple disciplines on the hospice care team is obvious: the dying and their families have multiple needs—physical, spiritual, psychological, legal, social, emotional, and economic—which no one discipline can satisfy or handle. The mutual needs of each discipline for the others to assist the client/family in this major crisis helps to create one crucial characteristic of a hospice team: a sense of equality among members where status differences are minimized, or perhaps non-existent. This means that the interdisciplinary team must have mature, self-confident members, sure of their professional capabilities. Only such persons can comfortably allow another professional to enter their territory and perform a function should the need arise. This overlapping of function is one of the strengths of the team approach. A sense of humor and the ability to be flexible and resilient are also critical.

Team Member Functions

Each member of the interdisciplinary team has his or her special knowledge and contribution to make to the client/family's care. The nurse may perform the following functions:

- admitting the client/family to hospice service;
- assessing need and making the initial care plan;
- symptom control and preventing complications of treatment (for example, preventing constipation which occurs with the use of narcotics);
- teaching the family or primary caregiver how to care for the client;
- listening to client/family expressions of needs and worries;
- monitoring disease progression and changing needs;
- communicating with the attending physician;
- consulting the hospice physician; and
- coordinating the work of all disciplines involved with a client/family unit.

The nurse is on 24-hour, seven-day-a-week call, and other team members may be on call too.

The social worker utilizes community resources to help the client/family as they need and desire help. The social worker also counsels with the client and the family during this most difficult life crisis to minimize stress, increase opportunities for growth and maturing, and increase coping mechanisms.

The home health assistants or aides give personal care under supervision, assist with food preparation and delivery, and do much active listening. The chaplain counsels the client/family regarding spiritual concerns. The dietitian consults with the client/family regarding diet, taking into account the client's desires, abilities and condition. The physical therapist helps clients remain safely mobile and independent as long as necessary. Even after the client has become bedfast, the physical therapist may modify goals and use active or passive range-of-motion exercises to increase comfort. The occupational therapist assists the client with activities of daily living and helps the client continue old or develop new diversional activities to give delight to each remaining day.

The language speech therapist is invaluable in cases of mouth and throat cancers where communication may become difficult and frustrating for client and family alike. Volunteers do everything—listen, play checkers, babysit, grocery-shop, pick up medicine—and often become virtual members of the family. Art therapists and music therapists also assist in the care of some patients.

As in all fields of knowledge today, hospice is constantly discovering new methods and approaches. It is obviously necessary for each member of the team to keep up with the expansion of knowledge through continuing education.

Coordination of Care

The nurse usually coordinates client/family care. The nurse visits the client/family with their knowledge and approval after receiving orders from the primary or attending physician, who is usually recognized by the whole family as the principal physician. Sometimes a specialist such as an oncologist or neurosurgeon makes the referral to hospice care. The nurse takes a history of the present illness and health history and performs a physical examination to establish baseline data.

The delicate question of the extent of client/family knowledge of the prognosis is best dealt with by listening to the family and by concentrating attention on feelings. In conference with the client and the primary caregiver (usually a family member, but sometimes a friend) the nurse then develops a plan of care and determines which team members are necessary to implement the plan. The client and caregiver may veto parts of the plan. For example, the nurse may believe that an occupational therapist would be helpful, but the client may refuse this assistance. Primary or referring physician agreement for all professional services is obtained. Sometimes the physician will prescribe all needed treatments, but sometimes the physician may not anticipate the assistance that physical therapy, for example, will provide in the home setting. It is then the responsibility of the nurse coordinator to inform the physician and secure an agreement.

Client/family needs and desires determine which services will assist them and for how long, including volunteer or non-professional as well as professional services. However, without being overly persuasive or coercive, the nurse must provide adequate information for the client/family to make an informed choice. The nurse must often explain the role and function of, for example, the social worker or the occupational therapist so that they can understand what they are choosing or refusing.

Team Conferences

If the interdisciplinary team is the center of the hospice program, the team conferences are its core. The conferences provide interchange of information on the client/family condition or events that have taken place. There is sharing of insights into the complex workings of human beings and groups. There is brainstorming about problems and solutions. There are suggestions for changes in the care plan. There is the explanation of technical medical information and care suggestions by the physician. There is coordination of action. Above all, emotional support among team members is essential.

Sometimes, these team conferences are held once weekly and combine all aspects of the team's work and needs. Sometimes they are divided so that one conference deals with medical-nursing problems and symptom control only, and a separate conference deals with both the client/family's and team members' emotional and/or psychological situations. In some hospices, conferences are daily, twice weekly, once weekly or every other week. It is impossible to do hospice work on an interdisciplinary team without interdisciplinary team conferences.

An interesting, necessary, and generally satisfying aspect of interdisciplinary team work is the decrease in feelings of territoriality and the blurring of distinctions between the work of the various professionals involved. One nurse was the only team member present when the client died, and suddenly, she found herself the chaplain when the family asked her to say a prayer over the body. She was able to meet their request and said some beautiful and appropriate prayers.

Social workers and home health assistants learn much about the use and side effects of various medications, and both become very skilled in reinforcing the nurse's teaching regarding the medication regimen. One home health assistant was particularly helpful when a client stopped taking around-the-clock medication for pain when his pain had been relieved. The home health assistant explained to him that if he stopped taking the medicine the pain would return and she went over all the reasons for the procedure again. He understood it better than when the nurse told him.

The occupational therapist may be the only team member present when the client feels like talking, and the information given later to the social worker or to the team as a whole may add greatly to the plan of care. The home health assistants almost always hear and see significant attitudes or actions which no other team member is aware of because they are usually with the client/family over longer periods of time. Their contributions to team conferences are invaluable.

For example, once a hospice team was working with a highly intelligent and very independent lady in her seventies. She had been divorced about 30 years, lost her only child and had supported herself and lived alone for years. She had taken excellent care of herself physically, and after intensive study in religion and philosophy she had come to believe in reincarnation. When colon cancer struck and rapidly metastasized to the liver and lungs, she faced it squarely: "I'm dying of cancer and I can't do anything about it. Everyone has to die of something." She did not feel that she needed the help of a social worker. She did accept physical therapy assistance in learning exercises to strengthen her failing legs. She refused to have anyone stay with her in her house as she became increasingly weak and short of breath. Numerous friends shopped, cooked and did laundry for her. She looked forward to the nurse's visit, chiefly because she wanted to know everything about her vital signs, her disease, its symptoms, its progression and procedures at death. Even so, she felt the nurse needed to visit only once or twice a week; and it was true that she had no pain, nausea, vomiting or other symptoms requiring titration of medications or change of medication regimen. The home health assistant went to her house every day to assist her with bathing, shampooing her hair, and preparing her meals. As the client became more and more dyspneic, weaker and increasingly helpless, and as she felt the end was approaching, it was with the home health assistant that she broke down and cried, "I wish this was all over," and confessed, "I hope it happens when someone is here with me." It was the home health assistant who heard her heartfelt wishes. Nevertheless, the client steadfastly refused to allow anyone to stay with her at night.

Volunteers on the Team

Similarly, the volunteers also hear and see many things unknown to the rest of the team. In team meetings their contributions often shed an entirely new light on a client/family situation that can be important to the professionals involved. For example, one hospice team was caring for an 85-year-old woman who had breast cancer which had metastasized to the lung and bones. The nurse, the social worker, and even the home health assistant saw her as an elderly lady of some remarkable achievements who was sweet, rather passive by this time, forgetful and sometimes depressed. They recognized that she was aware that her life was coming to an end, but accepting death after a full life as daughter, wife, mother and professional woman who had made significant contributions to the community.

Another view came from the volunteer, who visited her alone for several hours every Sunday for three months. She said, "She's not 85, she's not a day over 60. She's looking forward to her granddaughters' return from college at Easter. Before they come back, she plans to have the family history and the family pictures all in order for them. She's going to write a childhood history of her home county. She is so lively and full of plans. She's not ready to die, not by a long shot." Obviously the volunteer reached a part of that client known to no one else on the team and quite a surprise to them. This also illustrates the fact that while some elderly persons are ready or accepting of death, many are not.

One of the great joys of hospice work is working with a interdisciplinary team and fully sharing in the care of the client/family without the traditional professional discipline barriers.

The Mini-Team

Team members who are working with a particular client/family, the so-called *mini-team,* are also in very frequent communication with each other, sometimes every day. For example, while visiting a client and his wife, one nurse detected much anger from the client and fear from the wife. The nurse also became aware that the client possessed a gun and feared that in his angry mood he might shoot his wife, himself, or both of them. The social worker was contacted to meet with the family.

In another situation, a home health assistant observed the client having labored breathing and noted the appearance of cyanosis on the client's upper lip and mouth. She summoned a nurse, who came and stayed through the client's death.

There are many such situations which cannot wait for the information sharing and discussion of a team meeting. At the same time, many interventions may be made in client/family care by one team member alone who has the requisite knowledge and assumes responsibility. One nurse found that the client with superior vena cava syndrome was taking Lasix 40 mg. twice daily for reducing edema and had been having tonic muscle spasms. She contacted the physician immediately to discuss possible calcium or potassium depletion. Both mini-team and individual interventions and their results are then reported later to the entire team and discussed.

Bereavement

Hospice care does not stop with the death of the client, because family care must continue. Bereavement follow-up is an integral part of hospice care. It begins before the client's death with the observation by team members of anticipatory grief. Various team members help family members work through this grief. Often, just before or at the time of death, team members make written assessments of the family's ability to survive the loss in a normal manner. Grief is a normal and natural process experienced by all who suffer losses, but it is more difficult to go through for some than for others.

Who in the hospice team does bereavement follow-up varies. Sometimes it is the nurse, but often the nurse herself has suffered a significant loss with the death of the client and must work through her own grief with subsequently diminished ability to help others. Sometimes home health assistants or volunteers do bereavement work. It need not be someone who has been with the family during the client's illness. It needs to be someone who is at ease with the situation and attentive to the needs of the bereaved rather than to his or her own needs. The assistant or volunteer should be someone experienced in bereavement counseling who is an active listener, who can understand the shock and accept the expressions of grief, who can be sensitive to the depression, and who can accept the tears, cursing, and anger. Mourning is hard work and those who have to mourn need to be intelligently, skillfully, and compassionately comforted.

Funding for Hospice Care

In 1982, Congress amended Section 122 in the Tax Equity and Fiscal Responsibility Act. The legislation was motivated by the discovery that around 80% of the hospice patients nationwide were recipients or potential recipients of Medicare. Known as the Medicare-Hospice Bill, or just the Hospice Bill, it provides that Medicare Part A-eligible terminally ill persons, terminally defined as having a prognosis of six months or less to live, may choose to receive hospice care for two 90-day periods followed by an additional 30-day period.

If, however, a person elects hospice care, he or she must forfeit ordinary Medicare payment for curative treatment or therapies designed to *treat* the terminal disease. The bill does not, however, deny regular Medicare payment for conditions unrelated to the terminal illness (for example, the treatment of gallstones in a terminally ill cancer patient). A hospice patient may change his or her mind, however, and decide to resume regular Medicare coverage. If this is the choice, it is acceptable but the client must give up hospice coverage for the time remaining in the hospice period. For example, if Mr. Jones decided on hospice coverage and after 25 days wanted to revoke that choice, the remaining 65 days (90 days minus

25 days) of his hospice Medicare coverage must be forfeited. Mr. Jones may at a later date, however, resume hospice coverage, beginning with a new, second 90-day coverage period. Clients may also change hospices once in each of the two 90-day periods and the additional 30-day period without forfeiting any hospice care time.

Other benefits to the client and family include:

• payment for homemaker services;
• reimbursement for continuous care in the home during periods of crisis;
• payment for medical supplies and equipment at 100% of cost;
• reimbursement for medications used in palliative treatment of the terminal illness and its symptoms (with the requirement of a 5% or $5.00 co-payment per prescription, whichever is less, by the client);
• respite care of no longer than five days to relieve the family in an inpatient facility reimbursed by Medicare (except for a 5% co-payment by client and family);
• reimbursement at 100% of cost of inpatient care necessary for acute or chronic symptom control.

While the legislation makes it clear that the backbone of hospice care is home care, it also recognized the necessity for inpatient facilities when relief of intractable symptoms or respite for family caregivers is necessary. Of particular importance from the point of view of hospice philosophy is the waiving of the homebound requirement for clients. Hospice care seeks to make the remaining days of the client's life as satisfactory as possible. Activities which ensure client satisfaction often involve leaving the home, such as going to see the flowers in the park, visiting neighbors, or even choosing a cemetery lot.

With the regulations of the various components of the Hospice bill, published in the *Federal Register* in 1983, hospices found themselves faced with numerous difficulties. It was not news to hospices that the Hospice bill had a sunset provision: the "hospice benefit" is available only from November 1, 1983 through September 30, 1986 unless Congress acts to make a change. In August, 1983, Congress acted by passing House Resolution 3677 to raise the cap proposed by HCFA (Health Care Financing Administration) from $4,332 per patient per year to a more reasonable $6,500. Many hospices are concerned about the tremendous requirements the regulations impose upon them and question the possibility of fulfilling them. However, they want to operate according to high standards and with economic effectiveness to prove the viability of the hospice movement before the 1986 sunset.

Some of the difficulties in the regulations relate to finances. HCFA has designated four categories of hospice care:

• routine home care, reimbursed at $53.17 per day;
• continuous home care for crisis times, reimbursed at a maximum (for 24-hour care) of $358.67 or $119.56 (for eight-hour care);

- in-patient respite care, reimbursed at a daily rate of $55.33;
- general inpatient care, for acute or chronic symptom management reimbursed at $271.00.

Hospice personnel find these reimbursement amounts completely inadequate for the complex care hospice patients require. The total number of inpatient days used by Medicare hospice beneficiaries in any 12-month period must not exceed 20% of the total number of days of hospice coverage provided those beneficiaries. Medicare will pay the hospice which, in turn, will pay the inpatient facilities with which it contracts for bids. Hospices may thus amass staggering bills.

Difficulties with the regulations relate to equally fundamental but more philosophical concerns. For a patient to qualify for Medicare hospice coverage for the first 90-day period, the attending physician and the hospice medical director must both certify in writing that the individual's medical prognosis is that of a life expectancy of six months or less. Many physicians have indicated unwillingness to sign such a certification statement. Clients must fully understand that, in electing hospice, they are electing "palliative in lieu of curative care" (*Federal Register*, Vol 48, No 243, Friday, December 16, 1983, p. 56010, Section E).

Additional difficulties with the regulations relate to legal questions and the problem of turf. The hospice alone is given the right to "express authorization of any inpatient services" (*Federal Register*, December 16, 1983, p 56028, 418.566(2)). This authority is to be achieved through a legally binding written contract between the hospital and the inpatient facilities. Because this written document is to identify the specific services to be provided to the patient, one might expect difficulties to arise. The document states that services may be provided only with the express authorization of the hospice and that the services are to be coordinated, supervised and evaluated by the hospice. Under these rules, one might expect difficulties to arise. Such management in an inpatient facility by an outside health care provider raises many professional concerns.

Other difficulties raised by the regulations relate, as might be expected, to increased paper work and therefore increased costs. For example, the hospice would be required to keep records on the use made of volunteers and on the cost savings and expansion of care achieved by using volunteers. This process involves the volunteers in paper work—keeping records of mileage, time spent, activities—and hospice personnel will also have increased paper work and demands on time.

The problems mentioned above are only a few raised by the regulations which interpret the hospice bill. Some hospices decided to seek certification in 1983. Many others decided to seek certification at a later date after a lapse of time had allowed them to put in place those components of the hospice program required by the regulations. Some hospices will continue to choose non-Medicare hospice status and will not try to comply with the regulations nor receive Medicare payment under the hospice bill. All hospices, however, regardless of their choice regarding reimbursement under the hospice bill, will be needing far greater community support, both in dollars and in willing hands, than has ever been true before.

Summary

With home hospice care for the dying and their families, an old and satisfying method of dealing with one of life's most critical crises has been revived and given new life. Death has again been recognized as a natural part of life, and modern technological achievements have been made available to serve the needs and wishes of the dying and their loved ones. Once again there is talk of the *good death,* but exactly what constitutes a good death depends upon the dying individual.

Hospice care satisfies not only the needs of the dying and their families but of the caregivers as well. It enables the latter to exercise their special skills with the need defined partly by the client. Hospice care enables caregivers to work with other caregivers in a harmonious, non-competitive, mutually dependent, and supportive relationship. This relationship occurs because the focus of hospice care is not the professionals' exercising their skills, but the needs of the client and family. The client/family and their needs are the subject of conferences by team members. While the team members also have needs to be met, and these needs are neglected at the risk of compromising their ability to function in hospice care, client and family are at the center of hospice care. A recent increase in federal funding for hospice care will provide this type of care for more people.

REFERENCES

Saunders C: "Moment of Truth, Care of the Dying Person," Chapter 3 in Pearson L (ed.): *Death and Dying: Current Issues in Treatment of the Dying Person.* Press of the Case Western Reserve University, Cleveland, Ohio, 1969
Stoddard S: *The Hospice Movement.* Stein and Day, Briarcliff Manor, N.Y., 1978, p 73

BIBLIOGRAPHY

Berry I: "Pharmacy services in hospice organizations." *Hospital Formulary*, October 1982, pp 1333–38
Buckingham R W, Lupu D: "A comparative study of hospice services in the United States." *Am J Pub Health*, Vol 72, No 5, May 1982, pp 455–63
Burkhalter P K, Donley D L: *Dynamics of Oncology Nursing.* McGraw-Hill Book Company, New York, 1978
Caroline N L: "Dying in academe." *The New Physician*, Vol 21, No 11, November 1972
Corr C, Corr D (eds.): *Hospice Care: Principles and Practice.* Springer Publishing Company, New York, 1983

Da Ramon P B: "The final task: Life review for the dying patient." *Nursing 83*, Vol 13, No 2, February 1983, pp 44–49

Dobihal S V: "Enabling a patient to die at home." *Am J Nurs*, Vol 80, No 8, August 1980, pp 1448–51

Donovan M I, Pierce S G: *Cancer Care Nursing.* Appleton-Century-Crofts, New York, 1976

Eastman M: "Shattering myths about hospice care." *American Pharmacy*, Vol NS18, No 12, November 1978, pp 20–21

Garfield C A: *Psychosocial Care of the Dying Patient.* McGraw Hill Book Company, New York, 1978

Geltman R, Paige R: "Symptom management in hospice care." *Am J Nurs*, Vol 83, No 1, January 1983, pp 78–85

Giacquinta B: "Helping families face the crisis of cancer." *Am J Nurs*, Vol 77, No 10, October 1977, pp 1585–88

Hinton J: *Dying.* Penguin Books, New York, 1972

Isler C: "Approaching the final day." *RN*, Vol 41, No 4, April 1978, pp 63–65

Kubler-Ross E: *On Death and Dying.* Macmillan Publishing Company, New York, 1969

Kubler-Ross E: *Questions and Answers on Death and Dying.* Collier Books, New York, 1974

Kubler-Ross, ed.: *Death: The Final Stage of Growth.* Prentice-Hall, Inc., Englewood Cliffs, New Jersey, 1975

Lipman A G: "Drug therapy in cancer pain." *Cancer Nurs*, Vol 3, No 1, February 1980, pp 39–46

"Long-awaited hospice regs spark debate; House votes new pay limit." *Am J Nurs*, Vol 83, No 10, October 1983, pp 1467, 1480

Martin A: "Hospice nursing: Walking a fine line." *Nursing 81*, Vol 11, No 2, February 1981, pp 128–30

Maxwell M B: "How to use methadone for the cancer patient's pain." *Am J Nurs*, Vol 80, No 9, September 1980, pp 1606–09

McCaffery M: *Nursing Management of the Patient With Pain.* J. B. Lippincott Company, New York, 1979

McCaffery M: "Relieving pain with noninvasive techniques." *Nursing 80 Vol 10, No 12, December 1980, pp 55–57*

McNairn N: "Helping the patient who wants to die at home." *Nursing 81* Vol 11, No 2, February 1981, p 66

O'Connor A B: *Dying and Grief: Nursing Interventions.* The American Journal of Nursing Company, New York, 1976

Putnam S et al.: "Home as a place to die." *Am J Nurs*, Vol 80, No 8, August 1980, pp 1451–53

Saunders C M (ed.): *The Management of Terminal Disease.* Edward Arnold Ltd., London, 1978

Shneidman E: *Voices of Death.* Harper and Row, New York, 1980

Stoddard S: *The Hospice Movement: A Better Way of Caring for the Dying.* Stein and Day, Briarcliff Manor, New York, 1978

Thomas V M: "Hospice nursing—reaping the rewards, dealing with the stresses." *Geriat Nurs*, Vol 4, No 1, January-February 1983, pp 22–27

Wald F S: "Terminal care and nursing education." *Am J Nurs*, Vol 79, No 10, October 1979, pp 1762–64

West B A: "Understanding endorphins: Our natural pain relief system." *Nursing 81*, Vol 11, No 2, February 1981, pp 50–53

West B A: "Understanding your patient's pain." *Nursing 80*, Vol 10, No 9, September 1980, pp 26–31

West B A: "Patients shouldn't have to suffer—relieve their pain with injectable narcotics." *Nursing 80*, Vol 10, No 10, October 1980, pp 34–39

West B A: "Relieve your patients' pain fast and effectively with oral analgesics." *Nursing 80*, Vol 10, No 11, November 1980, pp 58–63

SECTION II
THE ROLE OF THE NURSE

CHAPTER 5

HOME HEALTH CARE: THE NURSE'S PERSPECTIVE

Marta Askew Browning

Nurses are uniquely positioned to assume leadership in what promises to be a significant shift of health care delivery from the institution to the home. This shift in locus of health care delivery is projected to continue through the remainder of this century because of the impact of federal legislation. Notable examples of such legislation include:

- Medicare and Medicaid, which provide reimbursement for home health services;
- prospective reimbursement for hospitals that promote early discharge of patients to home care;
- hospice benefits through Medicare for eligible beneficiaries who are terminally ill.

Home Health, Medicare, and the Nurse

Home health services for the population over 65 years of age are reimbursed primarily by Title XX: Federal Health Insurance for the Aged-Medicare. The Medicare legislation established specific regulations governing home health agencies. Within these regulations, the role of nursing is given much attention.

In "Conditions of Participation in Home Health Agencies: Federal Health Insurance for the Aged—Regulations" (12, 1968 Reg. 405.1220), the primary functions of a home health agency are as follows:

" . . . the provision of skilled nursing services and other therapeutic services on a visiting basis in a place of residence used as the individual's home."

To become certified as a home health agency, the agency must provide at least one other therapeutic service besides nursing. These other services may be physical, speech, or occupational therapy, medical social services, or home health aide services. Agencies may provide more than one therapeutic service, but the mandatory service is nursing. Without nursing, there is no certification. Thus, since the beginning of Medicare, nursing was established as the essential home health service.

The regulations identify seven major duties. The nurse:

- evaluates and regularly re-evaluates the nursing needs of the patient;
- develops and implements the nursing care plan for the patient;
- provides nursing services, treatment and diagnostic and preventive procedures requiring substantial specialized skill;
- initiates preventive and rehabilitative nursing procedures as appropriate for the patient's care and safety;
- observes signs and symptoms and reports to the physician reactions to treatments, including drugs, and changes in the patient's physical or emotional condition;
- teaches, supervises and counsels the patient and family members regarding the nursing care needs and other related problems of the patient at home;
- supervises and trains other nursing service personnel "Conditions of Participation," (12, 1968, 405.1228)

Over the years this general outline of professional nursing duties has been maintained. In addition, extensive updates have been added that specify the types, duration and frequency of treatments which may be provided by the nurse. It is important to note that the nurse is restricted in the development of the nursing care plan by these specific guidelines. Care that is not within the provision of the regulations is not reimbursed by Medicare.

Qualifications of the Home Health Nurse

Education and Licensure

The professional nurse delivering home health care through a Medicare-certified agency must maintain a current license as a registered nurse in the state in which she or he practices. The regulations recognize the value of experience and education by stating two preferred qualifications:

- one year of prior experience in professional nursing;
- qualification as a public health nurse who has completed a baccalaureate degree program or post-baccalaureate study approved by the National League for Nursing for public health preparation ("Conditions of Participation 12, 1968, 405.1228).

Personal Traits

The responsibilities of home health nurses are great. In addition to possessing desirable credentials—education, preparation, experience—these nurses should also possess certain personal traits. Among the most desirable of these are:

- ability to make independent decisions based on a sound theoretical and scientific knowledge base;
- assertiveness;
- ability to tolerate ambiguity and to function in an unstructured environment;
- willingness to assume responsibility for one's own actions;
- ability to organize and manage time efficiently;
- highly developed interpersonal skills and eagerness to work in and through groups to accomplish tasks;
- clear concept of the scope of professional nursing practice and a desire to promote the role of the nurse in delivering both present and potential services;
- interest in people and eagerness to work with a wide range of personalities;
- desire to encourage independence in consumers and staff rather than a desire to control their actions;
- patience and persistence in working with and through people to achieve change, often over long periods of time;
- ability to articulate clearly, both verbally and in writing;
- ability to stay calm in crisis situations, particularly since one seldom has immediate back-up support available;
- skill in conflict management;
- warmth, empathetic concern, and respect for other people;
- flexibility and ability to adapt quickly to changing situations or client care requirements.

Clinical Competence

Personality traits and education must be supplemented by one very important final requirement: *clinical competence.* Increasing fiscal constraints implemented to control soaring hospital costs (such as the introduction of prospective reimbursement and diagnosis–related groups to establish reimbursement ceilings) are forcing hospitals to discharge patients earlier. The home health agency is now expected to provide care not only for the chronically ill older client, but also for the older client still in some phase of acute illness. Tasks being performed in the home may be: administration of antibiotics, hemodialysis, chemotherapy by infusion pump, and supervision of intravenous chemotherapy techniques.

Complex patient–care procedures have prompted home care agencies to include staff nurses with advanced preparation or clinical specialities in fields such as gerontological nursing practice, enterostomal therapy, pulmonary care nursing, cardiovascular nursing, oncology, psychiatric nursing, and family nursing practice. At the present time, some of the most complex nursing care is being delivered in the home. With the exception of surgical and acute intensive care services, almost any nursing procedure can be accommodated in the home with some modification in technique.

Management and Supervisory Skills

For a home health agency to participate as a Medicare provider, the agency must designate a physician or registered professional nurse to supervise the agency's performance in providing home health services in accordance with the orders of attending physicians of the patients referred for care. The regulations express a preference for a public health nurse if a nurse is designated as a supervisor ("Conditions of Participation", 12, 1968, 405.1222). Currently, in most home health agencies, this supervisory responsibility is performed by a nurse rather than a physician. The organization may have a tier of nursing supervision starting at the top with an executive director who directs nursing supervisors who, in turn, direct team leaders who coordinate direct patient care by an interdisciplinary team.

In a number of states, state licensing laws indicate more stringent requirements for supervisory nursing personnel than do the federal regulations. Most often these include the requirement that a nursing director hold a master's degree, preferably in public health supervision or administration and have at least five years of public health experience, a portion in supervision. The requirements for nursing supervisors express a preference for a baccalaureate degree and a specified number of years of experience in public health nursing.

Home care nurses primarily responsible for the development and funding of programs and/or the supervision and direction of staff must move gradually away from clinical skill development to acquiring expertise in management. Home health is a highly competitive business. Nurses who currently hold management positions have generally risen to those positions because they were recognized and identified as excellent practitioners of nursing. Unfortunately, the skills that prepare one to be a fine clinician are not necessarily the same skills required to direct and administer the operation of a health care agency. Unless nurses develop administrative skills equal to those of successful corporate business managers, home care will be taken over by the non-nurse managers who are most able to operate efficiently in providing services demanded by consumers in a cost effective manner.

General Considerations for Nurses Employed in Home Health Care

The delivery of care to clients in the home and community is different from delivery of care in a highly structured and controlled institutional setting. In the institution, patients are brought to the nurse. They have entered the institution by referral from a physician or through the efforts of an active hospital marketing department.

In home care, the nurse must assume a more active role in the recruitment and retention of clients. As more reimbursement becomes available for home care, the number of home health agencies will increase, and competition among agencies will increase. For many nurses, functioning independently in a competitive environment will be a new experience. Consideration should, therefore, be given to selecting an appropriate employer, learning to operate in a competitive field, and cultivating referral sources to enhance agency business.

Selection of a Home Health Agency as an Employer

A home health nurse's first challenge is to choose a home health agency. Because home health care is provided by various types of agencies, these agencies have their own special characteristics and organizational goals.

The agency should have a written philosophy that supports a belief in quality care. Agency personnel should be able to identify ways in which quality care is defined, identified, monitored and evaluated. Job descriptions should be available. The duties described should be within the scope of nursing practice and include expectations beyond a minimum level of performance. The agency should provide an orientation and ongoing in-service education for employees. Such education should focus on keeping staff aware of the rapid changes in health care delivery and how new technology and treatments can be implemented in the home.

The nurse seeking an employer will wish to explore the qualifications of supervisory personnel and peers. It is important to obtain an accurate picture of the nature and extent of supervision and peer support available. Home care is provided in the home away from the direct guidance and support of other health professionals. At times the responsibility is awesome. The nurse must be able to count on back-up advice, direction and assistance by phone or by means of joint visits with colleagues.

Finally, the nurse seeking a position in home health should explore the funding and sources of revenue of the agency. With the rapid growth of agencies, it is important to determine whether the potential employer is fiscally sound and apt to be in business for a long time. In addition, the nurse will want to evaluate the philosophy of the agency regarding reimbursement for services. The agency should have definite plans for providing care for patients who need care but have exhausted their insurance benefits and/or private resources. The nurse must determine whether agency policies regarding types of patients served and financing of their care are compatible with the delivery of quality nursing care and if these policies are compatible with the nurse's own philosophy of nursing and home care.

Competition for Clients

As funding for home health increases, agencies will abound, each competing for a share of the marketplace. On the positive side, competition has the advantage of forcing agencies to operate efficiently and provide cost-effective services or go out of business; thus, cost of care will be reduced or at least restricted to a reasonable rate of growth.

On the other hand, competition can create an environment in which the consumer is tossed back and forth between agencies seeking to generate business and unscrupulous practices may develop in an effort to make a profit or obtain clients. For example, the term "dumping" is a familiar one to home care providers. This term refers to the questionable practice of admitting a client to service and providing care only as long as third–party insurance or personal finances are available for reimbursement. At the point that finances are exhausted, even though the client may still need care, he or she is "dumped" or terminated from service.

In many communities, there are no community-supported agencies for clients ineligible for insurance benefits but unable to pay for service. These clients are left without care. For those agencies that are the recipients of clients terminated inappropriately by another agency, the problems are enormous. Limited funds allotted to those needing financial assistance are strained; an influx of clients ineligible for reimbursement disrupts the agency cash flow position; agency staff must deal with the hostility and humiliation of the client who has been terminated from the former agency's service; and staff must cope with their own frustration of being unable to stop such practices.

Nurses are not generally exposed to competition or marketing techniques during the educational process nor during employment in institutional settings. They are, instead, nurtured in environments in which the patients come to them. It is, therefore, a challenge to the home care nurse to market his or her services to physicians, discharge planners, patients and other referral services. The need to market or explain one's services forces nurses and nursing organizations to identify and articulate clearly the benefits of nursing service. Those nurses who enjoy the setting in which they work and believe in the importance of the service they provide will be the best advertisement for those services.

Cultivating Referral Sources and Resources

Client referrals to the home care agency come from many sources. Indeed, almost anyone with whom agency staff interacts is a potential source of referral. Therefore, it is essential that all staff members become familiar with the specific programs and services of the agency and the methods used by the agency to establish and/ or negotiate fees.

When an agency provides services to elderly clients, it is particularly important for staff members to know current details about Medicare coverage. Staff members are continuously amazed at the lack of information and understanding elderly people have regarding the benefits of their Medicare insurance. Most are familiar with their right of reimbursement for hospital services, but are surprised to find that home care services are a covered benefit. This lack of awareness extends beyond the Medicare recipients to relatives and professional caregivers, such as the client's personal physician. Education, then, is the most important function in cultivating referral sources. People cannot use the service unless they know it exists and understand how it will benefit them personally.

Consideration should be given to some of the following groups as potential sources of referral.

Consumers Themselves

Older adults may be contacted through such groups as local units of the American Association of Retired Persons, professional groups of retired persons (teachers, postal workers, etc.), senior centers, agency on aging advisory councils and sub-units, church groups, local retirement villages, hotels, community centers, and any other gathering place for the elderly. At the time of initial contact, the client may not be in need of service, but during subsequent times of crisis the agency may be relied upon again.

Discharge Planners

Institution discharge planners usually are nurses or social workers who must identify alternatives for continued care in the community and present a choice of options to the patient. For example, a terminally ill cancer patient may want to go to a nursing home, enroll in a hospice program, or use a home health agency for support during the terminal phase of end-stage disease. It is important that the staff of the home health agency make frequent contact with discharge planners and keep them aware of changes or expansion in agency services.

Agency staff must be cognizant of the fact that the discharge planner will base subsequent referrals on how well the agency performed in the past.

Physicians

Physicians refer patients to the home health agency directly from their own private practice or from the hospital, through the discharge planner. Physicians are most often relieved to know that home care services are available to their patients.

The physician is concerned about the *quality* of home care supervision and will feel most comfortable when working in partnership with the nurse who acts as case coordinator for the physician's clients. Therefore, it is important for nurses to meet with physicians whose patients they care for, to establish professional credibility. Having made an initial personal contact, follow-up may be made through telephone calls or in writing:

- to communicate changes in the patient's condition;
- to provide periodic updates on patient progress in meeting treatment goals; and
- to suggest additional services and/or therapeutic approaches to care.

Inpatient Nursing Staff

Nursing staff delivering acute care services are often in a good position to identify those patients who will need follow-up services after discharge. If they are familiar with the services of the home health agency, they can suggest such services to the patient, the family, the physician, and/or the discharge planner.

Volunteers

Volunteers can be found in all sectors of the health care delivery system. Volunteers directly affiliated with the home health agency are a vital resource for educating the public on benefits of home care. These agency-affiliated volunteers may be board members, may provide direct client care support services such as "Friendly Visitor" or "Respite Care", may supplement clerical and administrative functions, and/or be involved in fund raising which subsidizes the cost of agency service.

However, volunteers with other health or social services connections must not be overlooked in obtaining referrals. For instance, a volunteer with Meals-on-Wheels is in an excellent position to identify the homebound elderly who would profit greatly from service.

Children and Friends of the Elderly

This group finds home health care agencies almost by accident. They may hear about the service by word-of-mouth or through civic, church and social organizations where educational presentations have been made. Occasionally, they contact the home health agency because they are familiar with a similar agency in another locale. For example, Visiting Nurse Associations have been well established in the northeastern section of the United States for almost a century. It is not at all unusual for an agency in one section of the country to receive a referral from a middle-aged daughter or son living in another section of the country who desires evaluation and, if appropriate, services for a retired parent living in that community.

The agency thus benefits from the fine reputation established by agencies similar in philosophy and organization. Maintaining contact with these long–distance referral sources is one of the greatest services a home health agency can offer family members. Fragmentation of the American family is reflected more by diverse residential locations rather than dissolution of the bonds of love and affection. When great distances separate family members, nothing is more reassuring than knowing that relatives and friends can receive help and service by caring professionals.

Social and Health Service Agencies

All agencies providing services to older adults within a community need to be informed about the availability of home care and will need to be educated regarding eligibility of clients for those services.

Agency-to-agency Referral

Home health agencies often refer clients to one another. Referrals can be made for a variety of reasons. Among these are:

Geographical location. Residence of the client is in the geographical location more easily served by a home health agency other than the one receiving the initial referral.

Availability of services. One home health agency has services needed by the client which are not a part of the programming of the agency that initially received the referral. Weekend nursing coverage, 24-hour call, or hospice volunteers are some examples.

Personal requests. Personal requests of the client, family or the physician for transfer from one agency to another.

Inadequate financial resources. Referral of clients who have exhausted financial resources to an agency which can cover costs of service with supplemental funding.

Inappropriate referral. This type of referral is the most exasperating for providers. The home care client, facing an acute personal crisis, is often desperate for help. The rapid proliferation of agencies and services available may prove confusing and overwhelming to the client. The consumer quite naturally may seek to manipulate the system to secure desired services. For example, the client may attempt to obtain a team of professionals and paraprofessionals whose personalities are compatible with his or her needs.

The client may try to use the services of a nurse from one agency and a physical therapist and home health aide from another. Or, the client may involve several agencies in the care, scheduling the delivery of services on different days so that the providers remain unaware of each other's involvement for several weeks until the third-party insurance payor denies reimbursement for duplicated services. Sometimes such manipulation of the system is calculated and deliberate. Most often, however, it is unintentional and is the result of an elderly client's misunderstanding of rules and regulations governing payment for home health services. At times such as these, cooperation between home health agencies is essential if the needs of the client are to be met in a fair and equitable manner.

Medical Equipment Suppliers and Pharmacists

Providers of durable medical equipment, supplies and medications are often prime referral sources. These providers become familiar with agency services and personnel in the process of performing their own tasks and duties. If contact with the home health agency is a positive experience, the relationship will develop into one of mutual benefit. Each provider will educate consumers about the services of the other and an effective word-of-mouth referral system will have been established.

Thus far, this discussion has centered around how the nurse can cultivate referral sources. By now, the reader has probably noted that the referral sources are also the community resources to which nurses and other disciplines refer their own client/family units for procuring specialized services or achieving specific health care goals. Thus, a reciprocal relationship exists.

The Delivery of Home Nursing Care

The Initial Home Health Visit

Often, the nurse will need to call the referral source to obtain additional information prior to scheduling a visit with the client. Consideration will also need to be given to the agency's policy regarding charges for an evaluation visit. In some agencies, an evaluation visit may be made for assessment of the client/family situation and environmental conditions with subsequent evaluation of appropriate eligibility of the client for admission to service. These evaluation visits are not charged to the client but absorbed in the agency's overhead costs. At other times, the initial visit will be ordered by the physician for the provision of treatment and will be reimbursable by Medicare.

Initial visits are generally lengthy, lasting from an hour to one and a half hours and include, but are not limited to, the following types of activities.

Establishing a Relationship With the Client and Family

This process can be initiated by introducing oneself and explaining one's role with the agency, expected role in delivering care to the family (for example, assessment visit only, follow-up care, or intermittent visiting to supervise the work of others), and the nature of the relationship between the nurse and the referral source. Here is one approach: "We work closely with Dr. Jones when he has home care patients. I will be contacting him after this visit to discuss the care needed. We will work closely together and with you to develop plans for care which meet your needs."

In addition, during this initial phase of contact, the nurse will want to elicit from the client and family the major problem and their view of what the nurse can do for them. Attempts to move forward with other nursing tasks will not generally meet with success until the client and family have the opportunity to share their perceptions of their current situation. For many elderly clients who are isolated from family, friends and support systems, this phase of the visit provides an opportunity to reach out, make human contact, and share one's frustrations.

Collection of the Health History

After eliciting information surrounding the client's/family's major needs, the nurse will want to refocus the direction of the interview to collect a health history and evaluate medications currently used by the client. It is important to ask to *see* all medications, both prescription and over-the-counter, being used by the client and to have the client and/or responsible family member describe what they think the medication is for, how often it is taken, and the response obtained from taking the drug. It is not unusual for elderly clients to be taking many medications prescribed by *different* physicians, or to be taking out-of-date drugs or drugs prescribed for someone else.

In addition, the elderly often adhere to the use of certain non-prescription, self-prescribed regimens, such as use of laxatives, analgesics and over-the-counter sedatives. The nurse will often identify medication problems and a need for client teaching regarding medication use. To further complicate matters, some elderly clients may be confused and are subject to undermedicating or overdosing themselves.

Performance of Physical Assessment

After the nurse has collected the health history, an evaluation of the physical status of the client is in order. This assessment should be systematic and planned carefully to avoid fatiguing the client. The nurse will want to evaluate carefully all physical parameters directly associated with the client's medical diagnosis. This careful evaluation of other body systems must also be done in the process of performing a physical assessment because the client may have physical problems unidentified by the referral source.

If the client uses a respirator, intravenous equipment, a catheter, oxygen or a dressing, the nurse will want the client and family members to describe the instructions they were given regarding the use of equipment or performance of procedures, and steps to take in an emergency. If appropriate, the nurse may also ask the client or family member to demonstrate the performance of procedures for which they have received prior instruction. This process gives the nurse a chance to observe an elderly client's comprehension, manual dexterity, and level of frustration related to expected self-care activities.

Summary of Major Client Problems

After the nurse has collected the health history and performed the physical assessment, he or she will want to identify the major problems. These problems need to be identified *with* the client and/or family to ascertain their priorities for intervention and to validate whether they perceive the same problems that the nurse has identified. No problem can be successfully dealt with until the client and family recognize that a problem exists and are willing to work to resolve the problem.

For example, the nurse may identify that a male patient, post-stroke, will need extensive personal care assistance. The nurse may believe that his frail, elderly spouse, suffering from heart disease, will be unable to carry out transfer activities, bed positioning, or range-of-motion exercises, or to provide assistance with these activities. The nurse may suggest the services of a home health aide and physical therapist. The client's wife may refuse these services because she feels that she will be able to manage her husband's care. Thus, the nurse may have to defer active intervention for specific problems until the family is ready to deal effectively with those problems.

Identification of Agency Services To Be Provided

After the nurse and client/family have identified the major health problems requiring intervention, the nurse will need to explain to the family the agency's role in meeting their needs. It will be important to explain the specific services that can be provided directly by agency staff (for example, nursing, speech therapy, physical therapy, occupational therapy, homemaker/health aide, social worker) and describe the services that can be procured by the agency but provided by other community resources (for example, transportation, Meals-on-Wheels, durable medical equipment, or respite care).

Family members will need instructions if they are expected to contact and secure services from any community resources. The nurse should also identify for the family the agency contact person who will be coordinating the services provided for them.

Identification of Ultimate Goals of Service

On the first home visit, the nurse must explain to the client and family that they will ultimately be expected to achieve self-sufficiency in meeting their own needs. The purpose of nursing, other therapeutic services, and support services, such as homemaking, are to aid the family in making a transition from the helplessness of an acute crisis to competency in making adaptations in life style or managing long-term care.

The client must understand at the beginning that the delivery of care is usually time-limited and that the agency staff are not permanent substitutes for family or community caregivers. This concept will need gentle reinforcement during the agency-client relationship to prevent development of dependency of the family unit on agency caregivers.

It is also important to discuss the *expected* length of time and number of visits which will be made before the client is discharged from service. These expectations will be based on the client's prognosis for improvement and financial situation. Defining goals in relation to expected length of service enables the family to establish target dates for acquiring competence in client care tasks. Target dates also reduce the anger and despair of a family who suddenly face termination from service without warning.

Evaluation of Fee Sources Available for Payment for Service

On the initial visit the nurse must explore the funding sources available to the client. The nurse will need to know if home care services are to be covered by third party insurance (private insurance, Medicare, or Medicaid), self-payment, or whether fee adjustments will be required. If a fee adjustment will be required, financial information must be collected which will enable the agency to determine the type of adjustment (for example, sliding fee scale) appropriate in the family's situation.

For agencies serving only those with private payment or third party reimbursement, they will need to refer clients elsewhere. Methods of fee setting and fee collection will need to be discussed fully with the client/family. The concept of covered and non-covered benefits under Medicare and/or Medicaid will need to be explained and the client/family will need to know what fees they will be expected to pay if they request and receive any services not covered as part of their Medicare benefit. Information regarding billing and payment for services may have to be repeated on subsequent visits because the older adult, and even middle-aged children, often find insurance regulations confusing.

Review of Consumer Bill of Rights

The nurse should inform the client/family regarding reasonable expectations related to agency performance. Furthermore, the client/family should receive information regarding procedures to be followed if they believe that the care received is inadequate.

Permission for Release of Information

In order to receive and transfer information among providers—physicians, discharge planners, home health agency staff, third party insurance payors—a permission to release information must be secured from the client/family.

Client/Family Teaching

The nurse has much to do on the first visit. The amount of material to be absorbed by the family is overwhelming. Therefore, client/family instruction is best kept to a minimum and focused only around needs which cannot wait until the next nursing visit.

Developing the Plan of Treatment

When the initial assessment has been completed, the nurse must establish the plan of treatment that will be authorized (signed) by the client's physician. Careful consideration must be given to the construction of the treatment plan, one that will not cause a denial of reimbursement.

This aspect of home care is fraught with frustration for nurses. The focus of professional nursing education has traditionally been to develop plans of patient care which consider the holistic needs of the patient and family. In most nursing schools, students are taught to identify *all* major needs of the patient and to consider all aspects of the patients' total situation when identifying patient problems appropriate for nursing intervention.

In the hospital setting, the nurse provides nursing care based extensively on the medical plan of care. However, in the home health agency, the nurse faces a dilemma. Elderly clients generally have limited financial resources. They are most often dependent on third-party reimbursement for coverage of services provided by the home health agency. Therefore, if the treatment plan requests services not covered by the insurance carrier, the agency staff will not be paid for those services.

Therefore, *the nurse is confronted with the challenge of developing care plans that provide for quality care that is reimbursable.* Careful consideration must be given to identifying services actually needed by the client. The nurse must avoid the temptation to provide desirable, but not crucial services. Reimbursement will be based on medical necessity and will be denied if services are not reasonable in relation to the client's health status. Primary prevention is not a reimbursable service, but concepts of primary, secondary and tertiary prevention can be readily integrated into the care plan of the client receiving intermittent nursing service.

However, even with careful planning, the nurse will be limited by types of service for which reimbursement is provided and the number of visits allowed by insurers for specific types of conditions. Nurses frequently are upset when care seems to be determined, not by the client's real needs, but by what is reimbursable. It is incumbent on the nurse, therefore, to advocate appropriate change in the range and scope of covered services through professional organizations and political activity.

When services must be limited, it is important for the nurse to assist the client in coping with the realistic limitations imposed by funding or by the progress of his condition. For example, the goal of the home health therapy provider is to promote maximum functioning within the client's physical limitations. Home health therapy services may be provided as long as the client is demonstrating progress. However, a day will come when the client reaches a plateau in performance. While he or she might want the therapist to continue visits, no further physical gain can be obtained from therapy services. The responsibility now is returned to the family.

In addition to identifying nursing services for the older adult, the nurse must also identify the need for services provided by other professional and paraprofessional staff (physical therapy, occupational therapy, speech therapy, social work, home health aides).

The nurse will list supplies and equipment needed by the client. When the plan of treatment has been developed, it is sent to the physician for signature. Upon receipt of the treatment plan, the physician may make adjustments in the proposed plan for management. Generally, changes are confined to aspects of medical management, such as alterations in medications, and the remainder of the plan is authorized as submitted by the nurse. Treatment plans are reviewed by the nurse and re-certified by the physician at least every 60 days.

Providing Ongoing Client Care Service

As nurses evaluate the suitability and application of suggested nursing care plans to a client situation, they should remember that:

- the method of implementation of care plans should foster independence of the client/family unit;
- client/family teaching is the most important function of the nurse;
- goals and plans for discharge should be developed at the time of admission, and progress should be reviewed with the client/family throughout the course of care;
- emotional support for the client is a "given" in health care, but the nurse must remember that in the home, support for the family caregivers is essential for maintaining the integrity of the family unit and to move the course of care toward the established goals.

Support for the Family

Many responsibilities undertaken by family members are strange and frightening, and fatigue can make tasks seem overwhelming. In addition, the nurse may need to accept the older adult's frustration with a system which he or she may perceive to be unfair.

For example, one older couple was surviving on a fixed income. The wife, the agency's client, was bedfast with severe Parkinson's disease complicated by heart disease. The responsibilities of the husband, as major caregiver, restricted him to the house. In order to provide them both with some contact with other human beings, the client's husband gently and tenderly transported the client to a local Senior Center for lunch three times a week. Dressing and performing wheelchair-to-car transfers was a laborious and painful process for this couple, but considered worth the effort because the end result relieved isolation and loneliness of both. However, the funding source denied Medicare reimbursement for this client because she was not "homebound". The husband, confronted with this ruling, was understandably angry with "the system" which presented him with a choice of remaining confined to home and receiving reimbursement for care or continuing to participate in a limited form of social activity and paying the full cost of care (which he could not afford unless depleting his entire life savings of $1,500) himself. Older adults, reared in a time when the work ethic was strong, may also have difficulty accepting their current limitations and resent having to rely on assistance (financial and personal) because they can no longer "pay their own way" and/or "take care of their own".

Records and Reporting

The nurse in home health, as in all other areas of nursing practice, is responsible for accurate, complete and timely documentation of client care activities on the clinical record. However, care must be taken that documentation includes facts that support the continuation of care which will be reimbursable by the third party payor, Medicare. Treatment plans and clinical records are routinely sampled by the Medicare fiscal intermediaries and payment for care may be denied if adequate and appropriate documentation is not present. Denial of reimbursement for care will cause the agency to take a financial loss. If too many denials occur, the agency comes under close scrutiny; all treatment plans are reviewed; and an increased proportion of the clinical records are examined in the entirety. This process is extremely expensive for the agency and, ultimately, for all taxpayers.

Private insurance payors may also ask for documentation of home care services that they reimburse. In addition, the clinical records are scrutinized by licensing and certification agencies to evaluate the quality of care delivered by agency staff and to ascertain the level of adherence to the medical treatment plan.

In home health, the nurse's responsibilities extend beyond the clinical record and involve the completion of other records and reports. Among these are:

- medical treatment plans for establishing service, reporting client progress, and requesting a recertification of care for an additional 60–day period if the client's situation is not resolved within the period covered by prior treatment plans;
- referrals to other professional disciplines within the agency and to community resources needed to meet client care goals;
- follow-up reports to discharge planners regarding the home situation of client/ family;
- discharge summaries for agency, physicians, other selected referral sources, and the utilization review committees of the agencies;
- financial evaluation forms for client/family and billing slips for services rendered and supplies ordered;
- mileage and expense sheets submitted to agency for reimbursement of personal expenses;
- time sheets used by the agency to determine productivity and to evaluate the time devoted to specified tasks.

Coordination of Services on an Interdisciplinary Team

In most agencies, the nurse coordinates the services of the interdisciplinary team in home health. This role may be performed when the nurse is the case manager and coordinates services for individual client/family units. Or, on a larger scale, the nurse acts as the team leader or nursing supervisor for an interdisciplinary group of professionals providing service within a specified geographical area.

Nurse Control of Client Services

The nurse coordinator controls access of the patient to the services of the other team members through the development of the treatment plan and identification of the services that will be used in meeting and resolving the client/family problems. Occasionally, the physician will refer patients to the agency specifically for physical or speech therapy; but most often, it is the nurse who identifies the need to involve other professional disciplines in client care. In addition, if care is to be paid for by Medicare insurance, the consumer must be receiving skilled nursing, physical therapy, *or* speech therapy before he or she is entitled to services of the occupational therapist, social worker, or home health aide.

Team Conferences

It is the responsibility of the nurse coordinator or supervisor to work with team members to establish goals of care for the client/family unit and to direct and coordinate the services of each discipline so that goals are met. To achieve this end, the nurse plans and schedules team conferences to allow team members to discuss and evaluate patient progress and determine strategies for dealing with specific client care problems. It is also important for the team members to synchronize services when the client is scheduled for discharge. For example, billing errors can occur when the nurse has closed the case and the occupational therapist or home health aide continues to visit. In the previous example, nursing closed the case, so services of the occupational therapist and home health aide are not reimbursable if they continue after nursing has ceased.

Supervision of the Team

Supervision of the interdisciplinary team is a special challenge for the nurse coordinator. The nurse knows professional nursing care and has usually had experience in supervising and directing the work of other registered nurses, licensed vocational (practical) nurses and nurse aides. Therefore, when working with other nurses, the nurse supervisor is on familiar ground. However, when coordinating the services of nursing with those provided by therapy and social work, nurses may not feel as secure. It is essential, therefore, that the home health nurse become thoroughly familiar with the job descriptions, professional philosophies and state licensing laws of all disciplines on the team.

Field visits to observe care being delivered by each discipline can aid in this process. The nurse will be able to see how a specific philosophy of care is implemented. A thorough respect for and understanding of the scope of service provided by each discipline is necessary to ensure quality of client–care delivery in a cost–effective manner.

Evaluation of the Team

Field visits are also an excellent method for the nurse supervisor to use in evaluating individual provider competency and in obtaining an overview of quality of care delivered by the agency. The nurse should evaluate the home health aides or other nursing assistants providing direct patient care. Home health aides work more independently than auxiliary nursing personnel in many other areas. Therefore, proper selection, complete orientation, realistic inservice education, and adequate supervision of home health aides are very important (Hogstel, 1983, pp. 107–123). Although nurse supervisors in the home usually are not primarily responsible for the selection, orientation or inservice education of home health aides, they have a responsibility for the observation, supervision and evaluation of these assistants.

Referral of Clients to Team Members

Specific therapeutic services can often be performed by more than one discipline. For example, range-of-motion exercises may be performed by the nurse, physical therapist, occupational therapist, and home health aide. However, only one discipline will be reimbursed for the service. Insurance companies will not cover duplication of service. Therefore, using knowledge gleaned in the evaluation of the client's health status regarding the extent and severity of physical disability, the nurse must decide which discipline can best meet the client's needs and at what point a specific discipline should be brought in.

In addition, the nurse must refrain from referring other disciplines unless such a referral is warranted. Often, there is a temptation to refer clients to everyone on the team for evaluation and possible service because they are available. Such a practice is costly for the client and, while not impacting his or her pocketbook directly, increases the total costs of health care for the taxpayer and public in general. Consideration of costs should not be taken lightly by the nursing case manager and/or team leader. Nursing must look first within its own professional resources before referring the client to others. "There are instances where less–costly modalities of nursing care are equally effective, compatible and feasible . . . and rely on sound nursing care measures that achieve the same ends". (SASMOR, 1981, p. 546)

Need to Hold Down Costs

Costs of agency care may also affect productivity of team members. When staff productivity is low, the number of units of service per person drops, and the revenue of the agency decreases. Activities of each discipline on the health care team must be thoroughly understood so that expectations regarding the number of families visited in a day are realistic in relation to the type of service provided by that discipline.

Making Client Assignments

The nurse coordinator or supervisor will wish to work with team members and schedule an appropriate number of daily home visits. Consideration must be given to the driving time and distance between clients' homes as well as the time each visit requires. For example, a nurse assigned to do three client admissions may have an extremely busy day as each visit will take one and a half hours of direct client contact time and a half hour to an hour of paperwork in follow-up telephone calls and other tasks. This nurse's production and revenue produced for the day will be low. Conversely, a nurse assigned one admission, a daily insulin injection, a dressing change, supervision of a colostomy irrigation, and supervision and teaching of a client with a Hickman catheter, will have made five reimbursable visits and produced much more revenue.

Management of Stress

Management of stress among team members is a significant task of the home health nurse coordinator or supervisor. The home health agency serves clients with serious acute care needs, chronic long-term conditions, and terminal illness. As a result, home care staff are prone to the same types of stress that lead to burnout among in-patient health care professionals.

In home care, however, the potential for burnout may be even greater. The home care staff become a part of the client's family and are integrated into their lives, often, as a special type of friend. When the bulk of a caseload is composed of older adults seriously ill and dying, and about whom one cares a great deal, the pressure on staff is enormous. In addition, there are often no magic cures on the horizon, no hope for a major miracle. The client has, quite simply, been sent home because everything possible has already been done, and now he or she must face the task of coping with a life of disability and/or confronting death with dignity. If the home care staff cannot create a support group for one another, burnout will occur.

Creation of a supportive environment for the team begins with the nurse-leader and filters outward to members. Nurses chosen for leadership positions must be those who value staff and are concerned about their personal needs and desires as well as the functions they perform within the agency. The nurse leader must remember that emotional support is a reciprocal process. In order to give support to others (clients), nurses themselves must feel supported. The staff member cannot give empathetic care to clients unless he or she has some source of support and reinforcement of self-esteem from significant others. Often, the only resource for that support must be other agency staff. Family and friends of agency staff members have not worked in home health and confronted the tremendous frustration of trying to meet the needs manifested by the ill and dying; therefore, it is often impossible for them to truly empathize or understand.

Thus, the nurse coordinator/supervisor will wish to become highly attuned to the special support needs of staff by:

- listening;
- relieving team members of responsibility for care of certain clients when they are emotionally stretched to the limit;
- relieving staff of less important duties so that they can spend some *quality* time with clients to whom they are especially attached during periods of crisis;
- remembering the power of "thank you, I appreciate the work you are doing", or other phases of positive reinforcement;
- appropriate use of touch in moments of stress;
- and provision of time for socialization and sharing of team members with one another.

In addition, team members must be encouraged to use these strategies and approaches with one another (Barstow, 1979, p. 1425–26).

Quality Assurance

The nurse supervisor should direct all activities toward the delivery of quality client care. It is important that care delivered in the home be based on sound nursing principles and in accordance with printed policies, procedures and standards of care established by the home health agency. Nurse supervisors will want to perform periodic audits of clinical records to evaluate the strengths and weaknesses of individual providers and overall agency service delivery. In addition, individual nurses and nurse supervisors will want to keep up with the trends in recommendations made by the Utilization Review Committee of the agency.

Evaluation of clinical records will identify potential problems in client care delivery and enable corrective measures to be taken before overall quality of care deteriorates. Conversely, evaluation can become a considerable source of pride, as successful approaches to client care are identified and noted.

Professional Development and the Promotion of Professional Nursing

Delivering nursing care in the home health environment is an extremely complex task. Continuing education is mandatory if the nurse is to keep up with clinical and legislative developments. Active membership in professional nursing organizations will enable the nurse to identify the role of nursing in such activities as client advocacy and participation in the political system to create change. As an example, legislation promoting co-payments and increased deductibles for health care can be disastrous because many elderly clients are living on fixed incomes and cannot afford the increase in out-of-pocket expenses. Additionally, legislation that promotes or focuses funding and support on institutional health care increases the likelihood that the older adult will be forced to leave home and seek help in a hospital or nursing home. These legislative trends are of pressing and legitimate concern to the home health nurse.

SUMMARY

The future appears bright for the delivery of health services at home. The potential for increasing demand and utilization of at-home services is steadily emerging because of consumer demand and the impact of federal legislation. Nurses who deliver care in the home need to be well qualified by education, experience and certain personal traits to meet the diverse needs in this role. There is much competition for clients, and the nurse needs to recognize that the concept of marketing is important in this field of health care. It is important, therefore, to utilize all possible resources for client referral.

During the initial home visit, the nurse should establish a relationship with the client and family; collect a health history; perform a physical assessment; identify the major client problems and agency services needed; and determine the possible sources of funding. The plan of treatment will be developed in coordination with the client's physician. Services are provided to the client/family based on the goals and plans made by the nurse.

The nurse also plays an important role in coordinating all of the services provided by the interdisciplinary team in home care. Supervision and evaluation of individual team members, many of whom are not nurses, will be a new challenge for many nurses.

Nurses in home health care should resist delivering care only when there is full reimbursement. Instead, they must focus on the services that should be provided to create and/or maintain a high quality of life for their clients. Once the crucial services are identified, nurses must seek to actively influence legislation or policy changes to ensure those services become a reimbursable benefit. Nursing has established a tradition of excellence in the delivery of home care. The profession should be proud of the standards established over many decades that serve as a guide for home health providers now entering the field.

REFERENCES

Barstow R E, Mullins A C: "Care for caretakers." *Am J Nurs*, Vol 79, No 8, August 1979, pp 1425–29

"Conditions of participation in home health agencies: Federal health insurance for the aged." *U.S. Department of Health, Education and Welfare*, Reg. 405.1228, August 27, 1968

Hogstel M O: *Management of Personnel in Long Term Care*. Robert J. Brady Company, Bowie, Maryland, 1983, pp. 107–123

Sasmor J L: "Dollars and sense: Looking at costs in patient care." *Am J Nurs*, Vol 81, No 3, March 1981, pp 546–47

BIBLIOGRAPHY

Clemen S A, Eigsti D G, McGuire S L: *Comprehensive Family and Community Health Nursing*. McGraw-Hill Book Company, New York, 1981

Leahy K L, Cobb M M, Jones M C: *Community Health Nursing*. McGraw-Hill Book Company, New York, 1977

CHAPTER 6

ASSESSING AND ADAPTING THE HOME ENVIRONMENT

Suzanne Dixson Thomas

One of the most difficult problems facing the elderly living at home is the gradual deterioration of the home environment and the increased difficulty for many older adults to maintain, repair or improve their homes. When these problems are combined with continuing chronic illness, the situation may become critical for the older adult and for the family. How can the nurse and the family best help the older adult to remain in the home? What adaptations can be made? What community resources are available, particularly when illness and/or disability occurs? These and similar questions are the focus of this chapter.

The Nature and Scope of the Problem

Rauckhorst, Stokes and Mezey (1980, p. 310) reported that when older people were asked where they most preferred to live, they replied that their first preference was to live in a single-family detached dwelling. The second preference was to live with someone of their same age and sex. Third, they would choose to live with or near family. And, predictably, their last choice would be to live in an institution (Rauckhorst, et al., p. 319).

These preferences reflect part of the American dream. That dream includes personal freedom, independent living through old age, living in a single-family home, and owning the home. Among older adults in the rural South, 81% of older women and 89% of older couples own and live in their own homes (Montgomery, Stubbs, and Day, 1980, p. 447). Moving from place to place is rare, and many people have lived in the same home for 35 years or longer. These facts are striking in contrast to income of the same group of people. Most report incomes at or below the poverty level. Reports of spending $200 or more in the last year to repair, maintain or improve their homes are rare, especially among single women. Yet, these homeowners report being fully satisfied with their homes in more than 95% of cases (Montgomery, et al., 1980). Although living in their own homes, these women could not afford to maintain them because of their low incomes. Their satisfaction seems to stem from ownership and independence rather than from the physical quality of the home environment.

Elderly people living in urban and suburban areas had similar preferences and concerns. Those living in the oldest neighborhoods faced another problem. Gentrification, or "the gradual resettlement of some inner-city neighborhoods by a younger, wealthier, better-educated elite" (Henig, 1981, p. 67), affects older people in another way. Faced with the higher prices generated by the renewed housing in their inner-city neighborhoods, and with younger generation people moving in, many older residents, especially those who do not own their own homes, are forced to relocate at a high toll emotionally, socially, and financially as well as physically. As property values increase, eventually property taxes increase; the cost of goods and services increase; and older citizens who own their own homes also may be forced to leave.

There is an interaction between the home environment and health of the older person that affects the nursing process. Adapting the home environment to enable the older person to reach higher levels of health is an essential role of the home health care nurse.

The Goal of Nursing Care in the Home Environment

The goal of nursing care in adapting the home environment for older adults is to assist them in maximizing the quality of life in their homes. When the interaction between home environment and health is improved, the quality of life is improved. An ideal outcome is for older adults to remain in their own homes, with assistance when needed, as long as they are able to maintain basic health practices and as long as they desire to remain in their homes.

The nurse's role in this process is shaped by the following factors: Who is the home owner? What does the person need from the environment? What does the person want? What is most important to the outcome of health care? What will the situation allow? What can the nurse do to help adapt the environment for healthy living?

In the next section, a framework for assessing needs is given to help the nurse and the clients understand what needs to be done and how to decide what is most important for promoting a positive interaction with the environment. Other questions must be considered by the nurse and the client at each stage of care.

A Framework for Assessment

Abraham Maslow's (1954) hierarchy of needs is a humanistic theory of motivation with a well-known structure for identifying and ranking human needs. The theory proposes that one's behavior is motivated by the individual's attempt to meet certain needs. A primary assumption of the hierarchy is that a human being's most basic physiological needs for survival must be met before higher level needs, such as safety, love and belonging, self-esteem, and self-actualization. Thus, the categories of needs are listed, as well as ordered. Identifying and prioritizing nursing problems is an important function of the nurse, especially during the assessment phase of the nursing process. In assessing the client's home environment, there are some special observations that can be made based on the needs of Maslow's hierarchy.

A tool for home assessment is presented in Table 6-1. It is designed to be used by nurses, clients and/or family members to help them identify and prioritize a number of specific housing needs of the elderly. The following section expands on this tool by describing how to make specific observations listed in the assessment tool. At the clients' request, the nurse could offer to perform these preliminary inspections. If problems are found, professional help should be sought.

Survival Needs

At the basic physiological or survival level of the hierarchy, one must have adequate heating and cooling, functioning plumbing, access to and through the home, equipment for the access to, preparation of, and storage of food, a bed, and essential clothing, furniture and space for carrying out activities of daily living. Some of these basic needs are not well met, especially by the isolated and indigent elderly who live alone. Although many of these people are satisfied in their meager surroundings, their health is often compromised because of inadequate shelter, dangerous extremes of temperature, and/or an insufficient quantity and quality of food.

Heating

Locate the heating system. Take a flashlight and inspect it. A central gas or oil heater will be found in the floor of a central hallway, sometimes in a utility closet, or behind a wall panel. Some are located in attics or basements. Look for instructions for lighting the heater and turning it off in summer. Determine when the equipment was last serviced by the appropriate service personnel. Heating equipment should be checked if it has been more than a year since it was serviced or if there are other potential problems. Check the condition of the filter where air flows into the system. Is it cleaned or changed monthly?

Locate the fuel source for the heating equipment. A gas heater will have a gas meter in the yard or attached to the outside of the house. Is there an odor or a sound of gas escaping? If soil is composed of clay, does the homeowner water the yard around the house all year long? If the soil is clay and the fuel pipes are underground or embedded in a concrete slab foundation, the yard around the foundation must be kept at a constant level of moisture year round to ensure a constant amount of pressure on the embedded pipes. Soil shifts result in leaky pipes and explosions which can destroy entire homes in seconds.

TABLE 6.1
Tool for Assessment of the Home Environment for the Elderly

I. Survival Needs
a. Heating
  1. Equipment in the home   yes _____ no _____
  2. Temperature reaches at least 70°F on coldest
     days   yes _____ no _____
  3. Equipment may be turned on/off/adjusted by
     older adult   yes _____ no _____
  4. Sufficient money available to pay for neces-
     sary fuel, equipment, repairs   yes _____ no _____
  5. Fuel is transported to the system without
     leaks or breaks in the system   yes _____ no _____
b. Cooling
  1. Equipment in the home   yes _____ no _____
  2. Temperature reaches at least 80°F on hottest
     days   yes _____ no _____
  3. Equipment may be turned on/off/adjusted by
     older adult   yes _____ no _____
  4. Fuel is transported to the system without
     leaks or breaks in the system   yes _____ no _____
c. Sanitation/sewage disposal
  1. Does the house currently have running water?   yes _____ no _____
  2. Does the house have:
        well water   yes _____ no _____
        city water   yes _____ no _____
        distilled water   yes _____ no _____
        water filtering equipment   yes _____ no _____
  3. Is there hot water?   yes _____ no _____
  4. What is the temperature setting?
        100°   yes _____ no _____
        120°   yes _____ no _____
        140°   yes _____ no _____
        higher   yes _____ no _____
  5. Is the plumbing working in the:
        bathroom   yes _____ no _____
        kitchen   yes _____ no _____
        utility room   yes _____ no _____
        yard   yes _____ no _____
        other   yes _____ no _____
  6. Is there regular trash collection?   yes _____ no _____
  7. Is the client able to prepare the trash for
     collection?   yes _____ no _____
  8. Are the city sewage services to the home
     adequate?   yes _____ no _____
  9. If in a rural area, is there adequate sewage
     and trash disposal?   yes _____ no _____

II. Safety Needs
a. Mobility and ambulation
  1. Is there easy access to the home and through
     the home?   yes _____ no _____

TABLE 6.1 *(continued)*
Tool for Assessment of the Home Environment for the Elderly

2. Are the halls and walkways uncluttered?   yes _____ no _____
3. Are there non-skid rugs and mats?   yes _____ no _____
4. Is the flooring and carpeting intact?   yes _____ no _____
5. Is there sufficient lighting?   yes _____ no _____
6. Is there equipment which aids with ambulation?   yes _____ no _____
7. Are the floors and walkways level?   yes _____ no _____
8. Is there lighting along the walkways at floor level?   yes _____ no _____
9. Are there orange reflective markers where the floor level changes?   yes _____ no _____

b. Protection from harm
1. Is there at least one smoke detector or alarm placed near the bedroom where the client sleeps?   yes _____ no _____
2. Are there strong locks on the doors and windows?   yes _____ no _____
3. Is there a communication alert system of some kind (for example, Telephone Speed Dialing)?   yes _____ no _____
4. Are the electrical outlets and appliances safe?   yes _____ no _____
5. If the home has space heaters, are they:
     permanently mounted   yes _____ no _____
     properly vented   yes _____ no _____
     covered with a grill   yes _____ no _____
     properly connected with fuel source   yes _____ no _____
6. Is the location of the client's home in a high crime area?   yes _____ no _____
7. Is there a crime prevention program or a neighborhood watch program in the area of the client's home?   yes _____ no _____

III. Love and Belonging Needs
a. Support
1. Are there close neighbors?   yes _____ no _____
2. Do the neighbors offer help to the client?   yes _____ no _____
3. Do friends and family visit in the client's home frequently?   yes _____ no _____
4. Do members from the client's church visit?   yes _____ no _____
5. Does the client have a pet?   yes _____ no _____

b. Communication
1. Is there a telephone?   yes _____ no _____
2. Is there a radio?   yes _____ no _____
3. Is there a television?   yes _____ no _____
4. Does the client subscribe to a newspaper . . . magazines?   yes _____ no _____
5. Are these methods of communication modified according to the clients' disabilities?   yes _____ no _____

c. Space
1. Does the client have adequate private space?   yes _____ no _____

TABLE 6.1 (continued)
Tool for Assessment of the Home Environment for the Elderly

2. Does the client like to keep personal items, such as purse or knitting, close by?   yes _____ no _____

IV. Self-esteem Needs
a. Is the house furnished comfortably?   yes _____ no _____
b. Are there mementos of past life experiences such as pictures, plaques, books, trophies?   yes _____ no _____
c. Are there religious oriented objects such as crosses, bibles, rosaries?   yes _____ no _____
d. Are the yard and house well kept?   yes _____ no _____
e. Is the client satisfied with the design, arrangements, and color of the home?   yes _____ no _____

V. Self-actualization Needs
a. Does the client have a vegetable or flower garden?   yes _____ no _____
b. Is there a workshop or sewing room?   yes _____ no _____
c. Is there evidence of products created by the client?   yes _____ no _____
d. Does the client appear to be happy in the home?   yes _____ no _____
e. Does the client invite the nurse to experience the sanctuary offered in the home environment?   yes _____ no _____
f. Does the client show the nurse the home and yard with expressions of satisfaction?   yes _____ no _____

If the client can afford the extra expense, an electrician can be hired to move a thermostat to a lower position, to set up a temperature control device that will ensure heat at the appropriate times and save money, and to check wiring and rewire as needed. Many older people have family members, friends or neighbors who would provide this service. For people who do not have these personal resources, utility companies may know of resources to help older people. The nurse could call the utility company for the client to obtain this information if needed. If the home was built with aluminum wiring, or if the wiring is over 25 years old, it is well worth having an electrician evaluate the adequacy of the wiring to carry the load of modern equipment.

Cooling

The assessment procedures for cooling are very similar to those for heating. It is essential that the person helping with the assessment carry out both assessments. Both of these systems are essential for the survival of older clients because of their decreased physiological ability to control body temperature.

An additional need for heating and cooling systems is that they be cleaned at least every season of use. Grass and shrubs should be trimmed away from an air conditioning unit located in the yard. The fans in the house should be cleaned without impairing their wiring to maintain their efficiency. Outside shade may be arranged over an air conditioning unit hung in a window to improve its working capacity. If it does not have to work so much to cool itself, it can cool the inside of the house better. The shade should not interfere with air intake or exhaust from the cooler.

Additional suggestions are regularly printed by utility companies and by home-owners' magazines and handyman manuals. If the system is working well and safely for the older person, no changes should be made.

Sanitation/Sewage Disposal

Most homes now have indoor plumbing, but it may not always work adequately. Water fixtures need to be checked for leaks. Water spills, constant dampness, and grating or knocking sounds may indicate leaks in the system. Sometimes a home-owner or a neighbor can determine the problem and repair it. If not, it may be necessary to call a plumber if the client can afford the cost of repairs.

Well water samples may be checked monthly by the local or regional public health department free or for a nominal fee. Filtering devices should be examined for proper functioning and, if they are the sort that soften the water, they may be adding a significant amount of sodium to the water. This is an important factor to determine because many older adults need to reduce their sodium intake.

Burn prevention is important for the older adult in the home. In a study by Baptiste and Feck (1980, pp. 727-729), people most likely to have serious burns from hot tap water were the elderly and infants. Burn accidents could be reduced in these age groups by reducing the hot water heater setting to 120° F for all uses. This temperature has been shown to be a safe water temperature for washing clothes and dishes. The lower temperature setting would also save money on utility bills.

Safety Needs

At the safety level, one must have protection from intruders, fires, electrical hazards, falls, weather, animals, traffic and criminals (Lawton, Nahemow, and Tsong, 1980). One must be able to use home machinery independently. Many elderly people isolate themselves in their homes because of the fear of crime and do not have the necessary funds to finance essential repairs.

Mobility and Ambulation

Some elderly people, especially those in their 80s and 90s, have special problems with ambulation. With reduced sensory capabilities, they are often less able to detect changes in their environments which may be hazardous. They also may have age-related changes in body systems that lead to poor balance, slow reaction time, and reduced physical capabilities to perceive, prevent and/or recover from an accident.

Elderly people account for a disproportionate number of accidental deaths in the home in the United States. Therefore, prevention becomes a top priority. The major causes of accidental deaths in the home for ages 75 to 84 are falls, fires and burns, ingestion of food or objects, and poisoning by solids, liquids or gases. After 85 years of age, death rates from falls increase (*Accident Facts,* 1981, pp. 80-83).

Given these statistics and the decline in bodily functioning, one must consider safe access to and through the home as an essential need of the elderly. Stairways should be checked for lighting, loose boards, sturdy rails, and objects on the steps or at the top or bottom of the steps. If there is a choice, older people should avoid stairways completely. Stairs can be extremely hazardous if there are problems with any of the factors previously listed.

There are many additional environmental factors that may affect health for older people. For example, older adults living in housing projects where the bathroom and bedroom are upstairs may stay in bed under the electric blanket until mid-morning, then arise, use the bathroom, and dress. They go downstairs, prepare a meal, and stay until nearly dark. Before dark, they climb the stairs, use the bathroom, and go back to bed. Their fear of the stairs, the cold, and the need for food are the parameters of their daily lives.

Doorways should be wide enough to admit a person in a wheelchair. The threshold to the doorway should be flat, flush with the floor, and not a barrier to crossing from room to room. Room connections and access to existing facilities should be arranged so that a person in a wheelchair can use them without danger of falls, fires, burns or accidents (see Figure 6-1).

Walkways must be kept clear. They should be cleared of water, ice debris, furniture, plants, clothing, loose carpets, or anything that might become a hazard. Many older people drag or slide their feet, so it is better not to have carpeted surfaces. Slick or smooth-soled shoes, as opposed to rubber-soled gripper-type soles, make walking easier for them. Both the carpet and the gripper soles trip people who slide their feet when walking. Highly waxed floors should be avoided because they are too slick for safety.

Lighting should be of the type that illuminates the surfaces to be viewed: the floor, the pathway to the bathroom or the kitchen, the front door, and the telephone. Glaring overhead lights should be avoided. Soft fluorescent lights offer even, widespread lighting that does not add a significant amount of heat to a room.

If any potential hazards are found in the environment of older clients, they need to be eliminated. Adding unfamiliar equipment or modifications may cause additional hazards in the environment of a person who has reduced vision, even though the changes may prove to be very helpful. The nurse should explain to the client that safety modifications need to be made and look for unexpected changes that might occur as a result of improvements. Additional checklists for safety may

FIGURE 6.1
Overcoming Barriers in the Home Environment

An elderly widow with diabetes, whose legs have been amputated, and who is also blind, lives in this home. Using the suggestions in Table 6.2 and this diagram, how would you modify this home to improve her mobility, safety and chances of survival? She sits in her wheelchair all day long. She is unable to move from room to room without assistance because of the doorway thresholds. And she cannot prepare her meals without assistance because of the arrangements in the kitchen.

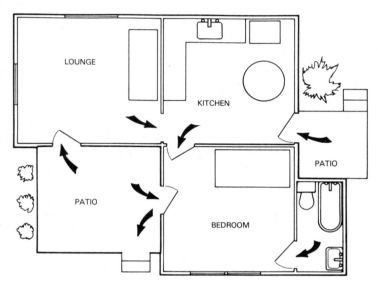

be found in the materials cited in the reference list (Pakov and Stephens, 1981; Siegel, 1982; "As Parents Grow Older," 1981, p. 227).

Changes often cost money and a way of paying for them needs to be found. The homeowner may seek some assistance from the U.S. Department of Housing and Urban Development. In certain political subdivisions, federal money is available at the local level and channeled through the states' block grants. The money may be used for grants or for low-cost loans at fixed rates for home improvement, and/or financial aid with high utility bills.

Specific information about financial assistance for home repair may be obtained from the U.S. Department of Housing and Urban Development, 451 Seventh Street, S.W., Washington, D.C. 20410. For more information clients should check with the local or regional office of Community Planning and Development. If an area is entitled to funds, the nurse should find out which sections of the community are targeted (communities having the highest number of sub-standard homes). It is worth applying for these funds, even if one does not live in a high priority target area. The applicant must be a resident home owner who plans to continue living in the home for which money is sought.

Protection from Harm

Clients and/or family members should be encouraged to purchase smoke alarms. In some cities, alarms have been available to the elderly through special city and/or federal funds. Because of decreased mobility in the elderly, it is essential that they have as much warning time as possible if a fire should start.

Sometimes, cities also have provided funds for elderly residents to purchase dead-bolt locks for their doors, an important safety measure in high crime areas. There are a variety of communication alert systems (Lifeline, telephone reassurance, and paging apparatus for family members) that help the elderly to feel safe and secure in their homes.

Need for Love and Belonging

One must have some sort of social network that will prevent social isolation, loneliness and withdrawal, conditions devastating to any person (Moustakas, 1961). The home environment may be adapted to facilitate having pets, visitors and one- or two-way communication with the outside world, such as a telephone, radio and television. Neighbors, family members, friends and church groups who visit the client in the home will also help to meet this need.

Self-esteem Needs

High self-esteem can be maintained in the home environment by living in one's own home surrounded by one's possessions, memories and accomplishments. They are sensory reminders of valued life experiences. Encouraging pride in the home and property by keeping the home clean and in good repair are also ways in which the home environment helps to meet the need for self-esteem. The design, arrangement and color of the home also may facilitate self-esteem.

Self-actualization Needs

Self-actualization in the home is fostered by assisting the individual to adapt to his or her own home and to change the home to meet personal needs. This increasing mutuality and satisfaction of needs and values fosters an environment of harmony.

Two Family Situations

The case studies that follow are included as examples of the principles and ideas that the nurse may use in assessing and adapting the home environment for older clients. The reader is encouraged to think of additional cases, ideas and principles.

CASE PRESENTATION: THE FRANK FAMILY

The Frank family has three children: Mike, age 10; Carolyn, age 14; and Tony, age 17. Recently, the Frank family decided to invite Mrs. Frank's parents, Mr. and Mrs.

Martin, to live with them, probably for the remainder of their lives. Mr. and Mrs. Martin could no longer live in their own home and take care of themselves independently, primarily because of increasing health problems. Mrs. Martin had advanced Parkinson's Disease, with poor emotional and social coping patterns, as well as advanced physical disabilities which made it difficult for her to carry out the most basic self-care activities. Mr. Martin was her primary caregiver until he developed congestive heart disease. His physician prescribed reduced activities such as lifting, carrying, and the type of physical care Mrs. Martin needed. Because of their needs for special diets and physical assistance, together with their increasing social isolation, the Martins asked for assistance from their children.

The Frank family discussed the need for physical care, the interpersonal relationships involved, the effect on the family finances, and the emotional impact of caring for the Martins. Mrs. Frank and the children agreed to take on the primary caregiver roles. Mr. Frank decided that the family could manage the extra financial burden, and that caring for the Martins would be a more financially feasible approach than others (Tesfa, 1982).

The Frank family needed help to anticipate the problems they would encounter giving care to the Martins. The family, with assistance from the nurse, made a list of home adaptations, equipment and supplies they believed would be needed. The list included ramps for front and back door stairways to accommodate Mrs. Martin's walker and wheelchair and a new television for the use of the Martins in their own rooms. The back bathroom was to be designated for the use of the Martins because it is the most convenient one to their rooms. However, the bathroom door was not wide enough for a wheelchair and there was a shower stall but no bathtub.

How should this list be ranked? What are the most essential items on the list for survival? For safety? What items would be classified as nice but not necessary? How would the family and nurse decide?

When setting priorities for planned adaptations, it is very important to determine the *minimum* changes that must be completed to begin this living arrangement. Expensive and time-consuming changes that would permanently alter the living space of the home should not be made until first trying the arrangements for a period of time. Somehow, the most important things fall into place with need, time and experience. Experiencing a living arrangement allows the people to test out their ideas and values on a realistic, day-to-day basis, and not on a hypothetical one. Many people cannot envision what something will be like until they try it because no one knows for sure whether or not it will work.

CASE PRESENTATION: THE CHAPMAN FAMILY

A second family, Mr. and Mrs. Chapman, were ages 78 and 77, respectively. They had three cats and two dogs. They lived in a seven-room house built about 40 years ago that was not insulated. There were steep stairs leading from the front porch to the front yard; the back porch and yard were similar, with about 12 steps to the ground. Mr. and Mrs. Chapman found that it was more and more difficult to get out and around because of their physical limitations. They had a working automobile as a reliable transportation and a telephone with an extension. They were no longer able to do much of the physical maintenance on their home. They were reluctant to hire someone else to make needed changes because of the expense.

At the same time, they did not want to buy a new home. They did not want to commit themselves to a new mortgage and high payments. Nor did they want to move to an apartment, a retirement village, or a condominium. They wanted to live in the comfort of and with the memories of their home where they had lived for 35 years and where they had raised their three children and four grandchildren. *Many older people would rather die in what seems like a miserable environment, than to leave their precious memories and their lifetime setting to go to an environment another generation has developed for themselves.*

Their living space was neat and clean, kept up as much as they could physically and financially manage. It was cold in winter, hot in summer, and damp all year long. Their children worried about whether their parents should stay there. Mr. and Mrs. Chapman had colds and flu every winter. One winter they had upper respiratory problems continuously from November through February.

The Chapman family illustrates a situation often encountered by the nurse in the home of older clients. This family was very attached to their home and they did not want to leave it or the associated memories, even though their interaction with the environment was beginning to threaten their physical well-being. How could their home be adapted to improve their interaction with it and not destroy their emotional and social interactions?

Frequently, elderly people live in old housing that is cold, damp and poorly insulated. Homes built more than 15 years ago were not insulated as well as newer homes. Homes built between World War I and World War II were built with technology and equipment that does not match what is available today (Montgomery, et al., 1980; Mayer and Lee, 1981; Lawton, 1981).

Both Mr. and Mrs. Chapman drank alcohol several times a week. This factor could affect their health in the circumstances described. In a study of the housing conditions of elderly adults in Denmark, Holma and Kjaer (1980, pp. 121-147) found that regular use of alcohol in the amount of three beers a day or its equivalent, accompanied by cold and damp surroundings, was a more important factor in the occurrence of upper respiratory diseases than was smoking. Alcohol appeared to give the person a feeling of warmth and well-being that masked the actual environmental conditions. Thus, older people became ill because they did not sense the temperature and their bodies' stress signals appropriately.

Family Conference

One of the most helpful things the Chapman family could do would be to have a family conference ("As Parents Grow Older," 1981). Because remaining in their own home was extremely important to the Chapman family, it was made clear at the time of the conference that moving away was not an alternative. The focus was on how to help adapt their home to make it a physical environment in which they could spend the rest of their days with all their memories around them, and without costing them an excessive amount of money. What types of changes would be most helpful? How could they be implemented? Who could do each one? When and in what order should they be done?

The Chapman family should have the last word on each decision. The children should proceed slowly, considering the anguish that people feel at the thought that they might need to be more dependent upon others for help. This role reversal often begins when a major catastrophe happens, such as a cerebrovascular accident (Lawton, 1981).

In one study, older people living with younger people reported better housing conditions, but these older people tended to be more dependent. Those who were more healthy lived alone and had poorer housing conditions. Lawton (1981, p. 64) hypothesized that the interaction between health and housing exists for both those living with family and those living independently. People who must live with family for health reasons benefit from the better living conditions. People who have better health and are able to live independently in poorer circumstances benefited from their continued independence.

Role Changes

Role changes in the older adult can create the same fears, sadness and grieving that moving into a dependent stage of living can at any age. Anger, sadness, reopening of old hurts and secrets operate together in the family conference. It is hoped that because of cooperative decision making, the family may also experience a sense of the future and a closer family unity than before.

Many times the reluctance of aging parents to allow their children to help them signifies the reluctance to move into the final stages of development in older adulthood. The family conference may be viewed as a crisis. The old ways of coping are not working. The future is uncertain. A power struggle is eminent.

Nursing Interventions

The nurse needed to assess coping styles and whether the Chapman family was in some stage of the grieving process because of moving into a more dependent place with their children. Tapia's (1982, pp. 252-258) model of family coping may be helpful to assess the family's needs and style of coping.

The family should be taught that a developmental crisis carries with it the same emotional and social stresses of any other type of crisis. Family members should be encouraged to be sensitive to one another's needs and ideas at this period of their lives.

Eventually, it is hoped, people will learn to plan early for housing in their old age as a part of retirement planning. For example, middle-aged couples could move from a large two-story or split-level house to a smaller one-story house, a condominium, or apartment after all the children have left home. A two-story house does not easily accommodate wheelchairs, crutches, or arthritic joints if these needs and problems arise in the later years. It is usually easier to make this move in the middle years while the family is financially and physically able to do so, rather than wait until a time when the change has to be made suddenly because of illness and/or disability.

Resources and Methods for Adapting the Home Environment

Availability of Equipment

For a complete listing of all types of equipment (for example, beds, wheelchairs, bedside commodes, disposable supplies) available for home health care, the nurse, the client, and/or the family should consult the many catalogues now available. For example, Sears, Roebuck & Company has a Home Health Care Specialog (1984) that lists and shows photographs of equipment for home care. Local equipment companies, medical supplies companies, and hospital supply companies also have home health care equipment. If necessary, the information could be located by going to the purchasing section of the nearest hospital to look at their catalogues.

Some of the common types of health care equipment that can be purchased or rented for use in the home are:

- manual or electric hospital beds (essential for long-term care to prevent caregiver fatigue and injury);
- manual, electric and geriatric wheelchairs (for use both in and outside of the home);
- walkers, canes, tripod canes, canes with small seats;
- trapeze bars (for bed or floor or bathroom);
- over-bed tables and trays;
- hydraulic patient lifts (for use with beds, chairs, commodes, and bath tubs);
- bedside commodes;
- bed pans and urinals; (If the client has been hospitalized prior to home care, this type of disposable equipment should be taken home with the client.)
- plastic mattress pads and covers;
- heel, ear and elbow protectors;
- disposable protective undergarments (encourage the family *not* to use the word "diaper");
- clothing and shoes with Velcro fasteners;
- stabilizing toilet guardrails;
- electronic blood pressure and pulse monitors.

It can easily be seen that almost all kinds of equipment and supplies available to give effective nursing care in the hospital setting are available for the home.

One company (KO-Z) manufactures clothing for people in wheelchairs and in beds that are both colorful and easy to put on: another suggestion is to buy patterns and make the clothing using materials most preferred by the client.

The Independence Factory, P. O. Box 597, Middletown, Ohio 45042, has published a set of ideas and gadgets in a handy volume called, *Make It Cheap.* The ideas are simple and easy to make and they help people remove their own home barriers. Examples include a telescoping light switch device, a pill tube which facilitates handling and self-administration of small tablets and capsules, a handle for a key ring, and an aid for removing a gasoline cap. An individual can order them from the Independence Factory, or can make them or have them made for a fairly reasonable price. Additional suggestions include those for modifying and/or building a house (see Table 6-2). Cars for the handicapped can be adapted to make driving safer with more ease and control. Other featured items will enable a person with physical handicaps, such as arthritis, to get into and around the house. Planning ahead for the purchase of a car or a house for future use is prevention; a little now pays rewards later when special needs arise.

Special Furniture Needs

Eldot (1982) suggested giving older people presents such as furniture to meet their special needs. "A sturdy chair with wide armrests and high back might make an ideal gift for some special elderly person. . . ." (p. 7c). One should be sure that the chair allows the hips to rest at the same level as the knees; feet should not be dangling; furniture should be strong enough and sturdy enough to support the person rising or sitting with the weight balanced on one arm of the chair. "Armrests should be flat and wide to give support without causing discomfort to brittle bones" (p. 7c). Firm, sturdy furniture is the key.

Exercise equipment may be improvised by making miniature sandbags for legs and arms to improve muscle strength. The client can be taught to lift the sand bags above the head with the hands, or lift them off the floor with the feet. It is important to encourage straight posture for balance and strength and for continuing function of body systems (Graves, 1981, p. 110). Furniture can be used to support proper alignment.

Beds should be firm, at about chair-seat height, but not so firm that they reduce circulation in older skin with poorer circulation and less fat. If a person complains of aching, throbbing, or burning feelings during rest periods, these problems may be a circulatory-neural indication that the bed is too hard. If older clients complain of being stiff, having difficulty turning, or difficulty rising, that may be a muscular indication that the bed is too soft. A soft bed can be "fixed" by placing a mattress-size ¼" plywood board for indoor use underneath the mattress. A hard bed can be "fixed" by adding more foam padding and covering it with blankets.

TABLE 6.2
Planning for Safety and Convenience at Home

Plan ahead for a home for an elderly client or for your own retirement and old age. A home can be designed or modified with these basics in mind:

Avoid stairways.
Avoid doorway threshold barriers.
Plan for low angle ramps leading to entries.
Build hallways, bathrooms and walkways wide enough for a wheelchair or a walker to pass and turn in the space.
Place knobs, handles, latches, and switches at a level you can reach while sitting or standing.
Build some cabinets and counter-top spaces at sitting level and some at standing level.*
Make the width of counter tops equal to approximately ½ to ⅔ the length of the adult's arm for best use of space with little counter-top storage. If counter top storage is needed, too, then add width accordingly.
Counter tops should extend outward to allow the person in the wheelchair to slide under the counter top to within 3-4 inches of the chest.
Cabinet doors can be made to slide sideways into recessed slides.
It is helpful to put sliding boxes in lower cabinets and turntables in upper cabinets. Both of these are available commercially. These are helpful to organize the contents and to allow the person to reach all items in the cabinets, and not only those in front.
Plan for lower level lighting, as well as ceiling fixtures, and lamps. It might be helpful to have these set up with lightmeters. Then they will turn themselves on automatically when the light level is low.
Plan for smoke alarms, fire exits in two or three places. Have a plan and rehearse your escape with every member of the household—including pets. Ask the local fire department to send an inspector to your home to help evaluate your provisions and to make suggestions. (*Make It Cheap*, 1976)
Plan for security systems, including: a telephone with an instant-dial feature; a buddy system with neighbors; burglar alarms; and a silent signal for help. The most important aspects of safety for older people are having people who check on them regularly, living in a neighborhood where there are many elderly people and few teenagers, and having some neighborhood barriers to strangers and excess traffic (Lawton and Jaffe, 1980).

*For work spaces that work for the whole family, both levels may be needed.

Other Home Adaptations

While assessing the home environment, the nurse should look at the home from the client's perspective. What barriers are there? What inconvenience? What would it take to be able to go to the bathroom without assistance during the night? Does the older person really have to use a wheelchair or remain in bed?

CASE PRESENTATION: MRS. IRONS

Mrs. Irons developed pneumonia and was admitted to the local hospital for treatment. She was accompanied by her youngest daughter. Using her Medicare benefits, Mrs. Irons was eventually sent to a convalescent center and remained there for nine months. Mrs. Irons reported that she stayed in bed there most of the time unnecessarily and developed a large pressure ulcer on her heel, which contributed to her lengthy stay there. She became disoriented, incontinent of urine and feces, and a retention catheter was inserted.

Mrs. Irons' older daughter, who lived in a distant state, found her mother in the convalescent center. She took her to her own home and asked for a referral for home health nursing services through the Medicare program. Mrs. Irons' pressure ulcer gradually healed; she regained her alert level of consciousness and was able to use the bedpan for toileting. Her older daughter, Mrs. Warren, and her son Joe, age 23, lived in a mobile home and they let "Granny" have the living room for her hospital bed, wheelchair and walker.

With encouragement from the nurse and the family, the determined Mrs. Irons re-learned to walk with the walker and began to move about the living room more independently. Mrs. Warren and Joe began to wish for more toileting indepen-dence for Mrs. Irons, as well. The urinary retention catheter was still in place. From the view of adapting the home environment, all that was needed—in addition to bladder training—was to move the kitchen table to the living room, remove the bathroom rug, provide night lights, and buy some toilet seat rails (see Figure 6-2).

FIGURE 6.2
Rearranging the Home Environment

Mrs. Iron's bed was in the living room of the mobile home. Her wheelchair would not pass through the space between the kitchen counter and the kitchen table. When the round table was moved to another place, she was able to reach the bathroom. What are some other ways to improve the home environment as it is shown here? What other barriers or hazards do you see? How might changes be made that would also be compatible with the life-styles of the daughter and the grandson?

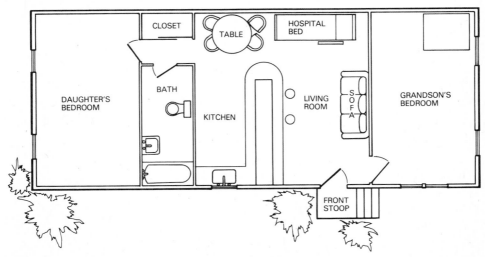

When the nurse and Mrs. Warren discovered these facts, there was great excitement in the home. At last, "Granny" was going to be more like her old self. Mrs. Irons, of course, was happiest of all. With more practice, smoothing out of details, settling of roles and functions, the goal of toileting *inter*dependence was achieved in a few weeks.

Helping Families With Equipment and Supplies

Creativity by the Nurse

Here is a chance for home care nurses to use one of their most important talents: creativity. Every home situation is a little different. So many things in a nurse's work are regimented—chart forms and format, required data for the auditor, counting mileage, clocking in and out of work. Here is one of those areas where creativity is greatly needed to help families.

Improvised Equipment and Supplies

Improvision is a form of creativity in home health nursing in which the nurse and the family members identify a need, sometimes for equipment or supplies, and then find a way to "use what we've got." In economic hard times, this becomes even more important.

Exercises to Stimulate Creative Thinking

Some exercises nurses can use to stimulate creative thinking for improvisation in home health care include the following: (These ideas are adapted from Torrance's (1974, pp. 8-15) tests of creativity.)

- Take three common household articles you have in your home. Using a notebook or some blank paper, *list* as many uses as you can for the articles in combination. Do not hold back any ideas. Do not attempt to evaluate them for feasibility, acceptability, durability or any other criterion. Just *brainstorm* and write it all on the paper.

- Make a list of the most common types of equipment and supplies used in the home for home nursing care by your clients. *List* as many common household articles that you can imagine which might be substituted for commercial items to meet the identified need. For example, a commonly identified need is absorbent pads for people experiencing incontinence. The nurse might begin with newspaper, sewing scraps, old blankets, old tee-shirts, or a cookie sheet full of kitty litter covered with a pad. These are simply examples of creative ideas that have not been validated for effectiveness. Do not attempt to evaluate your ideas for feasibility or for any other criterion while you are listing them. That will come later.

- Next, take the same commonly identified need, incontinence, and re-define the situation in as many ways as you can. For example, why is it called incontinence?

What would happen if we re-defined the whole idea? What if we dropped those cultural and social taboos about urine and feces? Think about biological functioning. Do not worry about laundry or odors. Now go to a place in your mind where you are a biological being functioning naturally, and think about urination and defecation. Think about yourself functioning in these ways. Shape what happens around what feels right and natural. As you return to the here-and-now bring that perspective with you.

- Using your perspective, think of (and write down) as many ways as you can to re-define this aspect of biological functioning. You may begin to see the problems and solutions in a different light.
- Incontinence can be re-defined as a normal biological function carried out in a socially unacceptable way. Remove the social wall and protect the person from damage from the waste products and what is left? A healthy person is there, functioning in a normal biological way. The person needs protection from harmful waste products and protection from social situations in which he or she might be stigmatized for incontinence.
- To what extent can the person render self-care unassisted? What is the best form of skin protection and cleansing? What are social situations in which special equipment, such as a condom catheter, might be needed? These are questions taken from a perspective of acceptance of biological functioning and not illness.
- Review your lists. Now look at them for feasibility, but do not let yourself return to the walled-in perspective. Will it work? Is it practical, safe, comfortable and effective? How and under what circumstances will it work? For example, will the idea to use newspapers for absorbent pads work? Yes, *and* (not *but*) they will need a covering of paper towels over them or a piece of cloth to prevent black ink stains.
- How will combined household items work as absorbent pads? Are pads really needed? Is there another way? One woman cut a hole in her mattress and box springs and kept a basin beneath the bed. She lay on her abdomen all night and then emptied the basin every morning. Her biological release of gastrointestinal waste products drained from a colostomy. A lack of necessary supplies proved to be socially confining for her. The United Ostomy Association volunteers helped her find a way to buy and use available equipment and supplies, freeing her from social isolation. If the improvisation is not as good as the purchased equipment, then focus nursing efforts on finding a means to purchase the equipment. If the purchased equipment carried with it a problem of stigmatization, such as having siderails on the bed for a semi-independent elderly person, then homemade improvisations may be the better choice. Listen to the client.

Using What Is Available In the Home

Other ideas that have evolved in home nursing include using:

- a small dinner bell for the client to call for help at night;
- two or more sturdy straight-backed chairs tied together and backed up to the bed for side rails;

- night lights along the route to the bathroom (red lights require the least retinal cell accommodation and are used in airplane cockpits for night flying and on some highways according to Forgus and Melamid, 1976, pp. 75-77);
- deep, wide pockets made of cloth for the wheelchair or walker;
- a backpack for the person who uses a cane or crutches. (A backpack will not swing separately when the person swings through the arc created by the crutches and stays on the back and swings with the person; thus it does not further interfere with the person's already impaired balance).

These devices enable the person to carry necessary items, making the person better able to care for themselves.

The nurses and family should weigh the cost of using household objects and adapting them to meet current needs against the cost of buying equipment. If the cost is equal, the time, energy and emotional implications to be expended should be considered.

Manufactured Equipment and Supplies

Specific information about buying or leasing equipment and supplies using Medicare, Medicaid or supplemental insurance programs change rapidly. The best source of current information is a vendor, a company that sells or leases medical equipment and supplies regularly.

When a client and/or family member purchases special medical equipment for the home, they usually pay the vendor directly for the equipment. Then the client files a claim form, which can be obtained from most vendors, with Medicare. The client will be paid 80% of the cost of the equipment by Medicare if the claim form is completed by the physician. Some vendors will allow the client to charge the item while waiting for the claim to be processed, about eight weeks on the average. Then the vendor receives the 80% payment of the total cost of the equipment and bills the client for the remaining 20%.

Medicare will not pay for all equipment the client might need at home. The client and/or family will need to provide for some of the equipment. Medicare and Medicaid will pay for durable equipment and some non-durable medical supplies. If non-durable equipment or supplies must be purchased by the client or family members, they should be encouraged to save copies of the prescriptions and receipts for income tax purposes later if desired.

Examples of durable equipment include "oxygen equipment, wheelchairs, home dialysis systems, and other medically necessary equipment that your doctor prescribes for use in your home" (*Your Medicare Handbook*, 1982, p. 35). No clear definition of "durable" or "medically necessary" equipment is stated in *Your Medicare Handbook* (1982). Vendors report a list of what is currently approved for funding based upon claims approved in the recent past of those not deemed necessary by the criteria of the Social Security Administration. Non-durable supplies or those deemed not necessary by the criteria of the Social Security Administration are those for which family members must pay. These are the items the nurse can help with, using creative approaches and comparison shopping.

Supplies on the market now have been developed over at least a 15-year period, since Medicare and home health nursing funded by Medicare began. If a nurse finds a need not met adequately by the existing supplies, it would be helpful to write to the manufacturers of home health supplies with a description of the needed item. For example, the technology of water sanitation lends itself well to the technology of catheter drainage tubing. Why not manufacture back-flow preventers on catheter drainage tubing? That would stop one course of bladder contamination and reduce the likelihood of infection in this vital system. And, back-flow preventers might be handy on intravenous tubing, too. The manufacturers can only make things as well as what they or nurses can creatively imagine. Because demand for home medical equipment is expanding, manufacturers will most likely be more interested in nurses' ideas than ever before.

Buy or Lease

The final decision about buying or leasing equipment rests with the family. The physician and the nurse usually offer guidance based upon their expectations of the client's prognosis. The physician must write a prescription for equipment if the cost is to be claimed on Medicare, Medicaid or an insurance program other than these two, and itemized receipts must be kept if medical equipment and supplies are to be claimed as deductible expenditures on income taxes. The prescription should include the following information: the client's social security number, name and address, including the telephone number, the name of the item; whether the item is to be permanent or leased; if leased, for what period of time; the purpose; the physician's signature and the date; the physician's printed name, address and telephone number. The prescription should be typewritten except for the physician's signature.

Many of the people served by home health agencies are those who have had debilitating physical illnesses that make it necessary for them to be homebound and in the care of others for the remainder of their lives. For this reason, these people may need permanent equipment such as hospital beds, wheelchairs, canes, walkers, mechanical lifts, and feeding and bathing equipment.

Purchase of durable equipment can be a stressful decision. It may evoke a developmental crisis for the affected person as discussed earlier. It may cause a crisis in the family. If parents have always been the ones who were sought for guidance and strength, it may be difficult for family members to accept their altered state. It is particularly difficult and somewhat depressing to think of that state as being progressivley worse or permanent.

Many older and handicapped people have permanent disabilities with temporary problems. For example, confusion is one of the common symptoms of illness in the elderly. If, for example, a person has had a stroke and usually functions very well with some help to walk and bathe, and suddenly becomes confused and cannot carry out the normal activities of daily living at the usual level of functioning, a physical problem, such as infection or electrolyte imbalance, may be the underlying cause. In this case, the family may have a temporary need for a hospital bed, side rails, bedside commode and oxygen.

Replaceable or Disposable

The family needs to decide whether they want to purchase replaceable or disposable equipment. Factors to consider in deciding include: the cost of the supply, the cost of maintaining the equipment, and the convenience and the cost in relation to income available for spending on these supplies. For some forms of equipment, such as sterile injection equipment, the safety factor involved in having the family re-sterilize, store, handle, sharpen, and use needles, syringes and solutions makes it impractical and even dangerous to attempt to re-use them.

Disposable supplies include syringes and needles, absorbent pads, bathing and cleansing supplies, sterile dressings, and any kind of sterile equipment or equipment which when once used may be considered contaminated or esthetically unacceptable to use again. Replaceable supplies include those items which, according to the manufacturer's instructions, are safe to re-use several times before discarding them. Some suggestions for replaceable items include: bulb syringes and feeding equipment, irrigation equipment for non-sterile irrigations, and in general non-sterile equipment and equipment which once used is acceptable to use again.

Summary

In spite of the deteriorating home environment and the changing physical status, older adults want to remain in their own homes for as long as possible. Helping a client remain independent has become a goal of home health nursing. Interventions focus upon improving the interaction between the older adult living at home with the home environment in order to maintain health.

A framework for assessing and prioritizing needs of the older adult living in the home is adapted from Abraham Maslow's (1954) Hierarchy of Needs. The case of the Martin family illustrates the need for a family living together to move slowly to adapt the structure of the home environment and to try adaptations that fit with their needs and values before making permanent changes. The case of the Chapman family illustrates the housing situation of many older adults living in their own homes: steep stairs, poor insulation, and poor heating and cooling equipment. The lack of desire to change the structure, together with the powerful need to remain in the setting in which they have lived most of their lives, also needs to be considered.

Both cases illustrate the importance of the family system to support older people through the developmental crisis of late maturity. These crises have as many potential and social problems as those of the earlier ages. They may be precipitated by a change in physical status, a change in living arrangements, or by the death of a spouse. The nurse is encouraged to intervene, determining the family's coping style according to the Tapia Model (1982).

In the second half of the chapter, the focus shifted to resources and methods for adapting the home environment. Ideas for existing products come from: the Sears Specialog (1984) *Home Health Care Catalog*, the KO-Z Company's pamphlets about clothing, and a catalogue published by the Independence Factory of Ohio, called *Make It Cheap*. Furniture seats should be parallel to the floor; sturdy, comfortable, firm, and padded well enough to promote adequate circulation.

Barriers to independence in the home can be numerous. In the case of Mrs. Irons, recovering more fully from a long illness to an interdependent level of functioning meant moving some furniture out of the way.

The home care nurse is encouraged to be creative, to think of the biological functioning of the person under care, and to broaden the perspective of needs beyond the walls of social and cultural taboos. The term "incontinence" is used as an example and is re-defined as normal biological functioning in a socially unacceptable way. Specific ideas for facilitating independence are given, and some criteria for evaluating creative new approaches are offered.

Manufactured equipment and supplies are considered for purchasing procedure, for sources, for durability or non-durability, for permanent or temporary use, and for replaceable or disposable use. Nurses are urged to be creative in identifying needs for new products and communicating those needs to manufacturers.

REFERENCES

Accident Facts, 1981. National Safety Council, Statistics Department, Chicago, Illinois, 1981

As Parents Grow Older—A Manual for Replication. The University of Michigan Institute of Gerontology, Ann Arbor, Michigan, 1981

Baptiste M S, Feck G: "Preventing tap water burns." *Am J Pub Health*, Vol 70, No 7, July 1980, pp 727-59

"Cheerful, Attractive, Reliable, Innovative, Needed . . . Garments . . . and Bedding," KO-Z's by Al-To, Inc., 7406 Clearhaven Drive, Dallas, Texas, n.d.

Eldot W: "The elderly have different furniture needs." *1982 Fort Worth Star Telegram*. Knight-Ridder News Service, Saturday, December 18, 1982, p 7c

Forgus R H, Melamed L E: *Perception: A Cognitive Approach*. 2nd ed. McGraw Hill Co., New York, 1976, pp 75-77

Graves M: "Physiologic changes and major diseases in the older adult," in Hogstel M O (ed): *Nursing Care of the Older Adult*. John Wiley and Sons, New York, 1981, pp 101-33

Henig J R: "Gentrification and displacement of the elderly: An empirical analysis." *The Gerontol*, Vol 21, No 1, 1981, pp 67-75

Holma B, Kjaer G: "Alcohol, housing, and smoking in relation to respiratory symptoms." *Environmental Research*, Vol 21, 1980, pp 126-42

Lawton M P, Nahemow L, Tsong-Min-Yeh: Neighborhood environment and the well-being of older tenants in planned housing. *Internat J Aging and Human Develop*, Vol 11, No 3, 1980, pp 211-27

Lawton, M P: "An ecological view of living arrangements." *The Gerontol*, Vol 21, No 1, 1981, pp 59-66

Lawton M P, Yaffe S: "Victimization and fear of crime in elderly public housing tenants." *J Gerontol*, Vol 35, No 5, 1980, pp 768-79

Make It Cheap. Vol 3. The Independence Factory, P.O. Box 597, Middletown, Ohio, 1976.

Maslow A H: *Motivation and Personality*. Harper & Row, New York, 1954

Mayer N S, Lee O: "Federal home repair programs and elderly homeowners' needs." *The Gerontol*, Vol 21, No 3, 1981, pp 312-22

Montgomery J E, Stubbs A C, Day S S: "The housing environment of our rural elderly." *The Gerontol*, Vol 20, No 4, 1980, pp 444-51

Moustakas C E: *Loneliness*. Prentice Hall, New York, 1961

Pavkov, Stephens B: "Special considerations for the community-based elderly." *Geriat Nurs*, Vol 2, No 6, November/December 1981, pp 422-28

Rauckhorst L M, Stokes S, Mezey M D: "Community and home assessment." *J Gerontol Nurs*, Vol 6, No 6, June 1980, pp 319-27

Sears Specialog, Home Health Care (Catalog). Sears, Roebuck, and Company, Chicago, Illinois, 60684, 1984

Siegel H: "Assessing an environment for safety first." *J Gerontol Nurs*, Vol 8, No 9, September 1982, pp 509-18

Tapia J A: "The nursing process in family health" in Spradley B W (ed): *Readings in Community Health Nursing*. 2nd ed. Little, Brown and Co., Boston, Massachusetts, 1982, pp 252-58

Tesfa A: "What does it take to let them go home?" *J Gerontol Nurs*, Vol 8, No 12, December 1982, pp 692-718

Torrance P E: *Norms—Technical Manual Torrance Tests of Creative Thinking*, Personal Press, Ginn and Co., Lexington, Massachusetts, 1974, pp 8-15

United Ostomy Association, Fort Worth Chapter, Fort Worth, Texas Whitten's Medical Supplies, Fort Worth, Texas

Williamson W: Personal communication regarding Fort Worth Home Improvement Loan Programs (HUD), March 1, 1983

Your Medicare Handbook United States Department of Health and Human Services, Social Security Administration, Health Care Financing Administration. Baltimore, Maryland, 55A Pub. No. 05-10050, January 1982

BIBLIOGRAPHY

Carrell A: *Super Handyman's Encyclopedia of Home Repairs Hints*. Prentice Hall, Inc., Englewood Cliffs, New Jersey, 1971

Coakley D, Woodford-Williams E: "Effects of burglary and vandalism on the health of old people." *The Lancet*, November 7, 1979, pp 1066-67

Cohen C I, Sokolvosky J: "Social engagement versus isolation: The case of the aged in SRO hotels." *The Gerontol*, Vol 20, No. 1, 1980, pp 36-44

Hall B: "Interest builds in city program for renovation." *1983 Fort Worth Star Telegram*, Saturday, March 5, 1983, p 3c

Lawton M P, Greenbaum M, Liebowitz B: "The lifespan of housing environments for the aging." *The Gerontol*, Vol 20, No 1, 1980, pp 56-64

Struyk R J: "Housing adjustments of relocating elderly households." *The Gerontol*, Vol 20, No 1, 1980, pp 45-54

Timan B, Goldfarb D, Curtis B: "Home safe." *Geriat Nurs*, Vol 3, No 6, November/December 1982, pp 399-401

SECTION III
MANAGEMENT OF HEALTH PROBLEMS AT HOME

CHAPTER 7

ARTHRITIS AND OSTEOPOROSIS

Mary Flo Bruce

The elderly frequently complain of pain and stiffness associated with movement. These discomforts are often caused by arthritis. In fact, the leading cause of joint pain and stiffness among the elderly is degenerative joint disease. Therefore, the nurse in the home needs to be aware of the prevalence, treatment and care of clients with degenerative joint disease.

More than 4% of all young adults are affected; 85% of those over 75 are afflicted. Rheumatoid arthritis has an incidence rate of .3% in young adults. The rate increases to more than 10% in those over age 65. Obviously these diseases affect a large proportion of the aging population. The community-based nurse should possess a thorough knowledge of the care of the individual with any of these degenerative joint disorders. It is equally imperative that the nurse realize that there are many acute diseases that cause pain and joint stiffness. Any client who complains of these symptoms who has not had a recent thorough physical examination should be urged to have one. It should not be assumed that all elderly clients who have these symptoms have one of the chronic degenerative joint diseases. Prompt diagnosis and treatment may prevent an acute disease from becoming chronic.

Once the diagnosis and treatment of the disease has been made, the home health nurse should educate and work with the client and family to manage it and any exacerbation of the disease.

This chapter discusses the pathophysiology of osteoarthritis, rheumatoid arthritis, and osteoporosis. It also discusses how a nurse can assess, plan, and intervene for a client with one of these degenerative joint disorders. Emphasis is placed on the need to work with each client as an individual. Drugs, nutrition, exercises and client education are included.

Overview of Chronic Degenerative Joint Diseases

The degenerative joint diseases that are chronic in nature can have mono- or poly-articular joint involvement and can be idiopathic in origin or secondary to other etiological agents such as drugs, trauma or other diseases. In order to differentiate between normal aging processes and degenerative joint diseases, the nurse must be aware of what musculoskeletal system function is lost in the aging process. Several changes occur in the system. Muscle fibers atrophy and decrease in number, while fibrous tissue increases and causes decreased muscle tone and flaccidity. Collagen is less resilient and cartilage has less elasticity. There may be a concurrent decrease in synovial fluid which compounds the problems encountered by the elderly client. Bone mass decreases and bones become more brittle because of the loss of bone mineral.

Osteoarthritis

Osteoarthritis is frequently referred to as degenerative joint disease because it is often noninflammatory in nature. It is the most common cause of chronic disability in the elderly. Pearson and Kotthoff (1979, p. 43) contended that 90% of the population over the age of 40 is affected to some degree by this disorder. Masi and Medsger (1979, p. 14) reported that 85% of those over age 75 are significantly affected. At this age, the incidence occurs almost twice as often in females as in males.

Osteoarthritis may be idiopathic or it may be secondary to trauma to the joints, obesity, neuropathic disorders such as diabetes mellitus, and immobility. Wear and tear on the joints as one ages is thought to be responsible for the development of the disorder. The disease may be mono- or poly-articular in nature. Mono-articular osteoarthritis is often a result of trauma.

The disorder is characterized by the wearing away of joint cartilage which leads to the exposure of underlying bone ends. Concurrently there is formation of new bone at the joint surface. The disease may be asymptomatic or symptomatic. Pain is always present if the synovial tissue becomes inflamed.

Normal cartilage changes are intensified. Localized areas of cartilage are softened with an accompanying disruption of the cartilage surface. Osteophytes, new bone formation, occur as a protuberance at the margins of the cartilage or within capsules or ligaments at the point of attachment. Advanced cases of osteoarthritis often display chronic synovitis.

The onset of osteoarthritis is usually insidious. Clinical manifestations include pain, stiffness upon rising, localized tenderness, crepitus and crackling upon joint movement, and associated muscle spasm. In the early stages, pain occurs only after joint use, is aggravated by prolonged activity, and is relieved by rest. The pain is diffuse and is described as an ache. As the disease progresses, the pain may occur during rest and, in severe cases, may awaken the client from sleep. Pain is caused by synovitis, capsulitis or by pinching, abrasion or pressure from the osteophytes.

Stiffness on awakening or after inactivity is usually of short duration and is dissipated as the client moves about and limbers up. However, with progression of the disease, motion becomes limited and weight-bearing joints may give away. Crepitus can be heard upon movement and is caused by cartilage loss and the osteophytes on the surface of the joints.

Heberden's nodes on the distal interphalangeal joint of the fingers are a common manifestation. These nodes are characterized by cartilaginous and bony enlargement of the medial and dorsolateral aspects with flexion and lateral deviation. When these nodes appear on the proximal interphalangeal joints they are called Bouchard's nodes. Women develop these nodes more frequently than men, and heredity is involved to some extent in their origin. The nodes may develop insidiously with little or no pain or the onset may be sudden with swelling, redness and aching, especially after use.

Osteoarthritis is characterized by one or two joint involvement. Occasionally, an individual develops poly-articular involvement which is referred to as generalized osteoarthritis. The pain and joint involvement is asymmetrical. The joints usually involved are knees, hips, lumbar and cervical vertebrae, and, first metatarsophalangeal, then carpometacarpal, and the distal interphalangeal joints of the fingers. Diagnosis is made by roentgenological findings of narrowing of joint space and marginal osteophytes. There are no diagnostic laboratory findings indicative of osteoarthritis.

Rheumatoid Arthritis

Rheumatoid arthritis is the most common chronic, inflammatory disease of joints. Rheumatoid arthritis can occur at any age, but the incidence greatly increases with advanced age and is two or three times more common in females than in males. It is a very serious systemic disease that causes severe pain, deformity and crippling.

The initial onset begins as an inflamed synovial membrane. The most common synovial joints involved are the knees and small joints of the hands, wrists and feet. Occasionally axial involvement occurs. Swelling of the soft tissues develops because of the accumulation of synovial fluid and periarticular edema. The swelling is usually symmetrical and uniform around the joints. Swelling is followed by formation of scar tissue and granulation tissue consisting of new capillaries and fibrous cells called pannus structures. The pannus structures intensify cartilage loss by destroying articular cartilage. At the same time, bone loss occurs due to regional osteoporosis which frequently accompanies rheumatoid arthritis. As the disease advances, bone reabsorption is further aggravated by the formation of articular erosions along the surface of compact bone.

Eventually, alignment of the joint is affected and joint deformity results from the inflammation and destruction of the capsule and ligaments, as well as shortening of the displaced tendons. Flexion contractures occur as a result of flexor muscle and tendon pull. However, scarring gradually develops and results in fibrous ankylosis. The disease is accompanied by rapid muscle atrophy and, at times, muscular inflammation. Many clients also develop subcutaneous rheumatoid nodules. These often occur in any area that has pressure, such as the back of the heel from shoes. These nodules also may develop in visceral organs and tendons.

The etiology of rheumatoid arthritis is unknown. It is a systemic, poly-articular degenerative joint disease that displays early manifestations of fatigue, malaise, fever and loss of appetite. Joint pain, stiffness and swelling follow these prodromal symptoms. The onset is usually insidious but an extremely acute onset of 48 hours or less can occur. The disease is characterized by remissions and exacerbations that have no given length of time. However, exacerbations do occur more frequently in the colder months (Williams, 1979, p. 467). Any exacerbation leads to further joint destruction and deformity.

Decker and Plotz (1979, p. 470) stated that the term "rheumatoid disease" is preferred over "rheumatoid arthritis" because this disease has many accompanying systemic manifestations. There seems to be no direct relationship between the chronic arthritis and the systemic manifestations. At times the systemic manifestations take precedence over the joint inflammation. The most common systemic manifestation is a normocytic, normochromic anemia. The degree of the anemia depends on how active the disease is at the time. Pericarditis also frequently accompanies the disease. It is usually asymptomatic except for pericardial friction rub. Rheumatoid vasculitis is a systemic problem for many of the clients. This is manifested primarily as skin infarction and ulceration, digital gangrene, and polyneuropathy. At times, there are also visceral and pulmonary changes. Many of the drugs used in treatment of rheumatoid arthritis also cause severe complications.

Diagnosis of rheumatoid arthritis is based on the inflammatory nature and the pattern of joint involvement. Laboratory tests show an increased erythrocyte sedimentation rate and a positive test result for the rheumatoid factor. Radiological manifestations include severe osteoporosis, bone reabsorption, and soft tissue atrophy.

Osteoporosis

Osteoporosis is the most common metabolic bone disorder and is characterized by a diffuse porosity of bone. It is found in one of every four females and one of every six males over age 70 (Masi and Medsger, 1979, p. 48). Osteoporosis occurs predominately in postmenopausal women. Some believe that elderly blacks are less prone to osteoporosis and the resulting fractures because their bones are genetically more dense (Goldsmith, 1971). There is an increased incidence in clients who have rheumatoid arthritis, as well as in individuals who are taking systemic steroids or who are chronic users of heparin. Decreased dietary intake of calcium or increased calcium excretion, immobilization and diabetes mellitus are also associated with increased incidence of osteoporosis.

Osteoporosis involves most bones of the body; however, the bones of the spine and pelvis are more severely affected. Quantitative decrease in bone mass results in decrease of body height, slumped posture, upper dorsal kyphosis, and increased susceptibility to fracture. These fractures may occur from trauma or they may occur spontaneously. Femoral neck fracture is the most serious and most frequent fracture that results from osteoporosis in the elderly.

Backache due to the collapse of the vertebrae is the most common sympton. The client may complain of back pain radiating to the legs. The pain may increase with coughing or sneezing. Other symptoms include muscle weakness and diminished sensation.

Diagnosis of osteoporosis is made radiologically and by ruling out other diseases such as leukemia, multiple myeloma, and hyperparathyroidism. Laboratory tests are found to be within normal range.

Medical Management

None of these degenerative bone and joint diseases present a life-threatening medical crisis in themselves. However, both a fractured femoral head and some of the concomitant systemic problems of rheumatoid arthritis can cause a life-threatening situation for some. In general, though, the medical management of these degenerative diseases is by preventive and/or palliative measures. Rehabilitative measures are an important component in the treatment of these disorders.

Preventive measures consist of educating the public about good health practices that will prevent or delay the onset of these disorders and education of the client and family to prevent further degeneration of bone or joints. Palliative measures include treatment of symptoms, alleviation of pain, and in some cases, surgery.

Osteoarthritis

Treatment of osteoarthritis consists of outlining a regimen of adequate rest for involved joints and proper exercise to strengthen the muscles. The drugs most commonly used are analgesics to relieve pain. At times, anti-inflammatory drugs are utilized. Intra-articular injection of adrenocorticoids are sometimes used to relieve pain and other symptoms. Surgical procedures are performed to correct misalignment and relieve joint stress. Surgery can also relieve pain and improve joint function. Regardless of the reason surgery is performed, the client must be fully advised about the expected results, the advantages and disadvantages, and the limitations of the proposed surgery.

Rheumatoid Arthritis

The medical management of rheumatoid arthritis must be aggressive because each exacerbation leads to further joint and cartilage destruction. The general treatment is very similar to the treatment of osteoarthritis. However, because of the systemic nature of rheumatoid arthritis, adequate rest is essential. The optimal amount of rest needed depends on individual factors and varies from client to client. Exercise is very important, but the exercise program must *minimize stress* on the affected joints. It is often difficult to develop a program that maintains range of motion and muscle tone without stressing the affected joints. Anti-inflammatory drugs are always used in the treatment of rheumatoid arthritis. While relief of pain is important, it is not as vital as the lessening of the inflammation.

Osteoporosis

The medical treatment of osteoporosis consists of alleviating the pain by use of analgesic drugs along with short periods of splinting or bracing. Active exercise is started as soon as possible. The exercise should begin cautiously and increase gradually. Immobility should be avoided if at all possible. The physician often prescribes a stool softener or mild laxative to prevent constipation and straining which increase back pain. Calcium tablets and intake of vitamin D are found to be beneficial. When these two drugs are prescribed, there should be monthly monitoring of serum and urinary calcium to prevent reactions to an excess of vitamin D. At times, estrogen therapy is initiated. However, the possible benefit of estrogen administration must be weighed against the possible increased risk of cancer. Sodium fluoride has been used as an agent that stimulates new bone formation. At present, it is not known if this remineralization produces a sufficient improvement in the strength of bone to justify its use.

Drug Therapy

Drug therapy is an essential component of both the acute and rehabilitative phase of management of bone and joint degenerative disorders. The nurse must have a thorough knowledge of the classifications, actions and side effects of various drugs. A broad knowledge base assists the nurse with client education. Because the full effects of some of the drugs are not immediately apparent, client education is needed to assure proper compliance in taking the drugs as ordered.

Both osteoarthritis and rheumatoid arthritis are treated with analgesics and non-steroidal anti-inflammatory drugs. After the initial onset of rheumatoid arthritis, remission-inducing drugs (for example slow-acting anti-rheumatic drugs) are often required. Included in this category are the organic gold compounds, anti-malarial drugs, d-penicillamine, immunosuppressants and immunostimulants.

Analgesics

Aspirin is probably the most widely used drug for bone and joint degenerative disorders. Aspirin is used in the treatment of osteoarthritis because of its analgesic effect. It is used in rheumatoid arthritis because it possesses anti-inflammatory and anti-pyretic effects along with analgesic effects. The analgesic action is based on the suppression of peripheral pain. The amount of aspirin needed to reach a therapeutic concentration varies greatly. Some individuals absorb aspirin poorly while others can suddenly absorb high concentrations with concurrent side effects. Characteristics of hypersensitivity to aspirin include anaphylactic shock, urticaria, angioedema and asthma.

Another severe problem with the intake of aspirin is the possibility of salicylate intoxication. Acidosis increases membrane permeability which leads to an increase in unbound salicylate. Therefore, an increase in total drug concentration results in severe symptoms such as respiratory depression, hyperpyrexia and convulsions. Serum salicylate levels are not definitive for the diagnosis of salicylate intoxication.

Tinnitus may be the first symptom of slight toxicity. In older adults this symptom may not occur because of hearing loss. Aspirin also tends to suppress hearing in some older adults.

There are a number of other side effects from the ingestion of aspirin that are not related to aspirin hypersensitivity or intoxication. Gastrointestinal side effects are probably the most common ones. Frequent symptoms are dyspepsia, nausea and vomiting. Aspirin damages the gastric mucosa which leads to gastric irritation and bleeding. The chance of bleeding is intensified because aspirin both inhibits platelet adhesiveness and aggregation and prolongs bleeding and prothrombin time. Roth (1980, p. 46) stated that asprin has another often unrecognized side effect of acting as a central nervous system depressant. These symptoms of depression in the elderly individual can result in an inappropriate diagnosis of chronic organic brain syndrome.

Both acetaminophen and phenacetin, aniline derivatives, are analgesics with slight anti-pyretic action. Besides aspirin, acetaminophen is the most commonly used analgesic. It is the less toxic of the aniline derivatives when taken properly. Overdose or high chronic doses can lead to hepatotoxicity and renal damage. Phenacetin can cause acute symptoms such as nausea, anorexia, dizziness, weakness and palpitations. Chronic use of high doses has been linked with nephrotoxicity and blood dyscrasias.

Narcotics or drugs that are under the Controlled Substance Act are not usually used to relieve pain caused by osteoarthritis or rheumatoid arthritis. Occasionally, narcotics are used during an exacerbation when there is severe pain. Darvon (propoxyphene) is used for short periods when other drugs do not provide sufficient relief. However, tolerance and dependency have been reported for this drug. When Darvon is utilized, the client needs to be aware of the fact that both alcohol and aspirin potentiate the effects of Darvon.

Nonsteroidal Anti-inflammatory Drugs

The nonsteroidal anti-inflammatory drugs most frequently used in the treatment of osteoarthritis and rheumatoid arthritis in the elderly include the indole series and the propionic acid series. Indomethacin (Indocin) was the first drug in the indole series and is still in widespread use today. Average doses range from 25–200 mg. each day. Numerous side effects are possible from this drug. Central nervous system side effects are dizziness, lightheadedness, depression, mental confusion, a feeling of detachment, and depersonalization. Part of the nurse's teaching plan should include instructing the client on the possibility of these side effects. The nurse should observe the client during the home visit for any change in emotional status and reassure the client that the symptoms are probably a result of the medication and are transient. The client should be encouraged to notify the physician if any of these feelings occur.

Indomethacin also produces gastrointestinal side effects such as dyspepsia, nausea, vomiting and diarrhea. It can mask the symptoms of peptic ulcers. Both the gastrointestinal and central nervous system side effects may increase with age, so the elderly individual is more prone to severe side effects. Indomethacin also potentiates the effects of the warfarin anti-coagulants such as Coumadin.

Two other drugs in the indole series frequently prescribed are tolmetin and sulindac. Both of these drugs have fewer side effects than indomethacin. Tolmetin has no potentiating effect with the warfarin drugs, and sulindac has less than indomethacin. The average dose of tolmetin is 200 milligrams given three or four times daily. Sulindac's average dose is 200 milligrams given twice daily. All of the drugs of the indole series are excreted by the kidneys.

There are several drugs in the propionic acid series that are in common usage. They are ibuprofen (Motrin), fenoprofen (Nalfon), naproxen (Naprosyn), ketoprofen, and alclofenac. These drugs have some gastrointestinal and central nervous system side effects. The occult blood loss is less than with aspirin; therefore, the chance of developing anemia is somewhat less. While both ibuprofen and ketoprofen appear to have no effect on the anti-coagulant drugs, naproxen has demonstrated some potentiating effect that has not been shown clinically significant. The effect of fenoprofen and alclofenac on the anti-coagulants is not known.

These drugs are excreted through the kidneys. They give symptomatic relief to clients with osteoarthritis and are used in the treatment of rheumatoid arthritis. The success of the drugs in the treatment of rheumatoid arthritis varies greatly with each individual client. These drugs and their average doses are shown in Table 7-1.

Efficacy of a particular drug on an individual client is entirely unpredictable. There is a great variation in the therapeutic results from one client to the other. The physician is often faced with the necessity of changing drugs every three or four weeks until the drug of choice is found.

Corticosteroids

The corticosteroids effectively and rapidly relieve many of the symptoms of rheumatoid arthritis. This is probably the reason that corticosteroids are still in

TABLE 7.1
Indole and Propionic Drugs Commonly Used in the Treatment of Arthritis

Drug	Dosage*
indomethacin (Indocin)	25–200 mg. daily
tolmetin (Tolectin)	200 mg. 3 or 4 times daily
ibuprofen (Motrin)	1200–3600 mg. daily in 3–4 divided doses
fenoprofen (Nalfon)	900–3000 mg. daily in 3–4 divided doses
naproxen (Naprosyn)	500–750 mg. daily in 2–3 divided doses
ketaprofen	150–300 mg. daily in 3–4 divided doses
alclofenac	3000–4000 mg. daily in 3–4 divided doses
sulindac (Clinoril)	200 mg. 2 times daily

* Dosages may vary from one reference to another and from one physician to another.

widespread use in spite of the many nonsteroidal anti-inflammatory drugs now available. Corticosteroids are very advantageous in acute periods of severe, painful symptoms and for short-term therapy. Prednisone is the drug most often used. The recommended dose for rheumatoid arthritis is 5 to 7.5 milligrams orally once daily. Adrenal corticotrophic hormones (ACTH) are occasionally given during acute exacerbations, but this treatment is not continued when the client is released from the hospital. Although not recommended, the fluorinated corticosteroids such as dexamethasone (Decadron) and triamcinolone (Aristocort) are used in the treatment of rheumatoid arthritis.

There are numerous side effects that can occur in any client who is administered corticosteroids. Two side effects that are not reversible after the treatment has been discontinued are osteoporosis and aseptic necrosis of the bone. Other side effects include increased risk of infection, gastric hemorrhage, intestinal perforation, pancreatitis, hypertension, edema, hypokalemic alkalosis, psychiatric disorders such as depression or euphoria, cataracts, glaucoma, impotence, glucose intolerance, acne, purpura, impaired wound healing, and obesity. Corticosteroids are contraindicated in clients who have osteoporosis, peptic ulcers, convulsive disorders, psychoses and severe psychoneuroses.

Client education is especially important for the individual taking corticosteroids at home. Besides being aware of the side effects, the client must understand the necessity of taking the drug exactly as ordered by the physician. The client must be educated about both the dangers of increasing the dosage in the hope of getting faster relief and the hazards involved if the therapy is suddenly discontinued. Because prolonged steroid therapy suppresses adrenal cortical activity, the client can develop adrenal cortical insufficiency.

Part of the client's instructions must include recognition of the signs and symptoms of adrenal insufficiency. The onset frequently begins with nausea and vomiting. These can be followed rapidly by tachycardia, hypotension and hyperthermia.

Electrolyte imbalances occur because of a deficiency of mineralocorticoids. The client becomes hyponatremic, hypochloremic and hyperkalemic. Hypoglycemia develops due to the decrease in glucocorticoids. Clients who are taking any corticosteroids should carry a card or wear a bracelet stating the name of the drug and the daily dosage. Then, in the case of a medical emergency, the health-care providers can realize the possibility of adrenal insufficiency.

Slow-acting Anti-rheumatic Drugs

Initially, aspirin and/or nonsteroidal anti-inflammatory drugs are sufficient to control rheumatoid arthritis. As the disease progresses, it may become necessary for the client to be started on one of the remittive drugs that pose a higher risk for side effects and toxicity. The remission-inducing drugs are slow to produce noticeable effects.

Organic gold compound therapy, chrysotherapy, is one of the earliest remission-inducing drugs to be used. Zvaifler (1979, p. 356) stated that out of every 100 clients who receive gold therapy, about one-half to two-thirds get some relief from the symptoms, one-fourth to one-third have toxic reactions, and about one-fourth receive no benefits.

Chrysotherapy is started during the active phase of rheumatoid arthritis, usually during the first two years. When the treatment is effective, the client notices a decrease in morning stiffness, less fatigue, and less pain. The erythrocyte sedimentation rate improves.

Chrysotherapy has numerous side effects which include gastrointestinal disturbance and agranulocytosis, transient albuminuria, dermatoses and urticaria. When the client displays toxicity, the drug is discontinued. Gold is not given concomitantly with other drugs which have the potential of suppressing the bone marrow.

Aurothioglucose, sodium thiomalate, and sodium thiosulfate are the gold preparations used in treatment of rheumatoid arthritis. The average dose is 25 to 50 milligrams a day, given in one dose, intramuscularly. Gold preparations can be used satisfactorily in the treatment of elderly patients. The mechanisms of action are not known. However, gold compounds do have anti-microbial and anti-inflammatory effects. Gold is excreted by the kidneys.

Anti-malarial drugs are used cautiously in the treatment of rheumatoid arthritis. The anti-malarial drugs are started within the first five years of the disease. They have a therapeutic effect that is compared to administration of gold compounds. However, the anti-malarial drugs have a serious drawback in that they cause retinopathy which is not reversible when the drug is discontinued. Other side effects include diarrhea, skin rash, nausea and hemolytic anemia. The drugs most commonly used are chloroquine and hydroxychloroquine. The average dose for chloroquine is 125 to 250 milligrams daily, and hydroxychloroquine is given 200 to 400 milligrams twice daily. When either of these drugs is used, the client should have a fundoscopic examination every four months.

D-penicillamine has demonstrated positive results in the treatment of rheumatoid arthritis. However, clients over the age of 60 do not often demonstrate a satisfactory clinical response, and the elderly tend to have an increased susceptibility to bone marrow depression. When d-penicillamine therapy is used with the elderly, the individual's nutritional status must be carefully evaluated and vitamin B_6 given if there is impaired nutrition.

D-penicillamine is contraindicated if the client is receiving the gold compounds. It is not to be administered to individuals who have renal insufficiency. Side effects include skin rash, pruritius, anorexia, nausea and vomiting. Two very serious side effects are bone marrow depression and renal insufficiency. Complete blood counts are done every two weeks for at least a six-month period. After that, they are done monthly. The first sign of bone marrow depression caused by d-penicillamine is thrombocytopenia. Urinalysis is done at least monthly. Proteinuria must be monitored closely and not allowed to exceed 2 grams of protein in 24 hours. Both bone marrow depression and nephropathy are reversible.

Client teaching must include informing the client to notify the physician immediately if an unexplained fever, a sore throat, or any bleeding occurs.

Both immunosuppression and immunostimulation are considered as "investigational" for the treatment of arthritic diseases (Steinberg and Decker, 1979, p. 387). When the nurse encounters a client who is taking immunosuppressant or immunostimulant therapy for rheumatoid arthritis, the nurse needs to investigate how the particular drugs work with the rest of the treatment plan.

The drugs used in the treatment of osteoporosis are calcium diphosphate, vitamin D, estrogen and fluoride. Calcium diphosphate is given in doses of 1 or 2 grams daily. Since many elderly clients have difficulty absorbing calcium through the gastrointestinal tract, vitamin D is often given to aid the digestion of calcium. Excess calcium leads to relaxed muscles, development of kidney stones, and deep thigh pain. Pathological fractures are a possibility. Monthly monitoring of serum and urine for excess calcium should be done, especially when vitamin D is given with the calcium. If the client is placed on tetracyclines, the nurse should instruct the client not to take the tetracycline at the same time as the calcium. There should be at least an hour between the two medications because calcium decreases the absorption of tetracycline.

Vitamin D is a fat-soluble vitamin absorbed in the gastrointestinal tract and stored in the liver. It is slow to metabolize and is excreted by the kidneys. The usual dosage for the client with osteoporosis is 25,000 to 50,000 units. Excessive amounts of vitamin D result in nausea, vomiting, diarrhea, exhaustion and urinary infrequency. Hypervitaminosis D leads to the removal of the calcium from the bones to the blood. Calcium may then be deposited in any tissues including the kidneys and heart. The elderly client should be counseled not to take vitamin D unless advised by the physician.

Fluoride is absorbed in the gastrointestinal tract. It has been found that fluoride has stimulated new bone growth in elderly clients with osteoporosis. The usual dosage is 25 to 50 milligrams daily. Fluoride should be taken only as prescribed because chronic excess leads to fluorosis which is the development of brittle bones.

The efficacy of estrogen in retarding osteoporosis has been demonstrated when it is prescribed immediately after an oophorectomy or within the first postmenopausal years. It is contraindicated in clients over 65 years of age.

Nutritional Needs

While it is necessary for the nurse to assess thoroughly the nutritional status of the client, it is equally important to realize that there is no known diet that prevents or helps either osteoarthritis or rheumatoid arthritis. There is no "arthritis diet."

Even though there is no arthritis diet, good nutrition is an essential part of the treatment regimen. The client needs to know what constitutes a well-balanced diet. Once this is established, the nurse needs to assess how the individual's culture, religion and/or economic situation may interfere with the client's willingness or ability to follow a nutritionally sound diet. The diet should have sufficient bulk and fiber to prevent constipation because straining can lead to increased back pain in the individual with osteoporosis or spinal involvement.

When the client is overweight, weight reduction is necessary to relieve strain on the weight-bearing bones and joints. After the client's activity level and eating habits are assessed, the nurse works with the client to plan an acceptable, nutritious diet with low or moderate caloric intake. If the client lives on a fixed, low income, it may be a challenge to assist the client in identifying foods both low caloric and affordable. Once the diet is begun, it is important to offer reassurance and emotional support to ensure that the individual continues to diet.

Middle age and older women often delete milk from their diet because they: 1) want to lose weight, 2) do not like milk, 3) think they do not need milk, and/or 4) have a lactose intolerance which causes milk to cause abdominal distention. The last reason is particularly true of black women. If older women cannot or will not drink milk, they should be encouraged to eat other foods containing calcium such as cottage cheese. The daily Recommended Dietary Allowance (RDA) is 800 mg, which can be met by taking two 8-oz. glasses of milk or milk substitute (Robinson, 1981, p. 223). Osteoporosis may be prevented and/or treated with dietary supplements of calcium and/or vitamin D if there is not an adequate intake of calcium in the diet.

Rest and Exercise

Both rest and exercise are very important components in the treatment of these disorders. A balance between rest and exercise, which allows the client to maintain joint mobility and prevent further disability, must be established. A more basic goal is to improve the individual's ability to function. Therefore, each program is developed keeping in mind the limitations of the individual.

The client may get excellent instruction in the hospital on the role of rest and exercise in the treatment regimen. Once home, the person may become discouraged and fail to follow the regimen, however. The home health nurse may have to re-educate the client and family.

A balance between rest and exercise is needed in the treatment of osteoarthritis, rheumatoid arthritis, and osteoporosis. However, the amount and type of exercise varies. The individual with osteoarthritis should rest the involved joints periodically during the day. Complete bed rest is seldom needed and is usually contraindicated. When the rest periods are divided throughout the day, the involved joints receive less damage. If the weight-bearing joints are involved, the client should rest in bed or on the couch. Use of assistive devices such as a cane or walker help to decrease the force applied to the lower extremities while walking. If only one side is involved, the cane or crutch should be held in the hand opposite the involved side.

Exercise is important, and the affected joints should be moved through their full range of motion several times a day. The exercise program should start with a couple of repetitions and is then gradually increased to 15 or 20 repetitions. The exercise should not be excessive because this only aggravates the pain and joint damage. When the discomfort continues for more than a half hour after the exercise session, the individual has exceeded the tolerance limit. It is important to stress that over-exercising can be as detrimental to the client as not exercising at all.

Because rheumatoid arthritis is an inflammatory disease, rest is essential. Occasionally, complete bed rest may be necessary during severe exacerbation. Rest is spaced according to individual need. In mild cases the individual is encouraged to rest at least two hours a day when fatigue occurs. The stiffness that follows the rest period discourages some persons from resting. The nurse should explain that the stiffness is part of the disease and, when remission occurs, the stiffness lessens. The rest period is important not only for the physical rest it provides, but also for the removal from psychological stress. Besides these general rest periods, the individual may have to immobilize the inflamed arthritic joints.

Range-of-motion exercises of all joints should be done at least once daily to maintain mobility. If increased mobility is desired, range-of-motion exercises are done three or more times daily. These exercises are done with the least possible movement. Each joint should be warmed up before placing it through the complete range of motion. The use of heat and/or massage of the joint before exercise lessens the stiffness, and the person is able to perform better. The nurse may also teach the client to exercise when the effects of the medications are optimal. Besides the range-of-motion exercises, the exercise program may include both isometric and isotonic exercises. It is important that the person follow the entire exercise program as ordered.

The person who is ambulatory and doing all the activities of daily living may feel that this is sufficient exercise. The nurse needs to re-emphasize both the purpose of and the need to follow the exercise program as prescribed.

Part of the client/teaching plan includes teaching proper posture while awake, while resting, and in bed. Faulty positioning leads to contractures. For instance, the nurse may need to explain that a pillow under the knee not only provides comfort but can cause flexion contractures of the hip, knee and ankle. The nurse can demonstrate correct posture in different resting positions and then have the client return the demonstration.

At times, splints and braces are used to provide comfort and prevent contractures. Splinting is also used after contractures have occurred and maximum correction has been obtained. When braces or splints are utilized, the nurse must ensure that the client and/or family know how to apply the device properly. The nurse can have the client put on the device and check to see that it is positioned correctly. The nurse should also find out if the client is using it only at the times needed. Because both splint and braces provide comfort, the individual may become dependent on the device and overuse it.

The individual who has osteoarthritis should remain as active as possible. Bed rest is contraindicated. When the individual must rest in the daytime, the person should be advised to rock in a rocking chair. Exercise is vital. However, the exercise should not consist of bending or lifting. Some people should not even open windows. Swimming, riding a stationary bicycle, and walking are excellent exercises in most cases. Occasionally, the physician may also advise the client to do specific exercises to strengthen the abdominal and back muscles.

There is increasing evidence that regular consistent exercise, even simple walking, may help to prevent and possibly reverse the process of osteoporosis (Richards, 1982, p. 102).

Heat and Cold Therapy

Superficial heat and cold are used to treat these disorders. Cold applications are used during an acute phase and heat is used to treat chronic conditions. Because the elderly have poor tactile sensitivity, the nurse should emphasize the importance of following specific instructions.

Cold is usually applied as an ice pack or ice massage. There are several methods of applying heat at home. The easiest method is probably the heating pad. However, moist heat is often more soothing for the arthritic client. Warm, moist packs can be applied to the joint. A warm tub bath in the morning is helpful for the client with generalized osteoarthritis. The bath removes some of the stiffness upon awakening. Some individuals find that a home whirlpool appliance set on a gentle cycle relieves pain and discomfort. Another modality occasionally used in the home is hot paraffin. Hot paraffin should be used exactly as prescribed. The nurse needs to observe the client using the heated paraffin treatment.

Surgical Interventions

Surgery is performed when it is thought that it may prevent further deterioration and/or deformities or ease the pain. The types of surgery performed for arthritic conditions include arthroplasty, arthrodesis, synovectomy, fusion, osteotomy and prosthesis replacement. The joints of the upper extremities that benefit from surgery are the shoulder, elbow, wrist and hands. Surgery is also done on the hip, knee, ankle, foot and spine.

Clients who refuse or hesitate to become active participants in their medical regimen are poor risks for surgery also, because total active participation of the client is an essential part of the post-surgical recovery phase. Recovery is slow, and the success or failure of the surgery often depends on complete commitment of the client to the treatment program. Any type of infection, serious respiratory or cardiac problem, and obesity may contraindicate surgery.

The home health nurse who is working with a client before surgery can clarify any misunderstanding about the surgical procedure, the risks involved, and the post-surgical regimen. If the person is hesitant about having the surgery, a second opinion may be sought. The client also needs to know how the pain will be managed once the individual has returned home. The client teaching plan should include any special help or equipment needed in the home, the post-surgical rest and exercise program, and any restriction to the activities of daily living, including restrictions on sexual activities.

Post-surgically, the home health nurse needs to ensure that the client and family understand and follow the complete regimen. The nurse should re-emphasize the need for compliance and active participation in the program. The client can demonstrate the exercises and any splinting or special positioning of the joint needed.

It is very important to teach the client and family how to look for infection. The nurse should explain the importance of alerting the physician at the first sign of even a minor infection because any infection can also infect the operative joint.

If the client does not receive written instructions as part of the hospital discharge plan, the home health nurse may write out all pertinent information such as time and duration of exercises and of rest, signs of infection, and times to take each medication. The nurse should be sure the client understands that overdoing can be as harmful as underachieving. The nurse inspects the home for any safety hazards and informs the client how to rectify these hazards. The nurse should also assist the client and family to identify any fears or anxieties that they may feel. This is easier if a therapeutic relationship has been established previously.

Psychosocial Aspects

The psychosocial aspects of a chronic illness are intensified when the individual also faces multiple problems associated with aging. Many older people are on fixed incomes and concerned about being a financial and physical burden to their family. Arthritis adds to the financial burden in the form of extra medications, treatments, equipment and transportation. Loss of function and deformities may result in the individual needing help with household chores, which becomes either an added expense or an added load for another family member. Both can result in the person losing some independence.

Depression frequently accompanies arthritis. This can be understood when one realizes that the individual faces exacerbations and remissions, along with pain, fatigue and deformities. The person and the family often go through the same stages of mourning as one who is dying. The nurse is in the position to assist the client and family to face the realities of the disease and to accept their feelings.

Sexuality of the elderly person is often ignored. However, this is an important aspect of one's life. The nurse should not assume that an individual is not sexually active just because the person is elderly. Sexual adjustments may be made with aging. With bone and joint diseases, the person may be unable to assume preferred positions or may be dysfunctional because of pain. After surgery such as total hip replacement, intercourse is contraindicated for several weeks. The nurse can play a vital role by assisting the client to discuss any questions or problems concerning sexual activities. A listening, nonjudgmental attitude can offer counseling to client and spouse. It may be necessary to refer the person to a sex counselor. Often however, the nurse can answer the person's questions or advise the person concerning positions that will not place stress on the affected joint.

Social isolation is often a problem for the elderly arthritic person. If the person is self-conscious because of loss of function and/or deformities, he or she may withdraw because of embarrassment. The individual should maintain as much activity as possible. The nurse should work with the client and the family to include the person in daily activities when possible. The nurse should help the client identify recreational activities in which he or she will be able to participate. For instance, the person could raise house plants which do not involve bending or lifting. Shelves can be placed where the person can conveniently reach the plants.

Fads and Quackery

Fads and quackery which take advantage of the arthritic person abound. The American Arthritis Foundation (1981) has estimated that arthritis sufferers spend $950 million annually on "quackery." One reason that a person with arthritis is so susceptible is that arthritis has periods of remission. A remission spontaneously occurs, and the person thinks that a cure has been found. There are numerous treatments for arthritis that have not scientifically demonstrated effectiveness. The danger of these treatments are twofold: 1) the treatment itself is harmful; and, 2) the person does not follow the prescribed medical regimen.

The nurse is in a position to gain the individual's confidence. It is important to listen to the person in a nonjudgmental manner. If the client reports the use of unorthodox treatment, the nurse must investigate to determine if the treatment is harmful. If not, it may be necessary to allow the person to follow the unorthodox treatment along with the medical regimen. The nurse should stress the necessity of completely following the physician's orders and not using the unorthodox treatment as a substitute. It is also important that the nurse not ridicule the client for these beliefs or practices. For instance, wearing a copper bracelet is not harmful as long as the client follows the total treatment plan. However, if the treatment is harmful, the nurse has the task of working with the client to discontinue the unorthodox treatment. This can be a difficult challenge.

Role of the Home Health Nurse

The nurse plays an important function when he or she assesses the client for a bone or joint disease. Early diagnosis may prevent loss of function and deformity. It is also important for the nurse to work with the client who already has a degenerative bone or joint disease.

The long-term goal for the client with osteoarthritis, rheumatoid arthritis, or osteoporosis is three-fold: 1) maintain or increase mobility; 2) prevent deformities; and 3) alleviate pain. Short-term goals are established to assist the client in attaining this long-term goal.

Assessment

Assessment of the client and family is one of the responsibilities of the home health nurse. The nurse may be the first health professional who sees the client having symptoms such as early morning stiffness, joint pain, and fatigue. These symptoms should not be accepted as "just growing old" but considered as possible early symptoms of some degenerative disease. A thorough assessment of the client should be conducted. The nurse can ask questions about the pain and/or stiffness while conducting a home visit. It is important to know when the stiffness occurs, its duration, and what helps relieve it. The same questions can be asked about the pain. When asking about pain, the nurse should have the client describe the type of pain and localize it.

The nurse should especially observe the client for any deformities, subluxation of the metacarpophalangeal joints or of the cervical spine, rheumatoid nodules, or wrist fusion which may indicate rheumatoid arthritis. Upper dorsal kyphosis and symmetric skin folds along the base of the thoracic cage are common in osteoporosis. Women with osteoarthritis frequently have Heberden's and/or Bouchard's nodes on their fingers. These nodes are less frequently found in men. The nurse should inspect for tissue induration which can be indicative of arthritic involvement.

The nurse should perform passive range-of-motion exercises of the joints. While checking for mobility, the nurse should inspect and palpate the joint and check for stiffness, ankylosis, muscle atrophy, and crepitation. The client's ability to perform activities of daily living (ADL) should be assessed, and any task that can not be performed should be noted. If there are any signs or symptoms of degenerative bone or joint disease, the nurse should urge the individual to see a physician. All of these disorders are chronic and progressive: therefore, early diagnosis and treatment are important.

When the client has already been diagnosed as having one of these diseases, the nurse must assess additional factors. The client's and family's knowledge concerning every facet of the disease process and the treatment should be assessed. This assessment includes information about the disease process, medications, diet, rest, exercise and any special procedures needed. It is important to have the client and family discuss their understanding of the disease process and the treatment program. Open-ended questions help establish their knowledge base. The nurse should clarify any misunderstandings or misconceptions the client and/or family have.

Therapeutic listening may help to get clients to reveal their attitude, anxiety and fears concerning the disease and the treatment program. A nonjudgmental attitude on the part of the nurse enhances the opportunity for the client and family to express themselves.

Interventions

Once the assessment has identified areas in which the client needs support or further teaching, the nurse can work closely with the client to ensure that the plan is being followed completely. If the client outlines the treatment plan and explains how it is being carried out, the nurse can evaluate any deficiencies or weaknesses.

Since denial often interferes with an individual's acceptance of a diagnosis of a chronic disease, the person's knowledge base may not be as complete as it first appears. The individual may be simply repeating what the physician has said. The nurse can ask open-ended questions that elicit how much the person actually accepts and understands. Myths and misconceptions may have to be clarified a number of times. The nurse should listen carefully to what the client says and does not say.

Medication plays an important role in the course of both osteoarthritis and rheumatoid arthritis. The client may need assistance in setting up a schedule for taking the medications, especially if the individual is forgetful or confused. Particular care should be paid to any medications that should not be taken together or with certain foods. Also, if the physician has advised that the client take an antacid with one of the medications, the nurse should emphasize the need to follow this advice because of the gastrointestinal side effects of many of the anti-arthritic drugs.

The client needs a realistic perception of when and what degree of relief to expect. If relief from the pain and/or stiffness does not occur as quickly as anticipated, the person may become discouraged and not take the medications as ordered. Another problem that occurs is that the effect of the drugs cannot be predicted from one person to another. The efficacy of the anti-arthritic drugs is variable. The drugs may have to be changed several times before an effective one is found.

The course and treatment program for osteoarthritis, rheumatoid arthritis, and osteoporosis varies greatly from one person to another. The nurse can evaluate any prescribed procedures by having the client demonstrate each procedure. Any family members who assist with the procedures should also show the nurse how they do it. This includes treatments such as exercises, splinting, bracing and positioning of affected joints. See the master care plans for arthritis and osteoporosis at the end of the chapter.

Chronic disease has a disruptive effect on the entire family. Therefore, the family should be included in any client teaching. The family needs to be involved in the care and not let the client isolate self from others. However, the client should do as much self-care as possible. If the nurse is able to develop a therapeutic relationship with the entire family, it is possible to assist family members with their anxieties and fears.

Community Education

One of the most important functions of the community health nurse is public education. Arthritis is a group of chronic diseases that extort a heavy toll annually in both human suffering and economic costs. There are numerous myths, fads and quack cures surrounding arthritis. The nurse can relay reliable information about arthritic diseases and the appropriate type of treatment for the disorder. Since early diagnosis and treatment is important, the public should be made aware of the arthritis warning signs. These signs are:

- persistent pain and stiffness on arising;
- pain, tenderness or swelling in one or more joints;
- recurrence of these symptoms, especially when they involve more than one joint; and,
- recurrent or persistent pain and stiffness in the neck, lower back, knees and other joints (*Arthritis—The Basic Facts*, 1981).

Summary

Osteoarthritis, rheumatoid arthritis, and osteoporosis affect a large proportion of the elderly population. In order for the home health nurse to care for clients with these diseases, the nurse needs to possess a broad knowledge base concerning the normal changes that occur with aging and a thorough knowledge about each of these disorders and their appropriate treatment. The client's care should be focused on the whole person and not just the particular diseases. It is important for the nurse to develop a care plan that takes into consideration the individual's entire life style.

If the nurse develops a therapeutic relationship with the client and family, they are more apt to follow the nurse's advice and guidance. Since these diseases are both chronic and progressive, there is a permanent impact on the life style of the client and family members. The elderly person has probably already had to make adjustments to this life style and may see the disorder as "too much" with which to cope. The nurse can assist the client in working through these feelings by using the person's coping mechanisms. It is important for the client and family to work through these feelings because compliance to the total program is necessary.

The nurse has to have a broad knowledge base about the disease process and the treatment regimen. Using this knowledge base, the nurse and client can develop an acceptable and workable plan. The nurse may have to do repeated teaching in each area before the client is able to follow the regimen. The nurse's main goal should be to assist the client to live as independently as possible and to realistically adapt to any limitations imposed by the aging process and the disease.

REFERENCES

Arthritis—The Basic Facts. American Arthritis Foundation, New York, 1981, pp. 6, 26

Decker J L, Plotz P H: "Extra-articular rheumatoid disease." *Arthritis and Allied Conditions*. Lea & Febiger, Philadelphia, 1979, p 470

Goldsmith N F et al.: "Bone-mineral estimation in normal and osteoporotic women." *J Bone Joint Surg*. Vol 53, 1971, pp 83–100

Masi A T, Medsger T A: "Epidemiology of the rheumatic diseases." *Arthritis and Allied Conditions*. Lea & Febiger, Philadelphia, 1979, pp 14, 28

Pearson L, Kotthoff E M: *Geriatric Clinical Protocols*. J. B. Lippincott Co., Philadelphia, 1979, p 43

Richards M: "Osteoporosis." *Geriat Nurs*. Vol 3, No 2, 1982, pp 98–102

Robinson N: "Dietary needs in later life," in Hogstel M O (ed.): *Nursing Care of the Older Adult*. John Wiley and Sons, Inc., New York, 1981, pp 223–224

Roth S H: "Drug therapy and the rehabilitation process: A necessary interaction," in Ehrlich G E (ed.): *Rehabilitation Management of Rheumatic Conditions*. Williams & Williams, Baltimore, 1980, p 46

Steinberg A F, Decker J L: "Immunoregulatory drugs," in McCarty D J: *Arthritis and Allied Conditions*. J. B. Lippincott Co., Philadelphia, 1979, p 387

Williams Jr. R C: "Clinical picture of rheumatoid arthritis," in McCarty D J (ed.): *Arthritis and Allied Conditions*. J. B. Lippincott, Philadelphia, 1979, p 467

Zvaifler N J: "Etiology and pathogenesis of rheumatoid arthritis," in McCarty D J (ed.): *Arthritis and Allied Conditions*. J. B. Lippincott, Philadelphia, 1979, p 356

BIBLIOGRAPHY

Alioa J: "Estrogen and exercise in prevention and treatment of osteoporosis." *Geriatrics*, Vol 37, No 6, June 1982, pp 81–85

Driscoll P: "Rheumatoid arthritis: Understanding it more fully." *Nursing 75*, Vol 5, No 12, December 1975, pp 26–32

Ehrlich G E: *Rehabilitation Management of Rheumatic Conditions*. Williams and Williams, Baltimore, 1980

McCarty D J: *Arthritis and Allied Conditions*. J. B. Lippincott Co., Philadelphia, 1979

Miller S: "NSAID's: Examining therapeutic alternatives." *Geriatrics*, Vol 37, No 3, March 1982, pp 70–73

Reich M: "Arthritis: Avoiding diagnostic pitfalls." *Geriatrics*, Vol 37, No 6, June 1982, pp 46–53

So You Have . . . Osteoarthritis. Arthritis Foundation, Atlanta, n.d.

Surgery—Information To Consider, Arthritis Foundation, Atlanta, n.d.

SAMPLE MASTER CARE PLAN FOR HOME CARE—

Nursing Diagnoses	Assessment	Planning
Potential joint contractures	• Unable to do active range of motion. • Muscle weakness. • Mobility restricted (walks with cane). • Pain in shoulders and/or knees.	*Short-term goals* Client will: • reduce pain • increase mobility • lessen muscle weakness • follow medical regimen • eat a well-balanced diet and reduce calories if indicated • socialize with family and friends
Impaired physical mobility	• Unable to walk without cane. • Unable to do complete range of motion. • Muscles of legs atrophied. • Pain when walking.	
Alteration in comfort	• Complains of pain and discomfort in affected joints. • Guards movement of affected joints.	*Long-term goals* Client will: • maintain or increase mobility • be free of deformities • be free of pain
Potential for physical injury	• Muscle weakness. • Mobility restricted (walks with cane). • Age (has some generalized muscle atrophy).	
Moderately impaired ability to perform ADL	• Unable to do household chores. • Impaired ability to prepare meals and/or dress.	
Depression and social isolation	• Withdraws from friends and relatives. • Refuses to do ADL that are within limitations. • Recently quit attending church. • Stares at T.V. most of day.	

OSTEOARTHRITIS

Intervention: Nursing Orders	Intervention: Resources and Support Systems	Evaluation: Expected Outcomes
• Have client explain disease process in own words; clarify misunderstandings and offer additional explanation. • Have client explain treatment regimen and purpose. • Set up schedule for medications. Explain each medication, purpose and side effects. • Have client explain purpose of balanced rest and exercise. Clarify misconceptions. Demonstrate each exercise to client and family. Have client repeat. • Work with client and family to set up treatment program. • Allow client and family to express feelings. • Work with client to set up schedule of ADL's. • Give client pamphlets from Arthritis Foundation. • Have client arrange times for social activities. • Investigate client's interests and have client set specific goals to do leisure/recreational activities. • Help client obtain housekeeping and/or personal care services.	• American Arthritis Foundation • Home Health Care Agencies • Meals-on-Wheels • Senior Centers • Church	*Client can:* • explain disease process • state prescribed drugs, the purpose of each, side effects, and times to be taken • plan well-balanced diet for week • demonstrate prescribed exercise and state when and what increases are needed • explain reason for rest periods, times per day, and duration • demonstrate functional position for affected joints • relate feelings to significant others • arrange social occasion for visiting with family and friends • make arrangements to be taken to church • read written instructions for each area of treatment regimen • read pamphlets from Arthritis Foundation: "Arthritis—The Basic Facts" "So You Have Osteoarthritis" • verbalize signs and symptoms of complications and tell when to call physician/nurse • verbalize knowledge of follow-up physician appointments.

SAMPLE MASTER CARE PLAN FOR HOME CARE—

Nursing Diagnoses	Assessment	Planning
Potential for joint contracture and/or deformities	• Joints inflamed, swollen, and painful. • Muscle weakness. • Paresthesias.	*Short term goals:* Client will: • reduce joint contractures • reduce pain
Alteration in comfort	• Movements guarded. • Complains of joint pain. • Complains of pain upon moving.	• lessen muscle weakness • follow rest and exercise regimen
Potential for physical injury	• Muscle weakness. • Movement limited due to pain and stiffness. • Muscle atrophy. • Safety hazards in home.	• eat a well-balanced diet • take medications as ordered • socialize with friends and family
Major impaired home maintenance	• Unable to do household chores. • Unable to open cans or packages. • Impaired ability to prepare food.	*Long term goals:* Client will: • maintain or increase mobility
Depression due to arthritis	• Withdrawal from friends and family. • Refuses to follow medical regimen completely. • Cries frequently and easily. • No longer attends church or Senior Center.	• be free of deformities • be free of pain
Social isolation	• Withdraws from family and friends. • Not attending church or Senior Center. • Stares out of window most of day.	

RHEUMATOID ARTHRITIS

Intervention: Nursing Orders	Intervention: Resources and Support Systems	Evaluation: Expected Outcomes
• Teach client concerning disease process; need for rest and exercise; medications and side effects; nutrition. • Have client demonstrate exercises. • Have client demonstrate functional position during activity and at rest. • Have client explain each medication dosage, time, and side effects. • Assess home for safety hazards. Work with client to correct hazards. • Work with client to arrange for home care aides. • Work with client to arrange for Meals-on-Wheels. • Allow client to discuss feelings concerning disease and regimen. • Work with client to identify a support system. • Help client set up visiting schedule. • Work with client to identify and utilize community agencies.	• American Arthritis Foundation • Meals-on-Wheels • Mental Health Association • Home health agency • Home aides • Local church • Telephone pals	*Client can:* • explain disease process in own words • explain need for balance of rest and exercise • state each prescribed medication, its purpose, side effects, and times to be taken • demonstrate each prescribed exercise and functional position • arrange visits with family and/or friends • Client will receive a written schedule for each area of treatment regimen • Telephone numbers of physician, agencies, friends, and family will be plainly written and in view

SAMPLE MASTER CARE PLAN FOR HOME CARE—

Nursing Diagnoses	Assessment	Planning
Alteration in comfort	• Low back pain • Complains of general aches and pains	*Short term goals* • Client will reduce pain • Client will increase mobility
Impaired physical mobility	• Walks with difficulty • Upper dorsal kyphosis • Atrophy of leg muscles	• Client will remain free from injury • Client will eat a well-balanced diet and increase calcium intake if needed
Nutritional deficit	• Poor muscle tone • Lack of information regarding daily requirements and proper foods	• Client will follow medical regimen • Client will socialize with friends and family
Potential for physical injury	• Muscle weakness • Walks with difficulty • Safety hazards in home • Lives alone and isolates self	
Moderate impaired home maintenance.	• Unable to open and close windows • Unable to lift and move even light objects	*Long term goals* • Client will obtain optimal mobility • Client will maintain optimal nutritive state
Social isolation	• Lives alone • Family seldom visits • Seldom goes out.	• Client will be free from pain

OSTEOPOROSIS

Intervention: Nursing Orders	Intervention: Resources and Support Systems	Evaluation: Expected Outcomes
• Teach client proper posture and alignment. • Have client wear low heels, sturdy shoes. • Work with client to identify when pain occurs. • Teach side effects of medications. • Have client demonstrate exercise regimen. • Teach client necessity of exercise and hazards of immobility. • Have client limit rest time in bed during day. • Assess home for safety hazards. • Work with client to correct hazards. • Help client to identify agencies that can be utilized. • Help client to identify a support system of family/friends. • Have client set up regimen for going outside of home.	• Senior Center • Local church • Meals-on-wheels • Neighbors and family • Telephone pals • Home health agency with aides.	*Client can:* • explain disease process. • state purpose of dietary regimen, purpose of vitamins and minerals, and plan a well-balanced diet. • state each prescribed medication, its purpose, side effects, and times to be taken. • demonstrate each prescribed exercise and relate the increments of increase. • demonstrate functional positions for rest and activities. • set up visits from friends and/or family. Client will receive written instructions for each area of treatment regimen.

CHAPTER 8

CARDIOVASCULAR DISEASE

Alice LeVeille Gaul

Cardiovascular disease is the most frequent cause of death in the United States, accounting for 44% of deaths in clients over 65 years of age (Yurick, 1980, p. 410). Atherosclerosis, an arterial disease, commonly affects the aorta, coronary arteries, and cerebral and femoral arteries, thus directly causing cardiovascular disease. The pathogenesis of atherosclerosis is not completely understood, but it is no longer considered a normal part of aging.

Fatty streaking of the arteries is noted as early as childhood but does not always turn into atherosclerotic lesions. Since development of pathological lesions takes between 20 and 40 years, research has centered on identifying risk factors. New risk factors are being discovered as research into the man-environment relationship continues. The known factors are listed in Table 8-1. Risk factors are not only cumulative, but also synergistic. That is, the more risk factors present, the more rapidly atherosclerosis develops, resulting in increased risk for a serious or fatal complication.

Prevention and Management of Cardiovascular Disease

Prevention and management of cardiovascular disease is accomplished through the interaction of exercise, diet and medication.

The Role of Exercise

The cardiovascular effects of planned exercises are depicted in Table 8-2. A specific exercise program for the elderly must be either prescribed by a physician or initiated after a physical examination. It must be planned and done on a *regular* basis. This does not imply strenuous exercise on a daily basis, but the same level of exercise done at the same time intervals. For the elderly client who is not

TABLE 8.1
Risk Factors in Pathogenesis of Atherosclerosis

Alterable	Unalterable
Serum lipids above normal	Age
Hypertension	Sex
Smoking of cigarettes	Heredity
Glucose intolerance	Race
Diet	
Sedentary life style	
Personality type	
Stress	

physically restricted, walking or swimming are ideal exercise forms which, if done regularly, will result in cardiovascular conditioning. For the physically restricted client, it is important to suggest exercise appropriate to the physical condition. This exercise may be as limited as walking around the room for a specified number of times at regular intervals to limited walks outside. Even a client who is confined to a bed or a wheelchair can participate in some active arm or leg exercises if there is no physical limitation that prohibits it. No matter how limited, the exercise must be *planned* and done on a *regular* basis.

Any person starting a strenuous exercise program needs to be instructed on the warm-up period, maximum safe intensity, and cool-down period. The warm-up

TABLE 8.2
Effect of Exercise on Cardiovascular Fitness

Increases	Decreases
Collateral circulation	Circulating lipids
Pumping efficiency	Glucose intolerance
Peripheral blood distribution	Obesity
Tolerance to stress	Arterial blood pressure
Prudent living habits	Heart rate
Joy of living	Vulnerability to dysrhythmia

period should consist of five minutes of light exercise, such as stretching, slow walking, or light calisthenics. The period of intense exercise should last 20 to 60 minutes, and the client should achieve a heart rate of 70 to 80% maximum (Luckman, 1982, p. 843). Maximal heart rate is generally 220 beats a minute minus the age in years (Underhill, 1982, p. 561). In a client with no existing cardiac compromise, that will generally be a pulse rate increase of no more than 20 beats per minute (McGurn, 1981, p. 59). The client should be taught to take the pulse before, during and after exercise. Five minutes after exercise the pulse rate should return to normal. The pulse of the elderly client may take longer to return to normal. The above guidelines are general. Each individual should seek clarification of these parameters from a physician or exercise therapist. The nurse in the home should encourage that this be done.

The cool-down period is essential to reduce vascular pooling in the dilated vessels and allow vascular resistance to return to normal. This period should last about five minutes and can consist of the same kinds of activities as the warm-up period. Clients should be instructed to discontinue exercise and consult a doctor if symptoms develop, such as dyspnea, chest pain, severe muscle cramping, palpitations, change in pulse rate or rhythm, or lightheadedness. *Isotonic* or active exercise is recommended. *Isometric* or passive exercises should be avoided because venous return may be impaired, thus compromising cardiovascular function.

The Role of Diet

The major goals of diet modification in cardiovascular disease are weight reduction, (if indicated) reduction of serum lipids, and reduction of sodium intake. Specific diets are prescribed relevant to the specific needs of individual clients. Prior to any *major* modification in diet, a physician should be consulted. Weight loss, if attempted, should be gradual because rapid weight loss may actually increase circulating lipids. The American Heart Association recommends a modified fat, low–calorie diet for prevention and control of coronary artery disease and achievement or maintenance of ideal weight. Sample meal plans and general guidelines are available from physicians, nutritionists and the American Heart Association.

Education and motivation are the keys to dietary modification. The nurse in the home must clearly explain, in a non-threatening manner, to the client the relationship between diet and cardiovascular disease. As much as possible, the client should be allowed choices of foods to eat within the prescribed diet.

Favorite foods should be encouraged but limited to permitted quantities. A variety of foods should also be encouraged. Obviously, cultural and ethnic preferences must be taken into consideration. Meals should be planned and prepared so that the family group can eat together if possible. Foods should be attractively prepared and seasoned. A variety of cookbooks are now available with recipes specially designed for sodium- and fat-restricted sites. One such book is Craig Claiborne's (Claiborne, 1980) *Gourmet Diet Cookbook.*

Clients should be taught to read the labels on packaged foods. Many food manufacturers are now marketing products with no added salt. This information greatly increases the kind and variety of canned goods available for the client on a sodium-restricted diet. Many foods are now available with lower saturated fat and cholesterol content such as "Egg Beaters," low cholesterol cheeses, low saturated fat margarines, and soy protein meat substances. Lo Calorie Entrèes™ and complete dinners, such as Weight Watcher™ entrèes and Stouffer's Lean Cuisine™, are of particular value to the client living alone. In all instances, the clients must read the labels to ensure the contents comply with the fat, caloric and sodium restrictions prescribed.

Limited income may be a factor in the older client's inability to comply with dietary restrictions. However, careful meal planning and education can overcome this problem. If the income is insufficient to provide the basic required diet, utilization of other community resources such as Meals-on-Wheels and food stamps could be obtained. Many restaurants are attempting to meet the dietary needs of the older client by offering smaller portions at reduced prices, with no salt added to foods, and low fat and cholesterol entrèes. The home care nurse could develop a list of community restaurants that offer this type of service.

The Role of Medication

Medication is a cornerstone of treatment and prevention of cardiovascular disease. Specific drugs will be mentioned later in connection with pathological disorders. The pharmacological action of most drugs requires that they be taken regularly in the prescribed doses. The older client is frequently on multiple medications, some of which look alike. Remembering to take a large number of medications correctly can be an overwhelming chore. Consequently, the medications are taken irregularly, inappropriately or not at all. As few drugs as possible should be prescribed for the elderly client (Mullen, 1981, p. 110).

The kinds and amounts of non-prescription drugs must be assessed and evaluated in terms of drug interactions and/or impairment of drug absorption. Food/drug interactions must also be evaluated. The nurse can assist the client by developing a list of all drugs taken, reason for taking them, time taken, and possible serious side effects. This list should be kept current and readily available to provide direction to the client as well as serve as an invaluable resource in the event of sudden illness and/or hospital admission.

Medications should be timed at specific intervals; for example, twice a day is non-specific while "upon arising" and "bedtime" are more specific. It is sometimes useful to relate the time a medication is due to an event in the day. The nurse could suggest that the client time medications by regular television or radio shows and other specific daily activities. For those on multiple medications, any type of graphic chart that illustrates when to take specific medicines would be valuable.

Two other factors influencing medication adherence are perception of illness and feelings of powerlessness. The client who does not perceive him or herself as sick or in need of medication will be unlikely to adhere to the medication regimen. This problem is particularly significant in hypertensive clients who usually feel well and in whom the medications may cause unpleasant side effects. The nurse must carefully explain the reasons why the client must take the medication. The nurse should frequently assess the regimen.

Problems of adherence to the medication regimen in the geriatric client can be individual or environmental. Diminished sight can make it difficult for the client to organize and take the required medications. Prescription labels are usually typed in the smallest print. The pharmacist can be asked to label drugs in large letters on stick-on labels. Childproof caps, while of great benefit in preventing accidental ingestion of drugs by children, are sometimes insurmountable barriers to the geriatric client. The client should be instructed to ask for regular caps.

Geriatric clients may not adhere to a drug schedule because they are angry at the disease and fear loss of control over their lives. They may perceive themselves as trying to live around a medication schedule that prevents enjoyment of life. Careful education and offering them an opportunity to ventilate their feelings may influence drug adherence. The nurse in the home should give the client choices of when and how to take their medications when possible.

Major Cardiovascular Conditions Affecting the Elderly in the Home

The major cardiovascular conditions of the elderly the home health nurse will most likely encounter are: angina pectoris, myocardial infarction, congestive heart failure, and hypertension.

Angina Pectoris

Angina pectoris is characterized by episodes of paroxysmal chest pain. Two types of angina have been described. These are typical angina, which includes both stable and unstable angina, and atypical angina, also known as variant or prinzmetal angina (Harvey, et al., 1980, p 246). The pain of either type is caused by a transient coronary ischemia which may be due to lodging of an atherosclerotic thrombus or a coronary artery spasm. The myocardial pain is temporary and the transient ischemia does not damage myocardial tissues.

Typical Angina Stable angina is characterized by paroxysmal substernal or precardial pain which may radiate to the left arm. It is precipitated by exertion or stress and relieved by rest and/or nitroglycerine. Attacks bear a similarity to one another in terms of precipitating events, onset, duration and intensity.

Unstable angina is, as the name implies, paroxysmal chest pain which is not predictably related to stress or exercise, varies in intensity and frequency and does not respond predictably to medication or rest. Either type may occur during the night. Unstable angina is sometimes called crescendo and pre-infarction angina.

Atypical Angina Atypical angina bears no relation to exercise or stress, has widely variant degrees of intensity and duration, and responds unpredictably, or not at all, to medication. It is theorized that this type of angina is due to coronary artery spasm. Unstable angina is rapidly progressive and frequently requires surgical intervention.

Etiology By far the most common cause of anginal attacks is coronary artery disease, but there is no numerical relationship between angina attacks and myocardial infarctions. Angina may develop post-infarction as well as in clients who do not infarct. Angina may serve as a warning device in that prior to a myocardial infarction there is usually an acceleration of anginal attacks.

Assessment Data

Pain. The nurse should elicit a description of the pain, including aggravating and relieving factors, location, intensity and duration (see Table 8-3). The pain of

TABLE 8.3
Comparison of the Pain of Angina Pectoris and the Pain of Myocardial Infarction

	Pain of Angina	Pain of MI
Description	Burning, squeezing aching Pain of each attack similar May be diffuse, less severe in elderly	Intolerable, oppressive, crushing, knifelike pain, or no pain
Precipitating Factors	Usually related to meals, emotional stress, extremes of temperature, exercise or activity	None identified May be related to exercise
Duration	15 to 30 minutes	Not defined, may continue until relieved by narcotic Often residual chest soreness
Relieving Factors	Relieved by rest Relieved by nitroglycerine	Requires narcotics for relief Not relieved by rest
Associated Symptoms	Apprehension Dyspnea Nausea Diaphoresis	Marked apprehension Nausea and vomiting Diaphoresis Dizziness Dyspnea* Mental confusion*

*May be presenting symptom in Silent MI

typical angina is described as squeezing, burning, choking and never knifelike or crushing. Often, it is located retrosternally and radiates to the left arm, although it may radiate elsewhere. Intensity of symptoms may vary with age of the client. Classically, pain precipitated by exercise, duration and stress rarely lasts over 15 minutes and is relieved by rest and nitroglycerine.

Associated symptoms. Depending on the severity of the attack, the client may describe symptoms of dyspnea, dizziness, sweating, palpitations and digestive disturbances.

Physical assessment data. Unless assessed during an attack, the physical examination will not generally deviate from the client's norm. During the attack, the nurse may auscultate a third or fourth heart sound.

Diagnostic data. The client with previously undiagnosed angina should be referred to a physician for suitable cardiac work-up including a 12 lead electrocardiogram, EKG stress test, and possible cardiac catheterization.

Nursing Diagnosis. The major nursing diagnosis in the anginal client is "alteration in comfort due to anginal pain."

Goal. Client will be able to relieve the pain of an acute attack. To relieve the pain of an acute attack, the client should immediately cease all activity and lie down. It is important that the client understand that the pain is a warning and that to ignore it could invite a more serious event. Besides resting, the client should take nitroglycerine tablets, if prescribed by a physician. The tablet is placed under the tongue and allowed to dissolve completely. Nitroglycerine should be taken at the first sign of an attack. Other persons residing in the same household should know where the nitroglycerine tablets are kept. Nitroglycerine has a very short shelf life and should be stored in a dark bottle in a dry place. All but a few days' supply, which is carried with the client, should be refrigerated. A cotton plug in the container will absorb some of the drug. The client should be told to check the prescription and expiration date because the average shelf life is three months (Rodman, 1979, p. 596). Nitroglycerine tablets with full potency should cause a transient burning sensation on the tongue and throbbing sensation in the head. Nitroglycerine tablets may be taken every five to ten minutes until relief is obtained. Generally, if pain persists after two or more tablets have been taken, the client should go to the nearest emergency room.

Other coronary vasodilators may be prescribed, either in place of or in combination with nitroglycerine (see Table 8-4). Nitroglycerine paste may be prescribed as a long-acting nitrate to promote coronary artery vasodilation. The client should be instructed to apply the paste exactly as directed, to avoid getting the paste on the hands, to rotate sites, and to ensure that the previous dose is completely washed off before applying the next dose. Inderal, a beta adrenergic blocker, may be prescribed to decrease the number of anginal attacks. By decreasing myocardial oxygen consumption, Inderal indirectly increases exercise/stress tolerance. If the client develops any signs of congestive heart failure, Inderal should be held pending immediate evaluation by a physician. However, sudden withdrawal of Inderal can exacerbate angina symptoms and should be accomplished over a two-week period (Rodman, 1979, p. 596).

Goal. *Client will identify precipitating and aggravating factors for angina attacks.* Exercise, stress, temperature change, meals or strong emotions may precipitate an angina attack. The nurse should assist the client in reviewing recent attacks and identifying the precipitating factors. A plan may then be formulated to adjust the precipitating activity to a reduced level that does not cause an angina attack. Reduction of stress and methods to improve coping skills in the face of anger or other strong emotions will aid in preventing attacks. If indicated, mild tranquilizing drugs may be prescribed. The nurse and client should be aware that a potential for impaired excretion in the geriatric client can lead to toxic accumulation of tranquilizers.

Weight reduction in these clients should be accomplished. Small frequent meals are less likely to cause an angina attack. The client should be encouraged to rest for a short period after meals. Because of the vasoconstrictive effect of nicotine, as well as increased carboxyhemoglobin in the blood of smokers, cigarette smoking is directly implicated as a cause of angina attacks. Smokers should be encouraged to quit, and both smokers and nonsmokers should avoid smoke-filled rooms. The client should avoid extremes of and sudden changes in temperatures. Exercise should be avoided when the temperature is very hot or cold. Concurrent medical problems and their relation to angina attacks should be evaluated and appropriately treated by a physician.

Goal. *The client will maintain activities of daily living commensurate with the prevention of angina attacks.* Planned daily exercise can decrease the number and severity of angina attacks. The level of exercise must be evaluated by a physician and the client so that an attack will not be precipitated. Short rest periods should be planned throughout the day.

The emotional implications of "heart pain" may be devastating to the client. A fairly common response is to cease all activity and become a "cardiac cripple" who is immobilized by fear. Careful evaluation and planning of activities of daily living so as not to precipitate angina is the first step toward helping the client understand that he or she may continue a productive life. If a necessary activity is known to precipitate an attack, nitroglycerine may be taken before initiating that activity. However, the nurse must guard against the indiscriminate use of nitroglycerine as prophylaxis because nitrate tolerance develops fairly rapidly.

If the client's life style involves travel, it should be encouraged. Nitroglycerine should be taken prophylactically during air travel, immediately prior to take off and landing. However, travel plans that involve significant change in altitudes should be evaluated by a physician because of the hypoxia encountered at high altitudes. This hypoxia may increase the incidence of angina attacks and could precipitate a myocardial infarction.

Myocardial Infarction (MI)

Myocardial Infarction by definition is cessation of the flow of blood and oxygen to the myocardial tissue resulting in necrosis of that area of the myocardium. Pumping efficiency is impaired, cardiac output may drop, and death may ensue. The pain of a MI is classically described as crushing, viselike or knifelike, and is usually accompanied by a feeling of doom. The client knows that something catastrophic is happening. The pain may be precipitated by exercise or stress but is not relieved by rest or nitroglycerine. The pain may or may not radiate and may be located underneath the xiphoid process which can cause the client to perceive it as indigestion. However, not all myocardial infarctions present in this manner. "Silent MI's," or painless infarcts, account for 20% of reported MI's, and the incidence may be higher as these clients do not seek medical attention. The incidence of "silent MI" increases with age (Harrison, 1974, p. 1230). Therefore, in the geriatric client, the presenting symptoms may be sudden confusion and dyspnea progressing to frank pulmonary edema.

Assessment Data

Pain. The nurse should elicit a complete description of the pain including precipitating factors (see Table 8-3). In general, chest pain not relieved by rest or nitroglycerine should be suspect. The paramedics should be called and the physician informed. Sudden confusion and dyspnea should be treated similarly. More than half the deaths from myocardial infarction occur outside the hospital within the first two hours after onset of symptoms (Underhill, 1982, p. 326).

Associated symptoms. Associated symptoms in the client with a MI are related to the catecholamine response and the decrease in cardiac output. Clients may be restless, thrashing about, wild-eyed, and report that something terrible is happening to them. Pallor may be present; skin may be cool and clammy; and shortness of breath to frank dyspnea is common. Nausea, vomiting and an urge to defecate may also be present. The client may also be lightheaded and dizzy.

Physical assessment data. The nurse should note the color and temperature of the skin and check for the presence of venous distention. The lungs should be auscultated for rales, giving careful attention to the bases. Heart sounds may be distant and the presence of an S_3 or S_4 heart sound may be detected. The nurse should carefully note the presence of any irregularities in cardiac rate and rhythm and report them to paramedics upon arrival. Blood pressure will generally drop. Serial monitoring of vital signs can provide valuable information regarding trends in the client's condition.

Goal. *Client will maintain sufficient cardiac output to maintain life.* The nurse or family member should notify the local rescue unit about location and type of problem. When in doubt, one should treat any episode of chest pain as an acute MI until proven otherwise. The client should be placed at rest in a semi-Fowler's position. Restrictive clothing should be loosened. Oxygen, if available, should be used. If at all possible, the nurse should stay with the person to provide reassurance and to encourage him or her to keep quiet, thus preventing increased oxygen demand to the myocardium. If family members are able to maintain calm, they may remain with the client. If not, they should be removed. The nurse should attempt to preserve normothermia for the same reason. Above all, the nurse should be prepared for and ready to initiate cardiopulmonary resuscitation.

Nursing management

Nursing diagnosis. Altered cardiac output due to myocardial infarction.

Goal. *Client will decrease the workload of the heart, maintaining individual optional cardiac function.*

Intervention. The nurse should assess knowledge of and adherence to the medication regimen. A variety of drugs may be prescribed post-myocardial infarction to increase cardiac function and minimize risk of complications. These drugs may include cardiotonics, coronary vasodilators, anti-arrhythmics, anti-hypertensive agents, and diuretics (see Table 8-4).

Cardiotonics or digitalis derivatives are drugs which act to increase the strength of myocardial contractions resulting in more complete systolic emptying, decreased filling pressures in the heart, and decreased venous congestion. Digitalis also has a direct effect on conduction velocity, thus affecting heart rate. Clients on digitalis should be able to count their pulses and recognize changes in rate and rhythm. Generally, a pulse rate under 60 or a regular pulse that becomes irregular or an irregular pulse that becomes regular requires withholding and notification of the physician. Early signs and symptoms of digitalis toxicity include nausea, vomiting, diarrhea, and visual changes, either a loss of acuity or a halo effect. Digitalis toxicity should be suspected in any patient who becomes ill while taking digitalis. Similarly, any marked deviance in cardiac rate and/or rhythm renders digitalis toxicity suspect. Because of potassium depletion, the risk of digitalis toxicity increases if the client is also taking diuretics.

Kidney and liver function should be continually evaluated as digoxin is excreted primarily through the kidneys and digitoxin is detoxified in the liver. A reduction in functioning nephrons by 50% is a normal part of aging. Cardiac disease can impair renal function even further, thus presenting a management problem for the geriatric client on digoxin. The nurse should ensure that the client makes and keeps regular appointments with the physician for evaluation. Refer to Table 8-4 for other potential drug/drug and drug/food interactions.

The majority of post-myocardial infarction clients are discharged on Coumadin anti-coagulant therapy. Points to elicit when assessing client's knowledge of anti-coagulant therapy include signs and symptoms of overdose, such as severe bruising, bleeding gums, nosebleeds, pink or red-tinged urine, black tarry stools, and development of headaches, visual and/or motor changes. Safety measures to emphasize include use of soft bristle tooth brushes, electric rather than safety razor, and avoidance of activities that could result in severe cuts or blunt trauma.

Aspirin is contraindicated. Green leafy vegetables and other foods high in Vitamin K will antagonize the effects of Coumadin.

Diuretics are frequently prescribed in the post–MI patient as well as for patients with congestive heart failure and hypertension. Because of the significance of diuretic/digitalis interaction, they will be discussed in depth in this section. A diuretic by definition is any drug that increases urine output. However, sodium and other ions such as potassium, chloride, and bicarbonate are also excreted. Different classes of diuretics (see Table 8-4) act in different parts of the nephron, resulting in a wide variance in the fluid and electrolyte abnormalities they can induce. It is incumbent upon the nurse to identify the class of the diuretic prescribed so that specific education regarding potential side effects can be presented to the client.

The total body fluid in the geriatric client comprises a lesser percentage than in the young adult. The older client taking diuretics must be evaluated for excess volume loss. Because of the decrease in skin turgor associated with aging, dehydration may be difficult to assess. Some signs to be alert for are increased urine concentration, thirst, fatigue, weakness and postural hypotension (Yurick, 1980, p. 485). Sodium excretion in the older client can lead to profound hyponatremia. The interaction of a sodium-restricted diet and diuretic therapy must be carefully evaluated for this reason.

If the client is taking a class of diuretics that results in excretion of large amounts of potassium, that potassium must be replaced. If the diet allows, the client should be instructed to eat foods high in potassium, such as oranges and bananas. Concurrent potassium supplement will usually be prescribed. Because most of these supplements taste unpleasant, it is not unusual for the person to continue taking diuretics and avoid the supplement resulting in severe potassium depletion. Because of electrolyte depletion, the client taking diuretics is at risk for developing metabolic alkalosis. Each individual should be encouraged to become aware of their individual state of well-being and to note and report any changes.

Anti-arrhythmic drugs (see Table 8-4) are prescribed to control cardiac rhythm disturbances. The specific drug is selected based on the rhythm disturbance presented. The client should be taught to assess the rate and rhythm of the pulse and report any change to the physician.

It is paradoxical that these drugs can cause a decrease in cardiac reserve and induce congestive heart failure. Clients taking these drugs should be assessed for early signs of congestive heart failure such as fatigue, disorientation, weight gain, and ankle edema.

Goal. *The client will participate in life experiences to the maximum extent possible.* Cardiac rehabilitation is begun as soon as possible; therefore, clients upon discharge will usually have a program of activity designed for them. It is imperative to assess the client's knowledge of signs and symptoms such as dyspnea, tachycardia, pain and/or change in cardiac rhythm that require discontinuance of an activity. Other symptoms requiring evaluation of activity are persistent sleep-lessness, syncope, fatigue and weight gain. If not already done, the activities of daily living need to be assessed in terms of adherence to the rehabilitation program. Isometric activities are not allowed, and the kind and amount of activity allowed will vary according to the severity of the cardiac deficit.

In severe cardiac disease, energy conservation must be stressed. If this is done, the client can participate, although minimally, in life experiences. Some methods of energy conservation are: 1) sit, if at all possible, while performing activities; 2) do the activity for no more than three minutes and then rest for at least five minutes; 3) rest frequently during the day; and 4) rest at least one hour after meals (McGurn, 1981, p. 464).

As a general rule, sexual activity with a familiar partner may be resumed after six to eight weeks. Sexual activity should not take place in extreme temperatures, after a heavy meal, following ingestion of alcohol, or if the activity is accompanied by emotional stress or tension (McGurn, 1981, p. 468). The superior position should be avoided during intercourse due to the isometric effect on the muscles of the arms and legs. However, if change of usual position for intercourse induces emotional stress, then it is probably better to retain old habits. Anginal pain that occurs during or after intercourse should be reported to a physician as should palpitations lasting more than 20 minutes. Because of the inherent diminished cardiac reserve that accompanies normal aging, the tachycardia that accompanies orgasm may persist for a longer period of time. If the cardiac disease is severe, sexual activity such as intercourse may not be permitted. In this instance, the client should be helped to utilize other forms of closeness, such as touching and stroking to meet this basic physiological need.

Congestive Heart Failure (CHF)

Congestive heart failure is said to be present when the cardiac output is insuffi-cient to meet the metabolic needs of the body. It is considered acute if it is insufficient at rest and chronic if it is sufficient at rest and insufficient with exercise. Some causes are myocardial infarction, constrictive carditis, valvular insufficiency, heart block, other arrhythmias, and chronic pulmonary disease. Clients with chronic congestive heart failure have diminished cardiac reserve. This is an important concept because many factors, such as infection, stress, change in altitude, and change in activity can initiate cardiac decompensation.

Pathologically, the underlying cause initiates incomplete emptying of the left ventricle with resulting congestion of the pulmonary and systemic circulation. By definition, congestive heart failure (CHF) implies lack of cardiac compensatory ability and cardiac reserve. This is even more devastating in the geriatric client who, through the process of aging, has a decreased stroke volume resulting in a cardiac output 30 to 50% less than a young adult (Ebersole, 1981, p. 104). Also, the elderly are more likely to have concurrent medical conditions that will aggravate congestive heart failure.

Congestive heart failure is a chronic incurable disease. Its symptoms vary depending on the compensatory ability of the heart.

Assessment Data Congestive heart failure is manifested in all body systems. Due to space limitations, only the cardinal symptoms will be discussed in detail. To generalize, it may be said that any deviation from the usual norm of the client with cardiac disease may be suspect as a symptom of congestive heart failure. McGurn identified several cardinal signs of congestive heart failure (McGurn, 1981, p. 327):

- Palpitations may occur and can be very frightening to the client. If they occur frequently, they will further compromise cardiac output.
- Dyspnea and/or hyperpnea may exist independently or together. Because of pulmonary congestion, the work of breathing is increased, resulting in shortness of breath, which may be accompanied by rapid respiration.
- Paroxysmal Nocturnal Dyspnea (PND) is the sudden occurrence of dyspnea due to reduced cardiac output and change in fluid dynamics caused by prone position during periods of sleep. It is a suffocating feeling often accompanied by confusion due to cerebral hypoxia. The client may throw off the blankets and do anything to get air. There is grave potential for injury in the often confused elderly client. More than one episode of PND may occur per night, preventing the client from getting vitally needed rest.
- Orthopnea and dyspnea on exertion (DOE) show the same dynamics as PND.
- Generalized and pitting edema of the extremities, jugular venous distention, and an S_3 heart sound are frequent findings in CHF.

Nursing Diagnosis The most useful nursing diagnosis is altered cardiac output due to CHF.

Goal: **Client will decrease the work load of the heart to maintain individual optional cardiac function.** The goal can be accomplished through the interaction of drugs that promote myocardial contractility such as digitalis, diuretics which promote excretion of excess fluid, and careful education of the client in reduction of cardiac work load. Digitalis and diuretics have been previously discussed under myocardial infarction and are presented in Table 8-4.

Nursing Management **The goal of nursing management will be to reduce the work load of the heart.** For the CHF client, rest and careful regulation of activities as well as a restricted diet will reduce cardiac work load: Assessment of the client's response to activity is the key to successful nursing management. Two of the earliest signs of cardiac decompensation are fatigue and anorexia. Unfortunately, fatigue and anorexia are considered by many to be normal for the elderly so clients do not report them as symptoms. Specific guidelines for interpretation of symptoms should be given to the client. For example, call the nurse or the physician 1) if your shoes become too tight; 2) if you cannot do your housework; 3) if you need extra sleep; or 4) if you get up at night to urinate more than normal. (McGurn, 1981, p. 334). The client must avoid anything which could initiate cardiac decompensation. The client should be instructed to get immediate medical attention if severe dyspnea, which signals pulmonary edema, occurs.

TABLE 8.4
Commonly Prescribed Drugs in the Treatment of Cardiovascular Disease.

This table gives a quick overview of cardiovascular drugs. Dosages are not given because of the wide ranges utilized. For complete information regarding dosage, actions and all side effects, consult a pharmacology book.

A. *Cardiotonics*

Drug	Side Effects	Precautions	Major Nursing Implications
Digitoxin (Crystodigin)	Due to overdose: GI: Anorexia, nausea, vomiting, diarrhea. CNS: headache, weakness, visual disturbances, depression, confusion. CV: serious disturbance in rate and rhythm.	Drugs that cause potassium or magnesium depletion or increase calcium may increase potential for toxicity. Any medications that interfere with gastrointestional absorption such as antacids, laxatives, or antidiarrheal medication may impair absorption of Digitoxin and thus lower blood level.	If concurrently on diuretics, K+ *must* be replaced. If concurrently on Quinidine, dosage should be reduced.
Digoxin (Lanoxin)	As above	Concurrent administration of Quinidine may impair the excretion of digitalis through the kidneys thus increasing the potential for Digitalis toxicity.	Niferidine may increase digoxin levels in presence of gastrointestinal upset or any signs of illness should suspect Digitalic toxicity. Digoxin should not be taken by clients with impaired renal function. Take same time daily. Check with physician before adding *any* drug. Client should check pulse and notify physician if rate or rhythm changes.

B. Diuretics

Drug	Side Effects	Precautions	Major Nursing Implications
Loop Diuretics Lasix	↑ BUN, serum glucose, nausea, vomiting, blurred vision, tinnitus, sweet taste, photosensitivity.	May cause rapid severe hypovolemia, alkalosis. Hemo concentration can cause circulatory collapse.	Similar to Thiazides plus potential for hypokalemia and volume depletion increased.
Edecrin	As above. Apprehension and confusion.	As above. Can cause severe hypoglycemia with convulsions, deafness. Potentiates Coumadin.	Similar to Thiazides and may cause rapid volume depletion. Clients with impaired glucose metabolism should not use.
Potassium—Sparing Diuretics Spironolactone (Aldactone)	Cramping, skin eruptions, ataxia, drug fever.	Neutralized by ASA Potentiates antihypertensives and other diuretics. Severe hyperkalemia.	Clients with impaired renal function may develop hyperkalemia. Concurrent use elevates Digoxin levels. Often used with Thiazide diuretic.
Thiazides	↓ K+ and Cl −, nausea, vomiting, bad taste, photo sensitivity, and constipation.	May cause metabolic alkalosis. Potentiated by alcohol, barbiturates. May cause severe hypokalemia without K + replacement.	Take same time daily—last dose no later than 6:00 PM.

(continued)

B. *Diuretics (continued)*

Drug	Side Effects	Precautions	Major Nursing Implications
Thiazidelike (Hygroton) (Hydromox) (Zaroxolyn)			Use potassium supplement. Report excessive fatigue and weakness. Dosage may require reduction during extremely hot weather. Do not add other drugs prescribed or over-the-counter drugs without notifying physician. Daily weight is the best measure of efficacy.
Triamterene (Dyrenium)	Nausea, vomiting, diarrhea, weakness, muscle cramps, photosensitivity.	Severe kyperkalemia.	Do not use with potassium supplements. Take after meals. May cause hyperkalemia.

C. *Antihypertensives*

Drug	Side Effects	Precautions	Major Nursing Implications
Rauwolfia (Raudixin)	Severe depression, hypothermia.	Diuretics potentiate. Concurrent use of digoxin and quinidine can cause arrhythmias.	Full effects not present until several days to two weeks. Action may continue 4 weeks past discontinuance.

Reserpine (Serpasil) (Sandril)	As above. Not frequently used now.	As above.	Not indicated for confused clients.
Guanethidine (Ismelin)	Orthostatic hypotension, reduced exercise tolerance, alopecia, inhibits ejaculation.	Alcohol and diuretics potentiate. Tricyclic anti-depressants antagonize.	Duration of action >4 days. Do not change dosages oftener than 5 to 7 days. Change from recumbent to upright position slowly. Hot weather, alcohol, and standing long periods can cause severe hypotension. Drug should be withdrawn two weeks prior to surgery or administration of anesthetics.
Prazosin (Minipres)	Tend to disappear with continued therapy.	Diuretics and other antihypertensives potentiate.	Take first dose at bedtime. Avoid sudden movements.
Metroprolol tartrate (Lopressor)	Bradycardia. Psychoneurotic depression, toxic psychosis.	May cause MI if withdrawn suddenly.	Do not discontinue suddenly—make sure enough drug on hand.
Cloridine (Catapres)	Sedation, fatigue, cardiac rhythm disturbances, dry mouth. Raynaud's phenomenon.	Antihypertensives, diuretics potentiate; potentiates depressant effect of alcohol, barbiturates. Tricyclic anti-depressants antagonize. Abrupt withdrawal causes rebound hypertension.	Do not discontinue abruptly—make sure enough drug on hand. Withdrawal of concurrent Inderal therapy can cause hypertensive crisis.

(continued)

C. Antihypertensives (continued)

Drug	Side Effects	Precautions	Major Nursing Implications
Methyldopa (Aldomet)	Sedation, loss of mentation, parkinsonian syndrome, nightmares, drug fever.	Levodopa, other antihypertensives, quinidine, and diuretics potentiate. Use with caution with anti-depressant, antipsychotic drugs.	Drowsiness common—do not drive etc. until tolerance develops. Move slowly from lying to sitting position. If dose increased, do so with evening dose.
Hydralazine (Apresoline Lopres)	Angina, headache, dizziness, acute rheumatoid state.	Antihypertensives and diuretics potentiate.	Consult physician if anginal pain. Move slowly lying to sitting position.
Beta Blocker Propranolol Hcl (Inderal) Used in treatment of angina and arrhythmias.	Bronchospasm, drowsiness, depression.	Withdraw slowly in angina patients—sudden withdrawal may cause a MI. Do not administer with psychotropic drugs.	Take with or following meals. Check pulse daily—report slow pulse. Caution when driving—drowsiness common. Do not withdraw suddenly.
Anti-arrhythmics Quinidine Sulfate (Quinidine Extentabs) Quinidine Gluconate (Quinaglute Duratabs) Quinidine Polygalucturonate (Cardioquin)	Cardiac arrhythmias, abdominal pain, diarrhea, disturbed hearing, vision, confusion.	excretion of Digoxin. Dilantin and Phenobarbital increase excretion effects with elevated K+ and with decreased K+.	Take with full glass of H_2O on empty stomach; carry ID card that names this medication. Do not discontinue without MD's knowledge. Use with caution with impaired renal function. Digoxin levels may be increased.

Procainamide Hydro-chloride (Pronestyl)	Cardiac arrythmias, bitter tastes, acute hepatomegaly rise in SGOT, neurologic disturbances.	Inderal has additive effect on cardiac cells. High K+ will exaggerate effects. Low K+ will depress.	Store in tight container in dry place—not refrigerator. Take on an empty stomach with full glass of water. Take pulse daily. Never allow more than six hours between doses.
Disopyramide Phosphate (Norpace)	Dry eyes and mouth; urine retention, constipation, dizziness, nervousness, edema, weight gain, hypotension, CHF	Effects of K+ are same as Quinidine and Pronestyl. Potentiates Coumadin.	Check voiding patterns. May cause urinary retention.
Verapamil (Isoptin)	Headache, hypotension, vertigo, heart block.	Beta blockers such as Inderal must be withdrawn 48 hours prior to Verapamil or severe hypotension and asystole may occur.	Do not administer concurrently with Inderal. Move slowly lying to standing position. May increase Digoxin levels.

(continued)

D. *Vasodilators*

Drug	Side Effects	Precautions	Major Nursing Implications
Nitroglycerin (Nitrostat) Nitrol Ointment Cardilate Tetranitol Erythrol tetranitrate Pentaerythritol tetranitrate (Peritrate) (Peritrate SA) (Duotrate) (Pentratol)	Headache, vertigo, postural side effects. As above plus skin rash. Temporary headache. As above. As above Rash, headache, transient dizziness.	Observe storing and carrying precautions. Alcohol may enhance hypotensive effect.	No alcoholic beverages. Do not discontinue suddenly. Timed release medication should be taken with a full glass of water on an empty stomach. Orthostatic hypotension can occur.
Isosorbide dinitrate (Isordil) (Sorbitrate)	Flushing, headache, dizziness, drug rash or dermatitis	Severe hypotension in sensitive clients. Alcohol enhances therapeutic effects.	

References:

Oppeneer J E, Vervoren T M: *Gerontological Pharmocology.* C.V. Mosby Co., St. Louis, Mo., 1983
"Giving cardiovascular drugs safely": *Nursing 79 Books.* Intermed Communications Inc., Harsham, Pennsylvania, 1979
Underhill S L, Woods S L et al.: *Cardiac Nursing.* J.B. Lippincott Co., Philadelphia, 1982

Hypertension

Primary hypertension is defined as elevation of systolic, diastolic, or both systolic and diastolic pressures. It is the most common cause of cardiovascular disease in Europe and the United States (Underhill, 1982, p. 601). Elderly Blacks are particularly at high risk for hypertension because of unknown hereditary factors. Stroke is the most common result (Underhill, 1982, p. 613). Absolute definition of pressure thought to constitute hypertension is controversial. One operational definition is blood pressure elevations associated with 50% mortality; BP 145/95 in males over 45 and 160/95 in all adult females (Underhill, 1982, p. 601).

There is even more controversy as to what pressures constitute hypertension in the aged client (Graves, 1981, p. 111). General consensus is that an increase in systolic pressure with accompanying diastolic increase will inevitably accompany the decreased vessel distensability and cardiac output of aging. Therefore, the diagnosis and treatment of hypertension in the elderly client is the individual decision of the physician (Ebersole, 1981, p. 104). When treatment is prescribed, blood pressure should be reduced slowly to avoid postural hypotension. Aggressive medication therapy is rarely utilized in the elderly client.

Nursing Diagnosis

Because hypertension usually is present without symptoms, the most useful nursing diagnosis around which to formulate interventions is: Potential for noncompliance due to inadequate knowledge of drug and/or diet therapy.

Goal. *Client will demonstrate adequate knowledge of diet and drug interaction in the control of hypertension.* Anti-hypertensive medications commonly prescribed are listed in Table 8-4. Common side effects of these drugs include dizziness, postural hypotension, and impotence. Clients should be educated to contact the physician for dose modification if these symptoms become disabling. Common techniques such as getting up slowly will minimize the postural hypotension and avoid a fall with possible fractures. Anti-hypertensive agents should not suddenly be discontinued because of possibility of severe rebound hypertension. Diuretics and restriction of dietary sodium are sometimes sufficient for control of hypertension. Weight reduction, if indicated, will positively affect blood pressure. Exercise, as previously discussed, will aid in the reduction of blood pressure. The client should be taught to take and keep a *daily* or weekly record of blood pressure. Specific parameters must be identified as indicating the need to report pressure variations. Physical signs of increased blood pressure such as headaches, nosebleeds, dizziness, and transient motor defects must be reported. Above all, the client must understand the need to comply with the regimen, *despite lack of symptoms.* If the client does not believe health is threatened, adherence is unlikely.

Careful non-threatening education is the key. Advantages must be emphasized and negative aspects of therapy minimized. The National High Blood Pressure Information Center of the National Heart, Lung and Blood Institute and the American Heart Association have many teaching aids available regarding low–sodium diets, drugs, and tips about living with hypertension (Underhill, 1982, p. 627).

Management of the Client with a Pacemaker

The majority of pacemakers are inserted in clients between 50 and 80 years of age. The insertion of a permanent pacemaker is a surgical procedure performed in a hospital and initial teaching should have been accomplished there. However, many factors, such as anxiety and reduction of hearing and/or perception, common in the elderly, may necessitate repeated explanations and teaching. Pacemakers are generally inserted for the management of heart blocks or other severe bradyar-rhythmias.

The two types in use are broadly classified as: 1) *fixed rate* pacemakers, which fire at a constant rate initiating every heartbeat, and 2) *demand* pacemakers which do not fire when a normal heartbeat is sensed. The procedure usually involves the suturing of the electrodes to the exterior surface of the ventricles or atria via a thoracotomy incision. The wires are then threaded through a subcutaneous tunnel to the generator which is buried in subcutaneous tissue either above or below the waist (Underhill, 1982, p. 539). The generator is charged by batteries that must be replaced or batteries that can be recharged transcutaneously. The nurse should ensure that the client has appropriate literature and management knowledge of the pacemaker generator.

Any client with a pacemaker must know the pacemaker rate and must be taught to take the pulse for a full minute at rest daily and record it. With a fixed or demand pacemaker, any decrease in normal rate may signify failing batteries. The pulse will not necessarily be regular but should not deviate significantly from the established normal. The following symptoms require counting of the pulse and possible notification of a physician: dizziness, syncope, shortness of breath, peripheral edema, palpitations, and confusion.

All clients with pacemakers should carry an identification card that contains the physician's phone and address as well as all pertinent information about the pacemaker, including type, rate, and date of implantation. Information books on pacemakers and identification cards are available from the American Heart Association.

Electromagnetic interference can render a pacemaker inoperative. Some of the newer models are shielded to keep out most interference, but in general the client should be given the following directions:
- Electric shavers are generally safe, but should not be used directly over the generator.

- Avoid or keep at least three feet away from microwave ovens.
- Gasoline engines and electric motors are sources of danger, so do not lean over either.
- Some antitheft devices in stores will interfere with pacemaker function. If the client becomes symptomatic while shopping, leave the store.
- Avoid completely any place where arc welding is done and large power transmitters or microwave antennas for radio, television, or radar are used.
- The metal in the pacemaker will trigger airport screening devices.
- If the client becomes symptomatic he or she should move five to ten feet away and count the pulse, which should return to normal (Underhill, 1982, p. 539).

Care of the area over the generator involves avoiding undue pressure, wearing nonrestrictive clothing, and accessing for skin breakdown. With proper instruction it is possible for the client with a pacemaker to live a normal life.

Arteriosclerosis Obliterans

Chronic arterial occlusion or arteriosclerosis obliterans is an insidious progressive disease that usually occurs in the fifth or sixth decade of life. The pathogenesis is atherosclerosis which leads to narrowing of the vessels resulting in chronic ischemia of the tissues supplied by the affected artery. Depending on the degree of occlusion and adequacy of collateral circulation, symptoms may vary from skin changes to gangrene; however, the classic symptom is intermittent claudication (Lewis, 1983, p. 830). Arteriosclerosis obliterans is a chronic progressive disease which can ultimately lead to loss of a limb. The intermittent claudication or ischemic muscle pain occurs in working muscle groups, such as calf muscles, and can be debilitating.

Assessment Data

History. The nurse should elicit from the client history of the pain including precipitating factors as well as chronology of aggravating and alleviating factors. The classic pain is described as cramping, tightness or aching in a muscle (Carnevali, 1979, p. 262). It is usually precipitated by a specific amount of exercise; for example, walking up one flight of stairs or walking two blocks. Repetition of the exercise will reproduce the pain.

The home health nurse can assess progression of the disease by comparing onset of symptoms to the activity necessary to produce them. As the disease progresses, pain may occur at rest. This pain is described as gnawing, severe and continuous. It occurs in the foot and is relieved by placing the limb in a dependent position. Severe dysfunction is present in 30% of clients (Lewis, 1983, p. 830).

Pulses. The classic data for arteriosclerosis obliterans is absent pulses distal to the site of occlusion. The site of occlusion corresponds to the site of claudication.

Skin changes. If the limb of a client with arteriosclerosis obliterans is elevated, a classic pallor or blanching will be noted. If the limb is allowed to be dependent, it will become dusky and red, often with a bluish appearance. The skin of an affected limb is generally shiny, hairless and cool to the touch. Nail beds are thickened. The beginnings of ulcers and gangrene are usually noted on the toes and feet. Trauma to the foot is usually the initiating event for the development of gangrene.

Nursing Diagnosis. The most encompassing nursing diagnosis for the management of a client with arteriosclerosis obliterans would be: Alteration in tissue perfusion due to arteriosclerosis obliterans.

Goal. Client will be able to perform activities of daily living with a minimum of pain. The client should undertake a planned exercise program of graduated walking. Even clients with pain at rest must be encouraged to walk at least four times a day. If walking produces pain, the client should be told to rest until the pain is gone and then continue walking. If obese, the client must be encouraged to lose weight. Smoking is absolutely contraindicated because of the added vasoconstrictive effect of nicotine.

Various drugs are prescribed for the treatment of arteriosclerosis obliterans including vasodilators, anti-coagulants, and anti-lipemics. The vasodilator used most often is cyclandelate (Cyclospasmol), which is effective in reducing claudication and other symptoms (Luckman, 1980, p. 1112). The use of anti-coagulants in arterial disease does not effectively prevent arterial clot formation. There is no documented evidence that the use of anti-lipemics will modify the course of arteriosclerosis obliterans. Their value may lie in reduction of serum cholesterol and prevention of coronary artery disease. When pain becomes persistent and severe, analgesics may be required.

Goal. The client will not impair skin integrity. Careful teaching regarding care of the feet and legs is mandatory. The skin and underlying structures are chronically ischemic. Minor trauma, such as stubbing the toe, may result in necrosis and gangrene. The direct application of heat to a lesion is contraindicated in patients with this condition.

Surgery may be recommended for the client with severe pain and/or development of gangrene. This decision in the elderly client is generally dependent upon the amount of concurrent cardiovascular disease. Sympathectomy may be done to improve circulation and relieve pain. In the elderly client, the development of acute arterial occlusion is grave with an approximate 40% mortality rate (Carnevali, 1979, p. 267).

Venous Insufficiency

Venous insufficiency is caused by valvular insufficiency and/or varicose veins. Assessment data differs from chronic arterial occlusive disease in the following manner. If pain is present, it is diffuse and dull, not the acute cramping type of pain. Symptoms are relieved by elevating the extremities. Edema and hyperpigmentation of the affected extremities are common. Ulcerations, if present, tend to occur in the pre-tibial area and around the ankles. The ulcerations, while extremely difficult to heal, rarely progress to gangrene.

Nursing measures previously described such as meticulous skin care and exercise are indicated in the client with venous insufficiency. Other measures include frequent elevation of the legs, elevating the foot of the bed, avoiding prolonged standing or sitting, changing position frequently, avoiding constricting garments and crossing legs, and wearing elastic support stockings. The client should be encouraged to be as active as possible. Signs and symptoms such as sudden sharp chest pain, shortness of breath, and hemoptysis require immediate notification of a physician because they could signal a pulmonary embolus.

Summary

The incidence of cardiovascular disease in the elderly is high. Although current research now indicates that atherosclerosis is not a necessary part of aging and risk factors have been identified, the elderly today are a product of the medical knowledge of the past generations. Cardiovascular disease is best treated by a combination of diet, exercise and medication. Promotion of adherence to the treatment regimen is the challenge of the home health nurse. If the client can adhere to the regimen, participation in an active life is possible because the goal of therapy is prevention of complications and returning the client to as active a life as possible.

Cardiovascular disorders are inextricably interrelated. The presence of one disorder in general promotes further disorders within the system.

Angina pectoris and myocardial infarctions are caused by partial or total occlusion of the coronary arteries by atherosclerotic plagues. Ischemia of the myocardial tissue produces pain and, in the MI client, tissue necrosis treatment is aimed at maintaining coronary vessel patency and sufficient cardiac output. The seriousness of these events in the elderly client is accentuated because of the diminished cardiac reserve that accompanies aging.

Congestive heart failure is present when the cardiac output is insufficient to meet the metabolic needs of the body. Drug therapy aimed at increasing cardiac output and removing excessive fluids is the cornerstone of therapy. Continual assessment of these clients is crucial because an increase in metabolic demand can cause irreversible failure.

Hypertension, the insidious progressive disease, is even more significant in the elderly client who has diminished vascular resistance because of aging. Therapy is aimed at reducing the mean arterial pressure and decreasing vascular volume. Drugs used to accomplish this have serious side effects.

Peripheral vessel disease, both arterial and venous, can be debilitating. Careful education regarding positioning, activity and prevention of complications is essential.

Management of cardiovascular disorders requires the home health nurse to be skilled at assessment and interpretation of data, planning for care, and evaluation of care. With skilled nursing management, the client will learn to cope with the condition and participate as fully as possible in life's experiences.

A sample master care plan for home care of the cardiovascular client follows.

REFERENCES

Carnevali D L, Patrick M: *Nursing Management for the Elderly.* J.B. Lippincott Company, Philadelphia, 1979, pp 262, 267

Claiborne C: *Gourmet Diet Cookbook.* Ballantine Books, New York, 1981

Ebersole P, Hess P: *Toward Healthy Aging.* The C.V. Mosby Company, St. Louis, 1981, p 104

Graves M: "Physiological changes and major diseases in the older adult," in Hogstel MO (ed.): *Nursing Care of the Older Adult.* John Wiley & Sons, New York, 1981, p 111

Harrison's Principles of Internal Medicine, 7th Ed. McGraw-Hill Book Company, New York, 1974, p 1230

Harvey A M: *The Principles and Practice of Medicine.* Appleton-Century-Crofts, New York, 1980, p 246

Lewis S M, Collier I C: *Medical-Surgical Nursing: Assessment and Management of Clinical Problems.* McGraw-Hill Book Company, New York, 1983, p 830

Luckman J, Sorenson K C: *Medical-Surgical Nursing: A Psychophysiologic Approach,* 2nd ed. W.B. Saunders Company, Philadelphia, 1980, pp 843, 1112

McGurn W: *People with Cardiac Problems: Nursing Concepts.* J.B. Lippincott Company, Philadelphia, 1981, pp 59, 324, 327, 464, 468

Mullen E M, Granholm M: "Drugs and the elderly patient." *J. Geront Nurs,* Vol 7, No 2, February 1981, pp 108-113

Price S A, Wilson L M: *Pathophysiology: Clinical Concepts of Disease Processes.* McGraw-Hill Book Company, New York 1979, p 338

Rodman M J, Smith D W: *Pharmacology and Drug Therapy in Nursing,* 2nd ed. J.B. Lippincott Co., Philadelphia, 1979, p 596

Underhill S L, Woods S L, Sivarajan E S, Halpenny C J: *Cardiac Nursing.* J.B. Lippincott Co., New York, 1982, pp 326, 444, 478, 486, 494, 495, 539, 561, 601, 613, 627

Yurick A G, Robb S S, Spier B E: *The Aged Person and the Nursing Process.* Appleton-Century-Crofts, New York, 1980, pp 410, 485

BIBLIOGRAPHY

Burnside I M (ed): *Nursing and the Aged.* 2nd ed. McGraw-Hill Book Company, New York, 1981

Daniels L, Gifford R W: "Treating and counseling older adults who are hypertensive." *Geriat Nurs,* Vol 1, No 1, June 1980, pp 37-39

Donahue E G et al.: "A drug education program for the well elderly." *Geriat Nurs,* Vol 2, No 2, March/April 1981, pp 140-142

Durgin S J: "The pharmacist's evaluation." *Geriat Nurs,* Vol 3, No 1, January/February 1982, pp 31-33

Eliopoulos C: *Gerontological Nursing.* Harper and Row Publishers, New York, 1979

Hayter J: "Why response to medication changes with age." *Geriat Nurs,* Vol 2, No 6, November/December 1981, pp 411-416

Kart C S, Metress E S, Metress J F: *Aging and Health: Biologic and Social Perspectives.* Addison-Wesley Publishing Company, Menlo Park, California, 1978

Kim M J, Moritz D A (ed): *Classification of Nursing Diagnoses.* McGraw-Hill Book Company, New York, 1982

Miller J F: *Coping with Chronic Illness Overcoming Powerlessness.* F.A. Davis Company, Philadelphia, 1983

Timiras P S: *Developmental Physiology and Aging.* The Macmillan Company, New York, 1972

SAMPLE MASTER CARE PLAN FOR HOME CARE—

Nursing Diagnoses	Assessment	Planning
Alteration in cardiac output due to myocardial infarction, congestive heart failure, or hypertension. Lack of adherence to prescribed regimen due to inadequate knowlege, teaching, or confusion. Potential volume or electrolyte depletion due to medication.	• Sitting and lying, blood pressures, headaches/visual changes, dizziness/syncope, distended vessels, orthostatic hypotension, shortness of breath, disorientation, confusion, irregular pulse. • Medication check/pill count. Check meal plans for a week. Evaluate use of other drugs, prescription and over-the-counter. • Excessive fatigue, decrease in urine output, concentrated urine, decreased skin turgor, eyeball tension, weakness, abdominal pain.	*Short-term goals* *Client will:* • maintain a cardiac output as demonstrated by increasing ability to perform ADL • maintain established parameters of BP, pulse, respiration in response to medication, diet, and exercise • maintain sufficient volume and electrolytes as demonstrated by adequate output, energy, and absence of symptoms of electrolyte disturbance *Long-term goals* *Client will:* • improve cardiac output and reserve and/or cardiac output will not deteriorate • through the proper use of diet, medication, and exercise control his or her own cardiac function and report deviations from normal • recognize and appropriately respond to volume and electrolyte changes

CARDIOVASCULAR DISEASE

Intervention: Nursing Orders	Intervention: Resources and Support Systems	Evaluation: Expected Outcomes
Teach client to: • take own blood pressure, pulse • intersperse periods of exercise and activity. • avoid sudden movements, prolonged standing. • take all medications as ordered • plan daily menus so as to comply with dietary regimen • do planned exercise and evaluate its effect. • know normal patterns of urinary elimination and report deviations • report to physician immediately headaches, confusion, chest pain unrelieved by nitroglycerine, severe fatigue, ankle edema, shortness of breath, change in BP or pulse	• American Heart Association for literature, teaching plans, menus • American Red Cross for individual and family instruction • Post-myocardial infarction self help groups • Medicare for equipment such as syphgmomanometers • YMCA or church groups for transportation to physician	• Cardiac output is monitored and cardiac function does not worsen. • Medications, diet and exercise are utilized to enable client to control own cardiac function and participate as fully as possible in life's experiences. • Possible reduction in the need for medications is accomplished through adherence to diet and exercise regimen. • Fluid and electrolyte volume is maintained and any deviation is reported to the physician. *Client can:* • verbalize signs and symptoms of complications • verbalize and demonstrate knowledge of medication schedule • state dangerous side effects for each medication • demonstrate ability to monitor own heart beat for rate and rhythm.

CHAPTER 9

CANCER

Patricia Bohannan

Cancer is a group of diseases characterized by the uncontrolled proliferation of abnormal cell growth. For unknown reasons, these abnormal cells escape normal body regulatory influences and grow in all directions. They may invade the blood and lymph systems and establish independent growth, or metastasis, at a distant site in the body.

Cancer generally increases with age. Some 75% of all cancers in men and 63% of all cancers in women in the United States are diagnosed at age 55 or older (Marino, 1981, p. 30). The probability of developing cancer is approximately 1 in 700 at age 25. However, this probability increases to 1 in 14 at age 65 (Butler & Gastel, 1979, p. 333).

Today more than 22 million Americans are 65 years of age or older. It is predicted that this number will more than double in the next 50 years (Peterson & Kennedy, 1979, p. 322). As life expectancy increases, the percentage of older people will increase and the incidence of cancer will rise, too.

The financial cost of cancer is difficult to judge. In 1976, cancer patients spent approximately $3.5 billion for hospital care alone. Several studies in 1977 suggested that cancer patient direct health care costs were in the $9 billion range. *Consumer Reports* estimated the average patient's bill to be approximately $20,000. Medicare paid for approximately 88% of the expenses of cancer patients who were over 65 years of age (*Cancer Facts*, 1983, p. 24). The costs of cancer in terms of loss of individual productivity and quality of life are not measurable, of course.

Major efforts have gone into programs to: 1) identify the cause of cancer; 2) develop new treatment modalities; and 3) develop screening mechanisms for early detection. As a result, more people are diagnosed early; treatment modalities are available; and people are cured or their life prolonged by inhibiting the growth of their cancer. These advances have not been achieved without paying a very high price. The financial burden for manpower, equipment and drugs has been and will continue to be great, both for the citizens of the United States and, most of all, for the cancer patient and his or her family.

Providing health care services to the cancer patient in outpatient settings and in the home offers the potential of reducing these health care costs. However, it is important that every effort be made to ensure that the quality of this care be maintained. Therefore, the purpose of this chapter is to: 1) review the effects of cancer on the elderly, 2) provide information on screening elderly people for cancer, 3) identify medical therapies utilized for cancer treatment and related nursing care, and 4) discuss the rehabilitative needs of the patient and family.

Effects of Cancer on the Elderly

Although it is clear that certain types of cancer occur with greater frequency in certain age groups, a specific age related cause-effect relationship is unclear (see Table 9-1). Several hypotheses suggest that aging is associated with a decline in immune function. Delayed hypersensitivity reactions in the skin have been demonstrated after the fifth decade of life. The levels of circulating thymosin may decline as early as the fourth decade of life, and there may be a decline in the production of thymus-derived (T) lymphocytes in people over the age of 70. Therefore, the development of cancer in later life may be related to the body's inability to recognize and destroy cancer cells when they develop (Horton and Hill, 1977, p. 195). Another hypothesis proposes that tumor growth in the elderly is related to a decline in hormone function (Horton and Hill, 1977, p. 195). Finally, in the very elderly, poor nutrition may contribute to the body's inability to produce antibodies in response to invading viruses that can cause somatic mutations which result in a cancerous growth (Burkhalter and Donley, 1978, p. 362).

Although many advances have been made in recent years in the treatment of cancer, the success of these therapies is dependent upon early detection of the disease. Early detection of cancer in the elderly presents some unique problems. Cancer frequently does not cause pain in the early stages. Older people tend to attribute mild pain to the aging process and do not seek medical attention. Many older people have visual problems that interfere with their ability to see symptoms such as blood in the feces or urine, enlarged lymph nodes, or small skin lesions. Many older people have a great fear of the diagnosis of cancer and so they deny or repress symptoms until the disease has progressed beyond the curative stage. Nurses caring for elderly clients in the home can play a major role in the critical effort to identify cancer early in order to provide curative therapy. Systematic assessment of all family members over the age of 45 on a regular basis by home health nurses could provide an effective screening program that would result in earlier diagnosis and treatment, higher cure rates, and better survival rates.

TABLE 9.1
Maximum Risk Ages for Cancer in the Elderly

Site	High Risk Age	Estimate New Cases for 1983	Death Rate 1983
Breast	40 to 50	114,900	37,500
Lung	50 to 60	135,000	117,000
Uterine	40 to 60	55,000	10,000
Colon/rectal	50 to 70	126,000	58,100
Skin	40 to 70	400,000	7,100
Oral	50 to 70	27,100	9,150
Digestive Organs (Exc. Colon/rectal)	60 to 70	76,400	57,100
Larynx	50 to 60	11,000	3,700
Kidney (Exc. Wilms)	50 to 60	15,000	7,300
Bladder	50 to 70	38,500	10,700
Prostate	50 to 80	75,000	24,100
Lymphoma (Exc. Hodgkins)	50 to 60	23,600	12,300
Myeloma	40 or older	9,600	6,900
Leukemia	All ages (10% children)	23,900	16,100

(*Cancer Facts*, American Cancer Society, 1983 and Rubin, 1978)

Once a person has been diagnosed as having cancer, the age of that person may have a direct effect on the effectiveness of the therapeutic mode chosen to treat the cancer. Older patients have a greater risk of complications during most major surgical procedures. Post-operative healing may be slower, and there may be a greater risk of infection. Their natural decline in immunity makes immunotherapy less effective. Radiotherapy and chemotherapy may be effective in treatment of the cancer, but the stress of the therapy and side effects may be less tolerated by the older client. Frequently, older clients have other chronic diseases which necessitate less aggressive therapeutic modes and cause more difficulty in controlling the disease.

The Western culture places a high value on youth. As we become older, society views us as less productive and, thus, less of a social contributor. For the older person who has been diagnosed with cancer, this social bias is doubled. Old age and cancer are usually viewed to mean termination of life. However, with the advances in medical therapy, cancer has become a chronic disease with all the problems of chronic disease. Older men and women with cancer experience the same threats to body image, self concept, and emotional instability that younger people with cancer do. A person living with cancer has described the state as limbo (Davis, 1966, p. 746). Cancer patients must live from day to day because they cannot predict the future. Many experience a withdrawal of friendships. The kind of life the cancer patient had before illness is often irretrievable. Nurses caring for the elderly cancer patient in the home can do a great deal to help the individual regain the fullest physical, mental and social life possible.

Cancer is a family matter functionally, as well as emotionally. The diagnosis of cancer has repercussions for all members of the family. Because of the illusive nature of the disease, ongoing adjustments are required of the patient and family. Some cancer patients may be up and about and assume the responsibility for their own care. Others may require a great deal of assistance with activities of daily living (ADL). The family often must assume this responsibility. In an urban society, this may pose demands and difficulties, especially for the elderly patient. Changes in roles and responsibilities cause disequilibrium in the family structure. The nurse caring for the elderly cancer patient in the home can assist the family to regroup, regain homeostatic balance, and reconstruct its own reality.

Screening the Elderly for Cancer

Two basic skills are essential for proper screening for cancer. A thorough health history will identify risk factors, and a complete physical assessment will detect early signs and symptoms. The following discussion will address risk factors and early signs and symptoms for common cancers seen in the elderly.

Skin Cancer

Although skin cancer is a very common form of cancer, most are basal or squamous cell types that are highly curable if diagnosed early. Individuals who have a light, ruddy complexion, blond hair and blue eyes are more likely to develop skin cancers than brunettes with dark eyes. However, dark-skinned people can have skin cancer on the palms of the hands, soles of the feet, and between the fingers and toes. Excessive exposure to the ultraviolet rays of the sun, exposure to petroleum products such as coal, tar or creosote, and exposure to ionizing radiation have been implicated in the genesis of skin cancer. In obtaining a health history, questions should be asked to determine if the patient is at high risk.

Two warning signs of skin cancer are a sore that does not heal and changes in a wart or mole. The majority of basal and squamous cell skin cancers occur on areas of the body that get heavy sun exposure. A firm cutaneous or subcutaneous mass or a persistent ulcer should be referred to a physician. Any mole that has variegated coloring, irregular borders, changes in surface characteristics, or an increase in size should be suspected for cancer.

When assessing the skin, good lighting is essential. In the home, outside lighting may offer the best view of the lesion. A small flashlight may also be used to enhance the view of the skin.

The best preventive measure is to avoid the direct rays of the sun. Clients should be advised to wear a hat and sun glasses when outdoors. Sun screen lotions with a sun screen factor of 15 or 30 are also helpful in deflecting the ultraviolet rays of the sun.

Head and Neck Cancer

The risk factors associated with head and neck cancer are tobacco use, alcohol consumption, chronic irritation from poorly fitting dentures, and poor oral hygiene. When obtaining a health history, it is important to ask about dipping snuff and chewing tobacco, as well as smoking cigarettes or a pipe. Frequently, heavy drinkers will deny the excessive consumption of alcohol. Often direct questions such as, "Do you have a drink every day?" or "Do you have four or five drinks every day?" will provide a better assessment than asking if they drink alcoholic beverages.

Warning signs associated with head and neck cancers include: hoarseness, persistent sore throat, changes in the symmetry of the face, hearing loss, an ulcer that does not heal, and the presence of a non-painful mass. Frequently, these signs appear and progress so slowly that the elderly client may be completely unaware of them.

When assessing the oral cavity, particular attention should be given to the buccal mucosa, the lower part of the mouth, and the under side of the tongue. If dentures or partial plates are present, they should be removed and the gums under them should be assessed for irritation. The neck should be assessed for enlarged lymph nodes, deviations of the trachea, and areas of distention. Any of these signs may be indications of cancer, and the client should be referred to a physician.

Equipment needed for assessing the oral cavity include a tongue blade and a flashlight. The use of a dental mirror can greatly enhance vision of inaccessible areas of the mouth.

Preventive measures should include good oral hygiene and decreased or abstinence in the use of alcohol and tobacco. Older people are often reluctant to change lifetime habits. Therefore, the nurse should encourage them to limit alcohol and tobacco if they are unwilling to stop their use. All older people who wear dentures or partial plates should be warned of the potential for oral cancer if these appliances cause irritation to the gums. A systematic program of daily oral hygiene can provide the older person with some protection against oral cancer.

Breast Cancer

One out of every 11 women will develop breast cancer in her lifetime (*Cancer Facts*, 1983, p. 15). Although no age group is exempt from breast cancer, the older a woman becomes, the greater are her chances of developing breast cancer. Other risk factors include: a family history of breast cancer, never having had children, having the first child after the age of 30, and chronic fibrocystic disease of the breast. If a woman has had breast cancer in one breast, she is at greater risk of developing breast cancer in the other breast. Indiscriminate use of estrogen replacement therapy has been implicated in the development of breast cancer.

The only early warning sign for breast cancer is a palpable mass. A very high percentage of cancerous lesions in the breast can be detected manually when they are only 1 to 2 cm. in diameter. This makes it very important for nurses to include personal instruction to the patient in self breast examination techniques. This instruction should include teaching the woman to do self-breast exams with her own hands (Marino, 1981, p. 190).

Educational materials such as films, pamphlets and posters can reinforce (but not replace) personal instructions. Return demonstrations of self-breast examination techniques by clients are also important. The American Cancer Society recommends monthly self breast examinations for all women over age 20. However, this practice becomes more critical at age 40. If the client is pre-menopausal, she should examine her breasts the first day after her menses stop. If she is no longer experiencing menses, she should examine her breasts on the same day each month. In addition to a lump in the breast, significant findings may include: nipple discharge, nipple retraction, eczema, dimpling, redness, or ulceration.

The elderly woman may be reluctant to tell the nurse she has these symptoms. She may be even more reluctant to allow the nurse to examine her breasts. However, the sensitive nurse who provides for the privacy of the client will be able to provide this teaching.

Examination should include inspection and palpation. Inspection should be done in the following positions: 1) sitting with arms at sides and hands in the lap, 2) with both hands on the hips turning from side to side, and 3) with both arms raised and hands pressing on the back of the head (White et al., 1979, p. 45).

Palpation should be done with the patient lying on a small pillow under the shoulder. The arm should be extended upward with the hand under the head. Using the pads of the fingers, the nurse compresses the breast gently against the chest wall using a rotary motion; then proceeding in a systematic clockwise manner around the entire breast. It may be necessary to make several circles around each breast if they are large. Palpation of the axillary and supraclavicular nodes should be done with each breast exam (White, et al., 1979, p. 44).

Although no special equipment is necessary to examine the breast, good lighting and privacy are essential. The client could view the breast examination if the nurse provides a large mirror.

The method of preventing breast cancer remains illusive. Identifying women who fall into high-risk groups, performing monthly self breast exams, and the use of mammography and/or thermography to identify early disease offers the best techniques available for early detection. The American Cancer Society recommends that every woman have a physician examine her breasts each year, and a mammography should be done annually on women over age 50 (*Cancer Facts*, 1983, p. 16).

Lung Cancer

Lung cancer is a most lethal type of cancer. It is most likely to occur in heavy cigarette smokers between the ages 50 and 70. Individuals who smoked heavily for 20 or more years, as well as having been exposed to coal tars or asbestos are also at high risk.

Warning signs of lung cancer include a persistent cough, recurring attacks of pneumonia or bronchitis, chest pain associated with breathing, blood-streaked sputum, and weight loss. Many lung cancers do not present with any symptoms. They are diagnosed secondary to some other health problem or upon a routine physical examination. Because lung cancer metastasizes so early in the disease, the client may present with symptoms associated with distant metastasis rather than the primary lung lesion.

Assessment of the elderly client should include a lifetime occupation history to determine exposure to carcinogenic pollutants. A respiratory infection that persists longer than two weeks while the client is on antibiotic therapy should be regarded as suspicious, and the client should be encouraged to return to the physician for follow-up care. Even the simple clinical symptom of unexplained weight loss, especially in a heavy smoker, should be considered significant, and the client should be encouraged to have a medical check-up and chest X-rays.

Authorities agree that the greatest preventive measure against lung cancer is cessation of cigarette smoking. Although the elderly may be reluctant to give up smoking, the most rational approach for the nurse is to inform the client of the hazards and provide information on organizations that conduct smoking-cessation programs. Individuals who refuse to stop smoking should be urged to decrease the total number of cigarettes they smoke to five or less a day, to switch to a brand with tar yields of less than 10 mg., and to smoke only half of each cigarette. However, nurses should make it clear to the client that these measures only reduce the hazards of smoking and are, at best, measures that may make cessation easier to accomplish.

Colon/Rectal Cancer

The incidence of colon cancer in the United States is exceeded only by lung cancer and skin cancer. Two out of three patients diagnosed with colon cancer are over age 50. A history of polyps in the colon or ulcerative colitis may place the person at greater risk to develop colon cancer. High fat, low-fiber diets have been implicated as a possible causative factor. A family history of colon cancer places the person in a high-risk group. Clients with a history of any of the above should have routine fiberoptic colonoscopy on a regular basis. The American Cancer Society recommends a stool guiaic slide test annually for all individuals over age 50. They also recommend colonoscopy every three to five years after two annual negative colonoscopies (*Cancer Facts,* 1983, p. 17).

Warning signs associated with colon cancer include bleeding from the rectum, blood in the stool, and changes in bowel habits. Many elderly people are very concerned about their bowel habits and often take laxatives regularly. However, they may have poor eyesight and be unable to detect blood in their stool. Assessment of the elderly should include a history of bowel habits and the use of laxatives. The Hemoccult slide test can be explained to the client who can prepare the slide in the privacy of the home. The Hemoccult slide test provides successful screening without a digital rectal exam (Richardson, 1977, p. 123). Nurses caring for clients in the home can play an important role in colon/rectal cancer detection by informing the client and his family of the risks and by using the Hemoccult slide test.

Other Types of Cancer

The elderly client is also at greater risk than a younger person for acquiring cancer of the reproductive system, the kidney, the bladder, and several other types of cancer. However, because of the frequency of occurrence, skin, head and neck, lung, breast and colon/rectal cancer have been discussed here. For more information on screening techniques for other types of cancer, see *Cancer Screening and Detection Manual for Nurses* by White (1970) et al.

Medical Therapies and Related Nursing Care

Four types of medical therapy are available for the treatment of cancer: surgery, radiation therapy, chemotherapy and immunotherapy. Usually the cancer patient will receive several of these therapies during the course of the disease. Occasionally these therapies are administered in combination. For the elderly cancer patient, the side effects can be as morbid as the cancer itself. However, these side effects are usually treatable. Therefore, the astute nurse who can recognize the beginning signs of complications can set up therapies. The following discussion will explain the medical treatment modalities and related nursing care.

Surgery

Surgical therapy may be recommended to effect a cure, to reduce the extent of tumor, to prevent future complications, to determine the extent of cancer metastasis, or to relieve pain or obstruction. Most surgical procedures for cancer are extensive and require long periods of anesthesia. Many elderly cancer patients have other physical handicaps that increase their risk of post-operative complications. Their nutritional status may slow down post-operative healing, and they tend to require a longer period of time to return to their pre-operative level of functioning.

Surgery is usually performed in a hospital and requires that the patient be hospitalized during the immediate post-operative period. Even though patients who have surgery may recover well from the surgery in the hospital, they may develop complications after they return home. Frequently the radical surgical procedures required for cancer therapy result in major functional and emotional adjustment when the patient returns home.

The problems of the cured cancer patient have been identified as: 1) cosmetic and functional deficiencies, 2) nutritional and/or malabsorption deficiencies, 3) sterility, 4) changes in family structure, 5) loss of social contact, and 6) tendency to develop a second primary site (Zubord, 1975, p. 267). The rehabilitation of many patients with cancer is related to: 1) the psychological and physical structure he or she brings to the situation, 2) the patient's and family's cooperation, 3) the patient's ability to accept the structural and/or functional changes that have been thrust upon him, and 4) the patient's ability to create a self-image that gives him the confidence to engage in those activities which he enjoyed in the pre-illness state (Hardy & Cull, 1975, p. 126).

The goals of nursing care of the elderly cancer patient recovering from surgery are: to reduce the patient's functional deficiencies, to provide adequate nutritional intake, and to encourage independent productivity. A master care plan that can be individualized to achieve these goals is included at the end of this chapter.

Radiation

Radiation therapy destroys cells by exposing them to high energy gamma or x-rays. These energy rays penetrate the cell wall and interact with chemical molecules causing a disruption in the chemical bonds. Because this interaction occurs on a chance basis, some cells will die immediately, some will die when they begin mitosis, and other cells will adapt and survive. Radiation therapy can be administered by exposing a tumor to a radiation source external to the body or by implanting a radioactive source into a body cavity. For radiation protection purposes, the patient who receives a radiation implant is hospitalized during therapy. Patients who receive radiation therapy from an external source may be treated with repeated small dose exposures daily over several weeks. Although the greatest lethal effect can be obtained by giving a single large dose, repeated small doses will produce accumulative damage with less severe side effects. Therefore, the patient will demonstrate more side effects near the end of treatment period and even two or three weeks after treatments have been completed. Radiation therapy may be used as a curative treatment, for palliation of symptoms, or as an adjunct to other treatment modalities. Over half of all cancer patients require radiation therapy sometime during the course of their illness (Marino, 1981, p. 260).

Reactions to radiation therapy can be classified as acute and chronic. Acute reactions can be seen during treatment and two to three weeks after the final treatment. Chronic reactions may not occur until several months or years after therapy. The acute reaction to radiation includes irritation, inflammation, and edema of the area exposed to the radiation. Chronic reactions include fibrosis and possible fistula formation in the area exposed. Injury to an area that has been exposed to radiation will always heal more slowly because of damage done by radiation.

Most patients receiving radiation therapy experience some degree of radiation syndrome, described as general fatigue, weakness, headache, nausea and loss of appetite (Leahy et al., 1979, p. 83; Marino, 1981, p. 273; Burns, 1982, p. 134). The skin covering the area being radiated may react first by developing erythema and progressing during therapy to a dark brown, dry desquamation stage. On rare occasions, the skin may peel off leaving a wet desquamation area present. Hematopoietic suppression may occur and blood counts are usually monitored during therapy. However, this side effect may not occur until after the treatments are completed. Additional reactions to radiation therapy are dependent on the anatomical location of the field, the size of the field, and the depth of the dose administered.

The goals of the nursing care of the elderly cancer patient receiving radiation therapy are to reduce functional deficiencies, to provide adequate nutritional intake, and to encourage independent productive activity. A master care plan that can be individualized to meet these goals is included at the end of the chapter.

Chemotherapy

Chemotherapy involves administration of toxic substances that systemically interfere with the life cycle of the cell and thus cause it to die. Although every cell in the body is potentially exposed to these toxic substances, the greatest kill rate occurs to cells that rapidly reproduce. Since most cancer cells have a short life cycle, they are more likely to die from this exposure. Chemotherapy is used when the cancer is not localized and the cancer cells are potentially anywhere in the body. Since chemotherapy is more effective when tumors are small, it is often utilized in combination with surgery or radiation therapy. The major types of toxic substances used as anti-tumor drugs include: 1) antimetabolities, 2) alkylating agents, 3) plant alkaloids, 4) antibiotics and 5) hormones. These drugs may be given singularly or in combination. They are usually administered intravenously but can be given orally, intramuscularly, intrathecally, and intracavity. Some patients will receive a total treatment protocol all at once while others will receive smaller doses over several days. Most patients remain on chemotherapy for an extended period of time to achieve remission of their disease.

Since all the cells of the body are exposed to these toxic substances, the normal cells that have a rapid reproductive cycle are affected by these drugs. Stem cells of the bone marrow, hair follicles, and the mucosal lining of the gastrointestinal tract are repressed, which results in mylosupression, hair loss, and mucositis. These reactions are generally not seen until five to ten days after the drugs are administered.

The most difficult side effects to manage are nausea and vomiting. These problems may occur immediately upon administration and usually continue for 24 to 48 hours. Nausea from chemotherapy may be related to: 1) direct irritation of the gastrointestinal tract, 2) stimulation of the chemoreceptor sites in the medulla oblongata, 3) stimulation of the vomiting center in the floor of the fourth ventricle, 4) anxiety or 5) a combination of these factors (Marino, 1981, p. 334). Nausea and vomiting can be so severe that the patient is at risk of developing severe fluid and electrolyte imbalance.

The goals of nursing care of the elderly cancer patient receiving chemotherapy are to reduce functional deficiencies, provide adequate nutritional intake, and encourage independent productive activity. A master care plan that can be individualized to meet these goals is included at the end of this chapter.

Immunotherapy

The most recent advances in cancer therapy have been in the area called immunotherapy. Immunotherapy is based upon the theory that the body can develop an immunological response to the cancer cells present in the body. Therefore, therapy which bolsters the patient's immune response may improve the way his body destroys cancer cells. The host immune response can only handle a limited number of cancer cells. A tumor that is one centimeter in diameter contains approximately one billion cells and has out-stripped the immune response. Therefore, a tumor that is clinically evident would require other modes of therapy. However, immunotherapy can be used as an adjunct to other therapies. Three types of immunotherapy are used: 1) active or specific cancer antigens, 2) passive or active antibodies, immune RNA, or transfer factor made outside the host, and 3) non-specific stimulation with various non-cancer antigens. Depending upon the type of immunotherapy given, the patient can develop erythema and ulcers at the injection site, nausea and vomiting, flu-like symptoms, and graft versus host disease.

Although immunotherapy is seldom used in elderly cancer patients, the home health nurse will need to understand this therapy because research is underway that has the potential for improving this therapy. The same general goals and nursing care that are used with other treatment modalities apply to the patient receiving immunotherapy.

Rehabilitation of the Cancer Patient and Family

The National Council on Rehabilitation defines rehabilitation as the restoration of the individual to the fullest physical, mental, social, vocational and economic capacity of which he or she is capable (Stryker, 1977, p. 13). The patient and family have been identified as essential members of the health care team that makes rehabilitation possible (Stryker, 1977, p. 16). Nurses engaged in the rehabilitation of the cancer patient must know the problems within the family in order to assist the maintenance of homeostatic balance (Mozden, 1965, p. 359).

Cancer is a chronic illness that may be expected to require a long period of observation, supervision and care. It requires ongoing adjustments for the patient and family as they must develop coping mechanisms as a means to minimize the problems and facilitate adaptation (Miller, 1978, p. 297). Factors related to the degree of adjustment are: 1) the amount of physical disability, 2) the visibility of the cancer or the degree of disfigurement, 3) the individual's previous coping capability, and 4) the family's interpersonal relationships (Leopold & Ramsden, 1979, p. 119). It has been suggested that rehabilitation programs should be directed toward helping the patient determine his own mode of living. Rehabilitation programs should be measured by: 1) the patient's ability to recognize and change destructive behaviors, 2) the patient's *attempts* to achieve goals rather than total goal achievement, and 3) the patient's ability to form goals and identify ways to achieve them (Anderson, 1977, p. 303).

Elderly cancer patients and their families tend to organize their lives around the illness. This results in the establishment of goals related to prevention of crises and the control of symptoms. If the home health nurse can assist with the achievement of functional improvement, the client and the family might be able to direct their attention to goals related to increasing social interaction, productivity and independence. The challenge in rehabilitation of the elderly cancer patient is to aid with dependent needs and at the same time encourage social interaction, independence and productivity.

Like any long-term illness, cancer is a major problem to the family. The patient's family must re-organize in order to maintain the necessary balance between family needs and the added demands of the patient. When the patient is at home, the responsibility of the day-to-day care rests with family members. There is a need to increase resources to these families and to teach them the skills necessary to provide this care. The home health nurse must identify these needs and provide for them.

Googe and Varricchio (1981, p. 25) identified the need to teach families about diet, pain control, sleep control, ambulation and elimination management. They also found that patients at home frequently needed special equipment, transportation to the physician's office, and skilled services such as intravenous therapy. Edstrom and Miller (1981, p. 50) developed a short course in which they instructed the family in basic nursing skills such as changing an occupied bed, how to use the bedpan, how to transfer the patient, and basic nutrition. Grobe, et al. (1981, p. 375) found that families are more likely to learn new skills when the patient is at home because they are more aware of the difficulties involved. These authors stressed the importance of emotional support for both the patient and the family.

Resources for the Client and Family

Nurses

A home health nurse is available through a home health agency or a Visiting Nurse Association. It is important that the nurse teach the family how to help with the activities of daily living for the patient. The patient should be encouraged to do as much for himself as possible. Special attention must be given to nutritional management, medications and ambulation.

Equipment

The American Cancer Society attempts to provide free equipment and supplies to cancer patients in many parts of this country. Hospital beds, bedside commodes, and wheelchairs often are loaned to patients without charge for as long as they are needed. They also have some dressings, ostomy equipment, and miscellaneous equipment needed for nursing procedures. The employees of the American Cancer Society are usually well informed about available community resources. Respiratory therapy equipment is sometimes available free through the American Lung Association. Most hospital equipment can be rented or purchased through a hospital supply company.

Medications

Some drugs may be available free through the Leukemia Society of America if the patient has a cancer of the blood-forming tissue. Otherwise, the family should be encouraged to price drugs at several pharmacies because prices vary considerably. Families should also be encouraged to keep records of drug expenses because they may be partially reimbursed through the insurance company or they may use these costs as a tax deduction.

The home health nurse must work very closely with the patient's physician to assure that the patient has the necessary routine medications as well as medications for potential problems that can arise. Most elderly cancer patients should have medications for mild pain, moderate pain, and severe pain. Woods et al. (1982, p. 36) recommends Tylenol for mild pain, Codeine or Percodan for moderate pain, and Methadone for severe pain. Families need to be taught how to assess the patient's pain to determine the type and form of administering the medication. Medications should be available for nausea, constipation and diarrhea. In addition, patients may be receiving routine antibiotics, steroids and many other drugs. The nurse must prepare the family for any synergistic effects that could occur. Families must also be aware that elderly people tend to metabolize drugs more slowly and may have toxic effects from accumulation of drugs in the body.

Activity

Remaining ambulatory as long as possible not only prevents complications but also contributes to the goal of productive activity. Frequently, elderly cancer patients can participate in some occupational projects such as hand work, sewing or painting. Sometimes they can help with small household tasks such as folding the clothes. If the patients are ambulatory, they should be encouraged to take walks daily, slowly increasing the distance.

Occasionally, the patient will be unable to walk. The nurse must teach the family how to assist the patient in moving from the bed to the wheelchair or bedside commode. This is especially important because of the possibility that family members may injure themselves.

Nutrition

No single factor seems to affect toleration of all types of cancer therapies as much as good nutrition. Neither is the family faced with a greater challenge. The relationship between appetite and cancer is still unknown. However, loss of appetite seems to be a problem for many elderly patients. Providing any food that the patient enjoys most when they are hungry seems most successful. Patients can often tolerate six small meals a day better than three large ones. However, eating meals with the family stimulates social interaction and should be encouraged. The family should be taught to increase protein in the diet and use high protein diet supplements.

Transportation

Occasionally the family will have problems transporting the patient to the physician's office or health care facility. The American Cancer Society and The American Red Cross often have vans available to transport patients. It is important that arrangements be made several days in advance and that appointments be coordinated. The patient and family should understand that this transportation system may require a waiting period because the vans will be transporting several patients at once.

Daily Records

A daily record of the patient's condition and activity can be most useful in assessing the patient's progress. The nurse can devise a simple form to aid the family in keeping an accurate record of the patient's daily progress. This record should be available for the home health nurse and should be taken to the physician's office. Figure 9-1 is an example of a simple record that could be used by the family.

FIGURE 9-1.
Patient Weekly Record

	Mon	Tues	Wed	Thur	Fri	Sat	Sun
Temperature Time—Degree							
Urine Frequency—Color							
Stool Amount—Color							
Fluid Intake							
Food Intake							
Activity							
Drugs (list)							
Other Comments							

Notify the physician if:

1. The temperature is greater than 101 degrees
2. Blood is present in the urine, stool, or from any site
3. The patient becomes disoriented or sleeps more than usual
4. The patient goes three days without a bowel movement
5. The patient has difficulty urinating
6. The pain is not relieved by the medication prescribed

Summary

The percentage of people older than age 55 is expected to increase over the next 50 years, and the incidence of cancer among this age group will also rise. To provide quality health care for the elderly in the home offers a possible solution to the high cost of health care. The home health nurse who is knowledgeable about early warning signs can help to detect cancer early. Providing care for the home-bound cancer patient is a challenge. The home health nurse can contribute much toward the goals of rehabilitation of the cancer patient. Finally, the home health nurse can support the family and help them regain homeostatic balance even when ongoing adjustments are necessary.

REFERENCES

Anderson N: "Rehabilitative nursing." *Nurs Clin North Am,* Vol 6, No 2, June 1971, pp 303–309

Burkhalter P K, Donley L: *Dynamics of Oncology Nursing.* McGraw Hill Book Co., New York, 1978

Burns N: *Nursing and Cancer.* W.B. Saunders Co., Philadelphia, 1982

Butler, N, Gastel B: "Aging and Cancer Management Part II Research Perspective." *Ca-A Cancer Journal for Clinicians,* Vol 29, No 6, November/December 1979, pp 333–40

Cancer Facts and Figures–1983, American Cancer Society, 777 Third Avenue, New York, 1983

Davis M Z: "Patients in limbo." *Am J Nurs,* Vol 66, No 4, April 1966, pp 746–48

Edstrom S, Miller M W: "Preparing the family to care for the cancer patient at home: home care course." *Cancer Nursing,* Vol 4, No 1, February 1981, pp 49–52

Googe M C, Varriccho C G: "A pilot investigation of home health care needs of cancer patients and their families." *Oncology Nursing Forum,* Vol 8, No 4, Fall 1981, pp 24–28

Grobe M E, Ilstrup D M, Ahmann D L: "Skills needed by family members to maintain the care of an advanced cancer patient." *Cancer Nursing,* Vol 4, No 5, October 1981, pp 371–75

Hardy R E, Cull J G: *Counseling and Rehabilitating the Cancer Patient.* Charles C. Thomas, Springfield, Illinois, 1975

Horton J, Hill J: *Clinical Oncology.* W.B. Saunders Co., Philadelphia, 1977

Leahy I, Germain J M, Varricchio G: *The Nurse and Radiotherapy.* The C.V. Mosby Co., St. Louis, 1982

Leopold R, Ramsden E L: "Rehabilitation Services," in Cassileth B R (ed.); *The Cancer Patient: Social and Medical Aspects of Care.* Lea and Febiger Co., Philadelphia, 1979

Marino L B: *Cancer Nursing.* The C.V. Mosby Co., St. Louis, 1981

Miller M W, Nygren C: "Living with cancer, coping behaviors." *Cancer Nursing,* Vol 1, No 4, August 1978, pp 297–302

Mozden P J: "Neoplasms." in Myers J S: *An Orientation to Chronic Disease and Disability* The Macmillan Co., London, 1965

Peterson B A, Kennedy B J: "Aging and cancer management part I clinical observations." *Ca-A Cancer Journal for Clinicians,* Vol 29, No 6, November/December 1979, pp 322–32

Richardson J: "Colonrectal cancer: Mass screening and education program." *Geriatrics,* Vol 32, No 2, February 1977, pp 123–131

Rubin P E: *Clinical Oncology for Medical Students and Physicians.* 5th ed. American Cancer Society, Rochester, New York, 1978

Skryker R: *Rehabilitation Aspects of Acute and Chronic Nursing Care.* W.B. Saunders Co., Philadelphia, 1977

White L N, Patterson J E, Cornelius Judkins A F: *Cancer Screening and Detection Manual for Nurses.* McGraw Hill Book Co., New York, 1979

Wood C A, Bailey L R, Yates J W: "Advanced cancer pain management in a community setting." *Oncology Nursing Forum,* Vol 9, No 1, Winter 1982, pp 32–36
Zubrod C G: "Successes in cancer treatment," *Cancer,* Vol 36, No 1, July 1975, pp 267–70

BIBLIOGRAPHY

May C: "Antibiotic therapy at home." *Am J Nurs,* Vol 84, No 3, March 1984, pp 348–49
Schaffner A: Safety precautions in home chemotherapy." *Am J Nurs,* Vol 84, No 3, March 1984, pp 346–47

SAMPLE MASTER CARE PLAN FOR HOME CARE—

Nursing Diagnoses	Assessment	Planning
Potential infection of the incision, the lungs, and the urinary tract resulting in inadequate healing and additional recovery period. Potential anorexia resulting in weight loss, poor healing and increased susceptibility to infection Potential immobility resulting in constipation, weakness, and increased susceptibility to thrombophlebitis and infections. Potential alteration of body image resulting in depression, fear and isolation Potential pain resulting in anxiety, depression, and fear of recurrence	• Observe for redness, swelling and drainage from incision. • Observe for lung congestion, productive cough, and temperature elevation. • Observe for frequency, burning, or other problems associated with urinary tract infection. • Assess the client's or family's ability to care for the wound. • Assess the amount of foods and fluids taken. • Assess the amount of physical activity the client participates in during the day. • Assess the characteristics of pain and the amount of drugs necessary to control pain. • Assess the frequency and ease with which the client is able to interact with family and friends.	*Short-term goals* *Client will:* • not get an infection • gradually increase physical activity • be pain free • take medications as ordered • have normal elimination patterns • take an adequate amount of foods and fluids • have normal healing of incision. *Long-term goals* *Client will:* • adjust to any necessary changes in lifestyle that might result from surgery • resume pre-operative role in the family • increase social interaction in groups such as church, support groups, friends

CANCER (POST-OPERATIVE)

Intervention: Nursing Orders	Intervention: Resources and Support Systems	Evaluation: Expected Outcomes
• Change dressing daily. • Encourage fluids to 3000 ml. per 24 hours. • Give high protein formula between meals and at bedtime. • Give vitamins as ordered. • Give pain medications as ordered. • Use relaxation techniques with pain medication. • Prune juice with breakfast. • Give enema/laxatives as ordered for constipation. • Encourage client to assume responsibility for self care. • Ambulate daily as much as possible. • Increase physical activity progressively. • Encourage client to express fears of recurrence. • Refer client and family to cancer resource groups.	• The American Cancer Society • The Ostomy Association • The Laryngectomy Association • Reach for Recovery • Cancer Support Groups • The American Red Cross • Church **Intervention: Teaching** • Teach client and family how to take medications. • Teach client and family how to care for incision site. • Provide family with recipes which will increase protein intake. • Teach family to monitor temperature, elimination, and foods and fluid intake. • Teach client and family any necessary alterations due to functional changes resulting from surgery. • Refer client and family to agencies that provide special equipment and transportation. • Teach client and family the importance of gradually increasing physical activity.	*Client:* • returns to normal activities as soon as able • receives assistance and support from family, friends, and other support groups • is alert to the need for continuing regular health assessment.

SAMPLE MASTER CARE PLAN FOR HOME CARE—

Nursing Diagnoses	Assessment	Planning
Potential nausea and vomiting resulting in anorexia, weight loss, and fluid and electrolyte imbalance. Potential malaise and fatigue resulting in inability to perform activities of daily living. Potential internal and external inflammation and edema of the radiation field resulting in complications that are dependent on the anatomical location of the radiation field (i.e. cerebral edema, esophagitis, pneumonitis, gastritis, cystitis). Potential dry and/or moist desquamation of the skin at the radiation field. Potential disruption in normal lifestyle because of daily appointments for treatments resulting in adjustments for the client and family.	● Assess food and fluid intake. ● Assess for changes in weight. ● Assess elimination patterns. ● Assess the skin of the radiation field for breaks, weeping, inflammation. ● Assess for any symptoms that may be associated with inflammation and edema of the radiation field (for example, gums, stool, urine). ● Assess the amount of physical activity the client participates in daily. ● Assess the client's and family's ability to adjust to the daily appointment for therapy.	*Short-term goals* *Client will:* ● have minimal weight loss ● have minimal desquamation ● maintain maximum physical activity ● experience minimal disruption in life style during treatment ● have normal elimination pattern ● take an adequate amount of foods and fluids daily. *Long-term goals* *Client will:* ● experience minimal side effect from radiation therapy ● resume pre-treatment role in the family ● resume pre-treatment social interaction in groups such as work, church, support groups, friends.

CANCER (RECEIVING RADIATION THERAPY)

Intervention: Nursing Orders	Intervention: Resources and Support Systems	Evaluation: Expected Outcomes
• Encourage fluids to 3000 ml. each 24 hours. • Give high protein, high carbohydrate formula between meals and at bedtime. • Give pain medication as ordered. • Use relaxation techniques with pain medication. • Encourage client to take short naps. • Encourage client to exercise daily. • Give anti-emetic 30 minutes before meals if nauseated. • Increase seasoning in food if client has taste changes. • Give prune juice or milk of magnesia for constipation or anti-diarrhea medication for diarrhea. • Advise client to avoid wearing tight clothing next to the radiation field. • Advise client to wash radiation field gently with water only being careful not to remove markings that denote the field. • Advise the client to avoid the use of perfumed agents because of possible skin reaction. • Advise client to avoid using a heating pad or hot water bottle on the field and to avoid exposing the field to direct sunlight. • Observe for blood in the urine and feces. • Encourage client to participate in family activities.	• American Cancer Society • American Red Cross • Church • Cancer support groups **Intervention: Teaching** • Teach client and family that radiation therapy itself is not painful, but inflammation that results from the therapy may cause some discomfort. • Explain that although the client is alone during treatment, he or she can be seen and heard by the therapist. • Teach client and family the importance of adequate and nutritious food and fluid intake. • Teach client and family how to care for the skin in the field. • Establish treatment times that best meet the needs of the client and family. • Assist with transportation to daily treatment appointments. • Teach client and family that generalized weakness may occur.	*Client:* • experiences minimal skin and elimination changes as a result of radiation therapy • regains full participation in family and social groups • seeks assistance if further complications develop.

SAMPLE MASTER CARE PLAN FOR HOME CARE—

Nursing Diagnoses	Assessment	Planning
Potential nausea, vomiting, diarrhea resulting in weight loss, fluid and electrolyte imbalance. Potential mucositis resulting in ulceration of the mouth, esophagus, stomach, bowel, anus. Potential alteration in the hemopoetic system resulting in possible anemia, infection, and hemorrhage. Potential alopecia resulting in changes in body image, withdrawal, and depression. Potential constipation resulting in abdominal distention, discomfort and possible obstruction. Potential cystitis resulting in urinary frequency, burning and urinary tract infection. Potential malaise and fatigue resulting in inability to perform activities of daily living.	• Assess food and fluid intake. • Assess changes in weight. • Assess elimination patterns. • Carefully inspect the mouth for any ulcerations or bleeding. • Observe the body for the presence of petechia or bruising. • Assess the insides of the lower eye lids for signs of anemia.	*Short-term goals* *Client will:* • have minimal weight loss • avoid exposure to infection • practice meticulous oral care • have normal elimination patterns • take an adequate amount of food and fluids • maintain some physical activity • experience minimal disruption in lifestyle during treatment periods. *Long-term goals* *Client will:* • experience minimal side effects from chemotherapy • resume pre-treatment role in the family • resume pre-treatment social interaction in groups.

CANCER (RECEIVING CHEMOTHERAPY)

Intervention: Nursing Orders	Intervention: Resources and Support Systems	Evaluation: Expected Outcomes
• Give anti-emetic 30 minutes before chemotherapy and every 4 hrs. for 24 hrs. After 24 hr. period, give anti-emetic 30 minutes before meds. • Encourage fluids such as Gatoraid, liquid jello, and fruit juice during first 24 hrs. after chemotherapy and then encourage fluids to 3000 ml/24 hrs. Rinse mouth with ½ H_2O_2 and ½ normal saline each time after eating. • Use salt on toothbrush unless bleeding of gums occurs, then just use above mouth rinse. • Take temperature daily in the evening. Notify physician if greater than 101°. • Avoid injections. If they are necessary, hold site for five minutes. • Give pain medication as ordered and use relaxation techniques. • Give high protein, high carbohydrate formula between meals and H.S. • Give anti-diarrhea medication for diarrhea. • Give prune juice or laxative for constipation.	• The American Cancer Society • The Leukemia Society of America • The American Red Cross. • Cancer support groups. **Intervention: Teaching** • Teach client and family the importance of taking anti-emetic regardless of the amount of nausea experienced. • Teach client and family the importance of fluid intake to prevent dehydration. • Have client squeeze a rubber ball 10 to 20 times, 6 to 8 times a day to build larger veins for chemotherapy. • Refer client and family to agencies that provide special equipment, transportation, and other support. • Teach the client and family to notify the physician if bleeding occurs anywhere. • Teach the client and family to notify the physician if the patient goes more than two days without a bowel movement. • Teach the client and family that chemotherapy will cause a drop in the production of blood cells and therefore it is very important that all follow-up appointments be kept so that tests can be done to determine blood counts.	*Client:* • adapts to routine of continued treatment if needed • regains strength to participate in family activities • receives continued support from family and friends

CHAPTER 10

MENTAL HEALTH PROBLEMS AND NEEDS

Linda M. Richardson and Rodney L. Lowman

The largest growing age groups in the U.S. are the very old—persons age 75 and above. (Butler and Lewis, 1982). The very old are especially vulnerable to psychological distress. Contributing to the large incidence of psychological difficulties among the elderly are the large number of stresses brought with age, combined with more limited resources for coping. A variety of psychological problems can be manifested among the elderly. The most common are: depression, paranoia and organic brain syndromes. It has been estimated that 15% or more of all older adults experience psychological distress of sufficient severity to warrant mental health intervention (Abrahams and Patterson, 1978–79; Kramer, Taube, and Redick, 1973; Report to the President 1978).

Treatment of mental problems among the elderly is certainly possible. However, few aged persons seek early intervention for psychological difficulties, as illustrated by their over-representation in inpatient mental health settings and their under-representation in outpatient mental health settings. Regardless of the stage and type of psychological intervention, the treatment goal is to maximize psychological functioning and to keep the elderly at home and functioning independently whenever possible.

This chapter reviews major psychological disorders found in aged persons living in their community. Interventions for these disorders will also be discussed, with an emphasis on home care. Even in cases of more severe psychopathology, requiring away-from-home treatment, the home health nurse can be helpful as a diagnostician and referral source and as a liaison between the mental health specialist and the client when the client might return home.

Developmental Tasks of the Elderly

Recent studies of adults have called attention to the need for theories specific to adult development. A taxonomy of the predictable stages of adult growth and development has yet to be reliably established. Fortunately, considerable advances have been made in this area in recent years as increasing research attention has been directed to the life stages of adulthood.

While in the past the elderly were usually considered a rather undifferentiated group, recently some gerontologists have suggested that classifying older persons by developmental stages is often more meaningful than grouping solely by age. Alternatively, the age span of later maturity can be subdivided into more homogeneous groups. An increasingly used differentiation, for example, divides the elderly into those who are "young-old" and "old-old." The former group is generally considered to include those from 65–75 years of age, while the latter is composed of persons 75 years of age and older.

An understanding of the developmental tasks of later maturity is essential for the nurse since these tasks provide a yardstick for gauging successful and problematic aging. Many classic theories of development (e.g., Freud's psychosexual stages) unfortunately do not cover the late adult years. Such theories often hold the view that little development occurs during this stage of the life cycle, or that adult development is largely predetermined in childhood. The three theorists to be discussed here—Erikson, Peck, and Havighurst—were early pioneers in offering theories of adult development, and their ideas still predominate present western thinking, although little research is yet available to validate these theories empirically.

Erikson was one of the first theorists to postulate that development continues throughout the adult years. He proposed that the final developmental issue in the life cycle, typically faced in later maturity, is the achievement of what he called ego integrity, versus its opposite condition, despair (Erikson, 1963). Those who are unsuccessful in reaching integrity are preoccupied with regrets about their lives and are saddened by the realization that it is no longer possible to begin life anew. Because of the dissatisfaction with life as it was lived, it is more difficult for despairing persons to consider or accept their inevitable death. Such persons may withdraw or may be avoided because of their negativistic attitudes (Jones, 1981).

More recently, Peck has elaborated Erikson's theory of development in later life by proposing three developmental tasks for older adults: ego differentiation, body transcendence, and ego transcendence (Peck, 1968). One task for older adults is to diversify their interests and activities, particularly if they previously were heavily invested in their work. This ego differentiation promotes the smooth transition from the loss of the work role into retirement and facilitates adjustment to the "empty nest." When alternate interests and activities are not developed, the individual experiences unresolved grief over the loss of the work role and may become preoccupied with this loss.

Secondly, Peck proposes the task of transcending one's body, all the ailments and physical pain associated with growing old, versus becoming somatically preoccupied. Older persons who are overly concerned about their bodies not only can miss out on many of life's pleasures but also can alienate their family and friends by their persistent concerns and complaints. Social isolation may occur as a result.

The third task identified by Peck is ego transcendence. He suggests that older adults who have accepted their lives as lived are able to face death without fear and desire to improve the world for future generations. Consequently, they devote their energies to such efforts and may also seek to contribute to others as a way of transcending death. However, those who are unable to accept their lives as they were are more likely to turn inward and become more isolated and alienated from the rest of the world; this may precipitate feelings of aloneness, fright and unhappiness.

The last developmental theory to be considered was formulated by Havighurst, who proposed six developmental tasks for older adults: 1) adjusting to declining physical strength and health; 2) adjusting to retirement and its reduction in income; 3) adjustment to the death of a spouse; 4) establishing affection within one's peer group; 5) adapting to a new social roles in a flexible manner; and 6) establishing satisfactory living arrangements (Havighurst, 1974).

Although these three proposed developmental theories are not exclusively psychological in nature, difficulty or inability in accomplishing the developmental tasks that each theory postulates for later maturity can result in psychological maladjustment. Most of these developmental tasks involve adjustment to losses or negative life changes, a process made more difficult by the older adult's declining physical and mental resources. Older adults who have broadened their sources of support and gratification beyond work and immediate family to peers, other relatives, and leisure interests or activities are more likely to successfully weather such changes. Mental health assistance may be necessary if the older adult experiences difficulty in achieving any of these developmental tasks.

Specific Mental Health Problems of the Elderly

The incidences of mental health problems increase with age. This phenomenon is due to the appearance of mental disorders in persons with no prior psychiatric history as well as the persistence or reappearance of mental problems in persons with a previous psychiatric history. Some of these mental disorders are found primarily in older adults, while others occur across the life span. This discussion will focus on three mental disorders of older adults: depression, paranoia and organic brain syndrome. These three were selected for discussion because they are the most common forms of mental disturbance among the elderly and because they are the problems most likely to be encountered by nurses caring for older adults at home.

Depression and Suicide

Because depression is the most common psychological problem experienced by the elderly (Whitehead, 1974), nurses need to be aware of its symptoms and appropriate methods of treatment. Numerous theories exist to explain why depression occurs in the elderly and other populations, but most psychological theories have in common an emphasis on loss and the perception of helplessness.

Because these two phenomena are the expected condition of the aging, it is not surprising to learn that surveys of the elderly have found that most older persons, regardless of living arrangement, report depressive symptoms (Gallagher and Thompson, in press).

The frequency of depressive experiences in the elderly means that nurses need to be especially familiar with the clinical symptoms of depression. Recognition of the indicators of depression, assessment of their severity, including suicide risk, knowledge of methods of intervening in the home, and awareness of the need for outside consultation or for hospitalization are therefore important areas of expertise required of the home health nurse.

Epidemiology Despite its apparent frequency of occurrence, depression in the elderly is a surprisingly difficult disorder for which to establish prevalence and incidence statistics. Recent changes in the psychiatric criteria for the presence of an affective disorder result in a probable underreporting even of clinically significant depression. The best epidemiological statistics available thus far concern the more severe forms of depression such as those requiring hospitalization. Studies estimate that about 1% of the elderly (65 years or older) are typically found to experience severe depressive disorders. Other estimates place the figure at 4 to 6% (Gallagher and Thompson, in press; Stenback, 1980). Most researchers consider psychotic depressive reactions to be relatively rare (Kay and Bergmann, 1980). Some 20 to 25% of older adults overall are thought to experience the milder "depressive states" (Stenback, 1980). If less severe isolated symptoms not constituting a diagnosable entity were tallied, the prevalence figures would probably escalate dramatically.

Older persons are also at relatively high risk for suicide. Unlike other age groups, the elderly rarely use suicide as a means for communicating a need for help or an expression of anger. Rather, their attempts at suicide reflect the desire to die (Busse and Pfeiffer, 1973). When the elderly attempt suicide, it is therefore more likely to be successful (Butler and Lewis, 1982). As in all age groups, males are more likely than females to commit suicide. The peak incidence of suicide for males occurs in the older years, especially in the 75 to 79 and over-85 age groups. Recent statistics show a rate of 41.4 per 100,000 for men and 7.2 per 100,000 for women in the over-65 age groups, compared to averages across all age ranges of 20.1 for men and 6.8 for women (Butler and Lewis, 1982). Suicide risk is especially high after the loss of a spouse (Lazarus and Weinberg, 1980).

Diagnosis Depression can be episodic or chronic and of differential severity, both in the elderly and other populations. Mild and transitory (a few days or less) depression is probably experienced by most elderly persons from time to time (Cohen, 1981). Such "bad days" can be in reaction to specific stressful life events (for example, the loss of peers) or can occur in response to concerns about the new limitations that accompany aging. More severe depression can be precipitated by reactions to similar events, or by more severe stressors (for example, loss of a spouse). Physical illnesses (Butler and Lewis, 1982) can also precipitate depression. In some cases, organic mental disorders can cause depression as a side effect.

Thus, depressive symptomatology differs in degree more than in kind. Differentiation of the severity of the depression may be made by evaluating the extent of an individual's withdrawal from usual daily activities, the presence or absence of the so-called vegetative symptoms (physical symptoms of depression such as sleeplessness and anorexia), and the responsiveness of the depression to such simple intervention as support, empathy and concern.

The Diagnostic and Statistical Manual of Mental Disorders, or *DSM-III* (DSM, American Psychiatric Association, 1980), classifies depression as an affective disorder and differentiates between major depressive episodes (unipolar and bipolar) and dysthymic disorders (or, depressive neuroses). Because both are considered generally to have initial onset early in life, they are therefore of limited usefulness in assigning diagnostic labels to the more transitory, subclinical (for example, nondiagnosable) depression of many older persons, although the elderly can certainly also experience such disorders. Symptoms in both *DSM-III* types of depression are similar except that a major depressive disorder is more severe and can have psychotic features, such as delusions or hallucinations, unlike the dysthymic disorders.

Almost all depressive disturbances share symptoms of withdrawal and disturbances of mood. The typical depressed individual has a sleep disturbance (sleeps too little or too much), a decrement in energy from prior levels, and is pessimistic and "down" in mood. Some persons express their depression through anger, crying, or problems in memory and concentration ability. Others have somatic preoccupations.

Gallagher and Thompson (in press), noted that the diagnosis of clinical depression requires depressive symptomatology of two weeks' or more duration, the presence of dysphoria, disruption of day-to-day functioning, and physical symptoms such as appetite and sleep disturbances. They also noted that over- or underdiagnosis can result from the practitioner not knowing how to properly interview elderly clients who are often not receptive to questions typically asked in a standard psychiatric interview, such as questions about their mental status, loneliness or fears. (Guidelines for psychological assessment of the elderly will be suggested later in this chapter.)

Treatment Many different treatment modalities have been suggested for the clinically depressed, including anti-depressant medication, behavioral monitoring of mood and behavior, and cognitive and other psychotherapies (Gallagher and Thompson, in press). The type of intervention used depends on the kind of depression manifested. Severe depressions often require inpatient treatment sometimes including electroconvulsive shock therapy. Criteria for hospitalization of depressed clients include extreme isolation and self-neglect, the need for care which cannot be provided (because of the unavailability or inappropriateness) at home, and the likelihood of a person's being harmful to himself (Bellak and Karasu, 1976). Brink (1979) suggested that uncomplicated reactive depression is usually responsive to brief supportive treatment, or to the temporary use of anti-depressant medication. Even when out-of-the-home treatment is employed, the home health nurse can provide adjunctive psychological intervention. Supportive listening may be of special value. The depressed person often feels cut off from his or her previous life supports and misunderstood. By making a sincere effort to understand the person's perspective and to empathize with the individual's realization of such phenomena as unrestorable losses (Stenback, 1980), the nurse can provide therapeutic assistance.

The nurse who cares for depressed clients must also distinguish between depression associated with losses of older persons compared with those of younger individuals. For the young person, the psychological task associated with losses is both grief and replacement by suitable new love objects. For the older person, the losses are often not remediable. The nurse who attempts to handle the older person's depression by encouraging actions to restore losses will, therefore, not necessarily be of help; simple listening and "being with" the individual may suffice.

Depression can also be precipitated by feelings of guilt and concern over past mistakes. Self-recrimination and the presumption that the person is to blame for his present life predicament may result in or exacerbate depressed feelings. The home health nurse does not have to be a psychotherapist to be helpful to such a client. The nurse can encourage the individual to accept past shortcomings, be more tolerant of failures, and more accepting of past accomplishments and strengths.

Some persons will require outpatient intervention by a trained psychotherapist who is a psychologist, psychiatric nurse, psychiatrist or social worker. The home health nurse should consider such a referral when: a) the diagnosis or extent of depression is unclear; b) mild symptoms are unresponsive to informal interventions; or c) the depressive features are very severe. When therapy is available in the community and the client is able to maintain present living arrangements while receiving such treatment, the nurse can help assure that the client attends the therapy sessions and can provide follow-up help in the home. This can include support in maintaining adherence to medication schedules, assistance to the person who angrily decides to drop out of psychological treatment, and explanations of what is to be expected in the psychological therapies.

The referring nurse should know that few studies yet exist to suggest which kind of psychological intervention works best with different elderly persons. In general, the uncovering, psychoanalytic methods seem to be less helpful to depressed clients than the more structured cognitive and behavioral methods. Many of the latter approaches require homework assignments between sessions that may increase the transfer of the therapeutic benefits to the home situation.

Paranoid Disorders

Like other forms of emotional disturbance, paranoid reactions differ in severity and age of onset. Reactions may involve suspiciousness and self-preoccupation, but the overt paranoid psychosis reflects a much more extensive interruption of normal cognitive and/or affective processes (including the presence of a thought disorder) and behavioral problems. While severe forms of paranoia, including those posing a threat to others or involving a rigid and intact delusional system, will generally require intervention by a mental health specialist, milder forms may be amenable to home intervention.

Paranoid disorders can be extensions or exacerbations of life-long patterns of withdrawal, suspicion and hostility, or may first be experienced in later life. The latter occurrence, when associated with severe symptoms, has been called paraphrenia (Butler and Lewis, 1982). Post (1980) noted that psychotic paranoid symptoms always involve hallucinatory phenomena, especially auditory ones. A subgroup of such persons demonstrates schizophrenic symptoms as well. Milder forms of paranoia may involve very circumscribed areas of the client's life, or behaviors which perhaps are tolerated by persons in the individual's environment.

Epidemiology The prevalence and incidence of paranoid disorders among the elderly is not well established, partly due to the lack of a generally accepted set of criteria as to what constitutes paranoia, and partly due to the rather haphazard differentiation made among various subtypes of paranoid reactions. Hayslip (1983) noted that paranoid reactions are the second most common psychological disorder among the elderly. Based on admissions to psychiatric and other hospitals, the prevalence of paranoid disorders as a primary diagnosis appears to be rather low; if more isolated symptomatology is included, the rate is considerably higher (Post, 1980).

Diagnosis Some forms of paranoia may develop from the aging process itself, although this is currently disputed (Post, 1980). For example, an uncorrected hearing loss may cause the person to assume that others are not speaking to him or her and then to believe that they are being avoided (Welford, 1980). One study showed a greater likelihood for persons hospitalized with paranoid symptoms to have uncorrected hearing problems than those who were experiencing affective disorders (Ray, Cooper, Garside and Roth, 1976). The loss of a spouse, or of close friends and relatives, also lends credence to a "conspiracy theory" view of the world. Indeed, paranoid symptoms may reflect an attributional process, a way of making sense of the disturbing things happening to the individual and to those in the environment. It must also be noted that apparently paranoid behavior is sometimes based on quite appropriate fears of loss of property by relatives attempting to exploit the person's helplessness or increased dependence. Others have noted the objective incidence of physical abuse of the elderly adult (Kirkham, 1981).

In determining the need for psychiatric referral, the nurse in the home should note the following: a) the apparent severity of the disturbed thinking; b) the consistency of suspiciousness, both in the person's present behavior and across the life cycle; c) whether the "paranoid" ideation may reasonably be true, or at least grounded in a legitimate fear; d) the disruptiveness to the person's life of the symptoms; and e) the likelihood of threat to others. Regarding the latter, the nurse should make note of the content of the client's paranoid beliefs, and inquire about the client's plans, if any, to act upon the belief system. A mental health specialist is recommended when there is doubt about the extent of the paranoia, because of the possibility of harm to others.

Treatment The most easily treated paranoid behavior or thinking that can be easily treated should first be ruled out and corrected, if necessary. For example, the person who is suspicious about what others are saying about him should be examined to rule out unsuspected hearing loss or an improperly fit hearing aid. Similarly, poor fitting glasses or clouded vision caused by cataracts or other eye disorders may also cause the client to invoke paranoid "explanations" for the changes.

In all dealings with the suspicious or paranoid individual, the home health nurse needs to be direct and honest, demonstrating respect both for the individual and for oneself. Paranoid persons are especially sensitive to the nurse who is not sincere or who does not set needed limits. When the individual is experiencing changes that may be anxiety provoking, such as sensory losses, clear explanations should be offered; when known, suggestions can be made on how to cope with the perceptual dysfunctions. Similarly, information that cannot be shared with the person should be withheld with a reasonable explanation of the need for non-disclosure. The consistent, caring expression of concern for the individual presented in a sincere, genuine manner, can do much to restore the human link so often absent in the paranoid disorders (Kaufman, 1979).

Interaction with paranoid individuals is often very difficult. They frequently offer no overt gratitude or appreciation to their helpers. The nurse needs to know that such persons are often, at least for the present, unable to be responsive to human help. The nurse must, therefore, be aware and supportive of all team members and assess them for burnout. The nurse must also be alert to possible verbal or physical abuse of the client by the professional worker or home health aide. Clients express their fears of intimacy by anger and hostility, attempting to keep people distant. Consistency of behavior and of help is of considerable importance, even when the nurse may not be feeling charitable to such an obstinate or hostile person. Unlike many psychological disorders, even minimal trust by the paranoid client may take months or years to develop.

The more severely disturbed paranoid individual may require anti-psychotic medications to relieve or temper the delusional system. Although such treatment will not usually be initiated in the home care setting, the nurse can still be influential through home visits to help assure that the client adheres to the medication regimen upon returning home.

Organic Brain Syndromes

Organic brain syndromes are among the most devastating illnesses both to older people and their families. This group of disorders, which includes both reversible and nonreversible forms, occurs with relatively high frequency in older adults. Because the incidence of organic brain syndromes in later life is high, it is important for home health nurses to be acquainted with the signs and symptoms of these disorders and intervention strategies. Given the severity of organic brain syndromes, it is also necessary for nurses to understand whether they should be treated at home or in the hospital.

Organic brain syndromes are a group of disorders characterized by global impairment of mental faculties caused by organic changes in the brain. The classic features of these disorders are impairment in memory, intellect and judgment, as well as orientation, and labile and shallow affect (Butler and Lewis, 1982). Causes of the organic brain syndromes include primary diseases of the brain, systemic illnesses that affect the brain, chemical agents that disturb the brain temporarily or permanently, and withdrawal of substances on which an individual is physiologically dependent (Butler and Lewis, 1982). This discussion will focus on the two most common organic brain syndromes in adults—delirium and dementia.

Delirium (which replaces the formerly used term, "acute brain disorders") results from widespread derangement of the cerebral metabolism and from neurotransmission disturbances (Butler and Lewis, 1982). Dementia, which corresponds to the previous term "chronic brain disorders," is a group of disorders that result from neurological changes in or death of brain cells. The more common forms of dementia in older adults are primary degenerative dementia with senile onset or senile dementia of Alzheimer's type and multiinfarct dementia.

Epidemiology It was once thought that aging was accompanied by inevitable mental decline. However, it is now recognized that severe mental decline occurs in only a small percentage of older adults even though age-related changes do take place in the brain. It is estimated that only 5% of adults 65 years of age and older are severely impaired due to organic brain syndromes and an additional 10% are mildly or moderately impaired (National Institute of Health, 1981). Thus, 85% of all older adults experience no such impairment.

The incidence and prevalence of delirium has not been documented, probably because of the multiplicity of etiologies and the frequency of misdiagnosis. While the true incidence and prevalence of dementia is also unknown, it has been estimated that approximately 6% of all persons 65 years of age and over have dementia (Wolanin and Phillips, 1981). Of those persons with diagnosed dementia, 50% or more have senile dementia of the Alzheimer's type and another 15–25%

have multiinfarct dementia (Eisdorfer et al., 1981). An additional 20% of those with dementia may have both senile dementia of the Alzheimer's type and multiinfarct dementia (Wolanin and Phillips, 1981).

The age of onset and prevalence by sex varies according to the type of dementia. Senile dementia of the Alzheimer's type has an average age of onset of 75 years and is especially common among persons over age 80. Moreover, it is found more frequently in women than in men though this may be confounded by the longer lives of women. The average age of onset of multiinfarct dementia is younger than that of senile dementia, 66 years. It is also far more frequent in men than in women, perhaps in part because of the higher incidence of hypertension in men.

Diagnosis The diagnosis of organic brain syndromes can be difficult because it must be made by exclusion. There are no definitive diagnostic tests for delirium or dementia. To ascertain organic brain syndrome, an extensive diagnostic evaluation must be performed. This should include a complete history and physical examination as well as a mental status examination. Because the client may be a poor historian, the assistance of a relative or friend may be needed. Delirium is ascertained by the discovery of a causative agent. Because there are no diagnostic tests for dementia and its cause is not known, the diagnosis is arrived at by eliminating all possible alternative diagnoses.

Delirium is a reversible form of organic brain syndrome with multiple etiologies. Some of the more common causes of delirium include circulatory diseases, nutritional disorders, infectious disorders, pulmonary diseases, drugs and other toxic agents, structural causes, such as tumors, and psychiatric problems (Eisdorfer, Cohen, and Veith, 1981). Typically, the symptoms of delirium have a sudden onset and can often lead to rapid deterioration and even death if treatment is not instituted promptly (Burnside, 1981). Delirium is of short duration, with possible outcomes being death, recovery or a chronic brain syndrome. The primary consideration in delirium is the determination of the underlying cause so that treatment can be initiated immediately.

The dementias are nonreversible disorders, the most common being dementia with senile onset or senile dementia of the Alzheimer's type and multiinfarct dementia. While the cause of senile dementia of the Alzheimer's type is unknown, the following have been proposed as possible causes: increased aluminum concentration in the brain; autoimmune disease; cholinergic system deficiency; genetic risk factors; and latent viral infections (Butler and Lewis, 1982; Wolanin and Phillips, 1981). On autopsy of victims of senile dementia of the Alzheimer's type, characteristic pathological findings are brain atrophy, senile or neuritic plaques which are degenerative parts of nerve cells that surround a core of fibrous material, and neurofibrillary tangles of fine nerve fibers twisted around each other and found in the cell bodies of neurons ("The Dementias," 1981). Both senile plaques and neurofibrillary tangles are found in the brains of normal older adults, but their numbers are higher in demented persons. The greater the number of plaques and tangles in an individual's brain, the greater the severity of the symptoms of dementia.

Multiinfarct dementia is associated with atherosclerosis and arteriosclerosis which result in restricted blood flow to the brain. The infarcts of multiinfarct dementia are cystic infarcts or lacunes which are located in the brain, arising from emboli lodged in the brain and resulting in the softening and death of brain tissue (Wolanin and Phillips, 1981). Lacunes are also found in the brains of non-demented older adults. The actual cause of multiinfarct dementia awaits discovery.

Once the presence of dementia has been ascertained, a differential diagnosis must be made as to the type of dementia. While there are no tests that differentiate between senile dementia of the Alzheimer's type and multiinfarct dementia, the clinical course of the two types varies. Senile dementia is characterized by a slow, steady, progressive decline in mental and physical functioning. Neurological signs and symptoms are global. In contrast, multiinfarct dementia typically has a sudden onset, the decline is intermittent and uneven, and there is evidence of focal neurological abnormalities. It is also associated with a history of hypertension and circulatory problems.

The signs and symptoms of dementia vary by the type and stage of the illness. The predominant signs and symptoms of senile dementia of the Alzheimer's type include: memory loss, particularly for recent events; impaired intellectual functioning including attention, learning, judgment, and abstraction deficits; apathy and withdrawal; decreased ability to adapt to the environment; language deficits; impaired social skills; disorientation; and loss of self care (Eisdorfer et al., 1982; "The Dementias," 1981). Ultimately, the person experiences extensive physical and mental deterioration culminating in death. These signs and symptoms are indicative of the global neurological abnormalities present in the disorder. The signs and symptoms of multiinfarct dementia are more variable than those of senile dementia because they are determined by specific focal neurologial abnormalities. Common signs and symptoms of multiinfarct dementia include confusion, impairment in memory, dizziness, headaches, decreased energy, and vague physical complaints ("The Dementias," 1981). Regardless of the form of dementia, it is important to clarify the nature of the cognitive impairments because they affect the person's ability to adapt to the environment and thereby affect the need for institutional care.

Treatment The treatment of delirium varies according to its etiology. Regardless of the cause of delirium, it is a medical emergency and usually requires hospital care. The major role of the home health nurse is to recognize the presence of delirium and make appropriate referrals for treatment (Wolanin and Phillips, 1981). Delirium is resolved either by recovery, death or a chronic brain syndrome.

This section will focus on the care of persons with dementia because the home health nurse is most likely to care for such individuals at home. Because the cause of dementia is not known, treatment is directed either at possible causes of dementia or at its behavioral manifestations. The goals for treating demented older adults at home are to maximize the client's functioning, promote independence, and maintain the individual at home as long as possible.

A variety of medical treatments may be initiated in the care of the demented older adult. Each is directed at resolving a possible cause of dementia. Diet therapy has been given to some individuals, the diet being high in materials that comprise acetylcholine ("The Dementias," 1981). Drug therapy has also been attempted. Demented adults have been prescribed drugs intended to prevent the breakdown of acetylcholine, drugs for improving memory, and drugs which bind aluminum to rid the body of excessive aluminum (National Institute of Health, 1981). None of these treatments has had demonstrable success in arresting or slowing the decline associated with dementia. To date, the most effective treatment of dementia consists of resolving all nonrelated physical and psychological problems, followed by management of the client's dementia-related problems.

Caring for the demented older adult at home can be a time-consuming and draining experience with few rewards. The home health nurse plays a critical role by: providing direct care to these clients; support and care to the daily caregivers as well as to other family and friends; information and referral to community resources; and by assisting in institutionalization when appropriate.

Most families prefer to keep their demented relatives at home as long as possible. The nurse can assist them by aiding in the creation and maintenance of a safe, structured home environment, by providing a consistent daily routine in individual exercise, and by offering opportunities for socialization and skill building (Eisdorfer et al., 1981).

The home health nurse may be more actively involved with the caregivers of the demented person than the client. The caregivers can benefit not only from information and advice on managing the physical and emotional care of their relative, but also from the support and encouragement that the nurse can offer. In addition, the nurse may suggest that the caregivers seek community support services, for example, a home health aide to assist in physical care, legal counsel to aid in managing legal and financial matters, a day hospital or day care to provide the client with opportunities for activity and socialization in a structured environment, and support groups for the caregivers themselves, available in community mental health centers, hospital-based clinics, or through voluntary organizations, such as the Area Council on Aging or the local chapter of the Alzheimer's Disease and Related Disorders Association.

Caregivers of demented persons find it most difficult to manage their loved ones when the disease process has reached an advanced stage. Behaviors that are especially difficult for caregivers to endure include incontinence, wandering, physical aggression, lack of recognition of familiar persons, and social unresponsiveness. Since the caregivers may be elderly themselves, the burden of caring for demented individuals may be especially great. Respite care can offer much needed rest and relaxation for the caregivers. Judicious use of medication may also assist caregivers in managing sleep disturbances, agitation and aggression; however, given the numerous side effects of most sedatives and major tranquilizers, they should only be employed when other management techniques have failed.

Ultimately, it may be necessary to institutionalize the demented older adult. Factors to assess when considering institutionalization include disturbances in thinking and affect, serious physical illness, harmful behavior to oneself or to others, and unavailability or inability of caregivers to provide the necessary care (Butler and Lewis, 1982). The decision to institutionalize is an individual matter because it depends on the client's condition and the resources of the caregiver.

Most demented persons live five to ten years following the onset of the disease. While dementia is always fatal, it is rarely the cause of death. Common causes of death include infections, malnutrition, injury or fluid and electrolyte imbalances (Wolanin and Phillips, 1981). Death of the demented person may come as a relief to the caregiver and other loved ones because of the burden they are shouldering. In addition, they may welcome an end to the physical and mental suffering of their relative. Given the drastic personality and behavioral changes experienced by demented adults, they may feel as though they lost the relative they once knew. While the rewards to caregivers of demented persons are few, they obtain satisfaction in the knowledge that they provided the best care possible to their relatives.

(For suggestions on managing specific behaviors commonly exhibited by demented persons, see Burnside, 1981.)

Home and Community Health Care Interventions with the Mentally Disturbed

As the emphasis on home health care of the aged has increased, so has the number and variety of services available to community-residing aged with mental health problems or needs. Some of these services can be provided in the client's home, while others are offered in the community. The target of these services also varies. Typically, the focus of the service is the individual, couple or family with actual or potential mental health problems. However, the recipient of services may also be the spouse, sibling, child, grandchild or other relative or friend who is providing care or support. The more common services offered to caregivers and to older adults with psychological needs will be reviewed in this section. The goal of all such interventions is to minimize the dysfunctional effects of mental health problems, to maximize independent functioning, and to avoid or delay long-term institutionalization whenever possible.

Obstacles to Mental Health Care of the Aged

The aged person, as a potential recipient of services, the mental health professional, as a potential health care provider to the older adult, and the social milieu of the elderly, all can act as obstacles to older adults obtaining the mental health care they need (Gaitz, 1974). Many elders are reluctant to seek mental health services because of their lack of information about mental health problems, their fear of the stigma of mental illness, their lack of awareness of mental health services, their belief that mental problems are untreatable, and their inability or reluctance to admit their mental health difficulties and their consequent need for assistance (Sparacino, 1978–79). Even if older adults recognize the need for help, they may resist seeking it because of lack of confidence in the benefits of treatment, vulnerability, fear of change, and belief that available services are poorly suited to individual needs.

Another barrier to mental health care of the aged is the mental health professional. Few persons in any of the mental health disciplines have been prepared to work with older adults; among the untrained, few have had experience working with this population. Moreover, many mental health professionals may hold negative attitudes toward the aged, stereotyping them as dull, uninteresting, of low conceptual ability, dependent, lacking in energy, unproductive and having limited ability to change (Davis and Klopfer, 1977).

Other reasons mental health personnel avoid working with older adults include: fear of arousing the therapists' own anxieties about impending old age; difficulties they may have maintaining distance from the problems of the aged; fear that older clients may die during the treatment; frustration with the sometimes slow progress in therapy; unconscious over-identification with the elderly, especially if they are physically disabled; discomfort with the potentially unpleasant or threatening prospect of witnessing and sharing in the pain that many older persons experience; and arousal of conflict with "parental" figures through contact with persons of similar age to their own parents ("The Aged and Community Mental Health," 1971).

Even if professionals have positive attitudes toward older adults, they may question the treatability of this age group or believe that treatment would be a poor investment given their few remaining years. The therapists who choose to treat older adults are unlikely to receive much support from their colleagues, their efforts instead being greeted with curiosity, puzzlement, or even hostility. Sometimes such therapists may be advised to redirect their energies in "more fruitful" directions ("The Aged and Community Mental Health," 1971; Kastenbaum, 1964; Lawton and Gottesman, 1974).

The social milieu also serves to hinder older adults from obtaining needed mental health services. Many aged adults lack the financial resources to pay for mental health care. Given that a large number of the elderly are retired and living on fixed incomes, they are sorely pressed to obtain home necessities and thus cannot afford such "luxuries" as mental health care. Preventive mental health services are almost never covered by insurance or other reimbursement plans. Medicare, the major form of health insurance for most older Americans, currently provides a maximum of $250 per year for outpatient mental health care (Herman, 1980). Some state Medicaid programs offer supplemental assistance, but the nature and extent of such programs varies widely. Private health insurance, as well as Medicare, often encourages costly and stigmatizing hospitalization by providing much better benefits for inpatient than for outpatient mental health care. As a result, older adults may be priced out of the market for mental health care, even if they are receptive to such intervention.

Yet another obstacle to older persons' obtaining mental health services concerns their attitudes toward psychological intervention. Most of today's elderly were raised in eras when self sufficiency was regarded as extremely important. Asking *anyone* for help, much less a mental health provider, was seldom encouraged. Older adults, therefore, may avoid any services perceived to be psychological in nature.

Types of Mental Health Services for Elderly in the Home

There are many forms of intervention for older persons who experience psychological problems. A recent review article by Hayslip (in press) discussed general treatment considerations, specially for clinic- or hospital-based interventions. An entire issue of *Psychotherapy: Theory, Research & Practice* (Gottsegen and Park, 1982) illustrated the diversity of psychotherapeutic approaches to the aged. Other authors have recommended psychotherapeutic strategies to be used in treating specific disorders (for example, Butler, 1975; Gallagher, 1981; Gallagher and Thompson, 1982).

While such work makes valuable contributions to the psychotherapy of the aged, it is not the primary concern of this chapter. Rather, the authors' interest is in addressing the types of mental health interventions that can be provided or coordinated by the home health nurse and which do not require specialized training in mental health. Therefore, this chapter will focus primarily on interventions that can be provided in the home, or those of a preventive nature in the community that can be coordinated by the home health nurse.

Mental Health Assessment

The nurse in the home must first know how to make a mental health assessment to determine the present mental and psychological status of the client and the type of treatment or referral which is needed. Such assessments can be brief, or more protracted, but should focus on the older adult within the context of his familial, social, cultural and community environments because behavior can only be meaningfully evaluated when considered within the circumstances in which it occurs.

Prior to initiating the interview, attention should be directed to the interview setting. It should be private, free of noise and distractions, comfortable and conducive to the establishment of trust and rapport (Hayslip, 1983). In addition, the purpose of the interview and the uses to be made of the data collected should be explained to the older adult before beginning the assessment. The interview itself should focus on evaluating the concerns of the older adult, his mental status, his personal and environmental resources, and his limitations—physical, emotional, financial, social and environmental. Blake (1980) suggested that a psychological assessment of the older adult should cover the following areas: a detailed problem description, including associated problems and symptoms; patterns of sleep disturbance; bodily functions and mental status; past health history; drug history; family and marital (including sexual) history; current activities; and other topics relevant to the specific client.

A physical examination should be performed as part of the assessment. Obviously, to collect all this information may take more than one interview, depending on the client's attention span, physical health, alertness, verbal facility, and other factors. Additionally, it may be desirable to interview significant others in the older person's life, to determine their understanding of the situation and the client's present functioning, as well as to obtain a historical perspective.

Nursing personnel not familiar with procedures in a mental status examination may want to make use of a structured instrument such as the Mental Status Questionnaire (Kahn, Goldfarb, and Pollack, 1960), a brief screening tool consisting of questions concerning the client's orientation to person, time and place. While this measure is highly accurate in detecting cognitive disturbances, some of the items may have little relevance to older adults, (for example, knowledge of the exact date).

The nurse also needs to be aware that such assessments must be artfully performed. A depressed patient, for example, may disguise mood disturbance by giving answers of "I don't know" to many questions. The skilled interviewer seeks to separate the responses of those persons who truly do not know from those of individuals with insufficient energy to respond. In addition, hostile or suspicious individuals may require extreme skill, tact and patience on the part of the examiner to obtain a thorough assessment of their present functioning. The assistance of relatives or appropriate informants may need to be judiciously utilized with such clients. Finally, multiple brief visits may often be more desirable than one or a few very long encounters, to better establish rapport, to gather an adequate baseline of the problematic behavior, and to avoid exhausting or alienating the client.

Interventions

Having established the specific psychological problem the client is experiencing, or the need for referral to obtain assistance in diagnosis, the home health nurse often has several intervention strategies from which to choose. These can be categorized into those services that can be provided in the home and those that are community based.

For those clients who reside in the home, are home bound, lack transportation, or live in rural areas, a number of services are available. One of the most common and longstanding of these is home health care. Such services include the care provided by health professionals, such as nurses; hot meal programs; telephone reassurance programs; and home visitor services. Many such programs rely on the participation of volunteers.

Health professionals may provide care to older adults in their homes whenever these individuals are unable to seek such care in the community. These health care providers give their usual services in the client's home rather than in their offices. Mental health care has been delivered primarily by nurses and social workers (Butler and Lewis, 1982). Typically, aged clients are initially visited by home health nurses for the purpose of assessing the client's mental health needs. In some instances, the nurse may consult with a mental health professional regarding the nature of the client's difficulties, the most appropriate intervention, and effective methods for its implementation. Such consultation may include a home visit to the older adult to assess the situation first hand. If mental health intervention in the home is warranted, the nurse or the social worker is likely to be responsible for delivering the service or assuring its implementation. These interventions may be directed to the prevention of mental health problems or to their amelioration, the specifics being tailored to the individual client's needs.

Another service which can promote the client's psychological well-being is home food service, such as the Meals-on-Wheels program. For aged persons unable or unwilling to cook for themselves or who do not have proper nutrition, this service can be beneficial because an inadequate diet can contribute to mental health problems, potentially exacerbating symptoms of depression or dementia. While not all persons using the home food service are satisfied with it (some complain about the cost, the lack of choice over the food, the time of day the meal is served, or its temperature on arrival), it does ensure a well-balanced meal (Murray, Huelskoetter, and O'Driscoll, 1980).

Telephone reassurance programs hold much promise as a fairly inexpensive way of reaching the elderly. In most such systems, the older adult calls a designated person, or is phoned by a volunteer. Such contact is usually on a daily basis, providing a social outlet and offering reassurance that someone is concerned. This form of intervention allows access to home-bound persons, and to those with relatively minor mental health problems not requiring either institutionalization or a service like medication. This service is also useful for the client who may resent more intrusive face-to-face contact. A variation of this approach is a program initiated by some communities involving companionship or visitor programs for older adults. Such visits are face-to-face and keep the older person actively involved with others. Approaches such as these may help the elderly remain in their homes.

Community-Based Interventions

In addition to services offered in the home, many communities offer mental health services to the elderly. Some of these address direct intervention in mental health problems, while others emphasize prevention and accomplishment of the developmental tasks of later maturity discussed above.

Such care can be provided in a variety of locations. Community mental health centers are a common site, as are outpatient hospital-based clinics. Relatively few older adults receive mental health services from private practitioners, largely because of the cost of private care.

In many communities, there are a number of programs for older adults whose primary purpose is the maintenance and promotion of health and concomitantly the prevention of physical and mental decline. Two types of programs will be discussed: those whose main focus is health prevention and those whose primary emphasis is health maintenance.

Among the most common community programs for older adults are Senior Centers. Typically these centers provide a range of educational and recreational activities as well as health screening and counseling services. Possible activities include cards, bingo, arts and crafts, woodworking, book clubs, exercise and cooking. Services include blood pressure screening, tax preparation, vision screening, legal aid, and nutrition counseling. Such centers also serve as meeting places for older adults, providing opportunities for sharing of common interests and companionship. In most centers, meals, usually lunch, are served. For those who lack transportation to the center, rides may be provided by community agencies or center volunteers. Sponsors of Senior Centers include nonprofit organizations, for example, United Way or churches, private donors, and government agencies. The activities and services available in Senior Centers provide physical and mental stimulation to adults and thus encourage them to function at their maximum potential. As a result, Senior Centers can serve as a preventive mental health intervention by promoting socialization and the development of new friendships, and by encouraging the development of new interests and skills and the refinement of others, thereby offering new sources of satisfaction and self esteem.

Preventive Intervention Through Volunteer and Self-Help Programs

Volunteer programs provide another type of community-based intervention for the elderly. Older adults volunteer their services, either without pay, or for a small remuneration. Such programs provide an outlet for those elderly who want to remain active and productive, or to help others. Examples of such programs include Foster Grandparents, Retired Senior Volunteer Programs (RSVP), the Service Corps of Retired Executives (SCORE), and the Senior Companion Program. The Foster Grandparents program is a federally funded program which employs low-income retired adults to work with children in a variety of institutional settings, such as children's hospitals, juvenile correction centers, psychiatric wards, and state schools for the retarded. Program participants are paid a small salary for their services. The R.S.V.P. program provides volunteers to work in a wide range of community settings commensurate with the volunteers' skills and abilities. Settings vary with the needs of the community but may include day care centers, hospitals, courts, schools and nursing homes. The Service Corps of Retired Executives coordinates the services of retired executives and the needs of small businesses requesting assistance. Finally, the Senior Companion Program is a federally sponsored program that employs low-income older adults to give care and provide companionship to other older adults, typically persons who are home bound or institutionalized (Bruce, 1981). All of these programs provide older adults with opportunities to share their talents and skills with others and, therefore, promote positive feelings of self esteem and may reduce frequent causes of depression, particularly among those who were productive citizens prior to their retirement. Such programs can serve to deter the development of mental health problems by providing opportunities for activity, productive achievement, fulfillment, socialization and involvement through helping others.

Older adults may also seek opportunities for self-improvement or for improving life for the aged as a group. Two recent programs designed to enhance the self-development of older adults are Elderhostel and Senior Actualization Group Experience (SAGE). Elderhostel is a program that provides educational experiences for older adults. Typically, these courses are offered at local colleges and universities over short time periods, for example, one to two weeks. Course offerings vary from leisure subjects (quilting or music) to intellectual topics (current American politics or nuclear arms debates). Participants in these courses welcome the opportunity to continue their learning in a noncompetitive atmosphere with peers as fellow students. SAGE is a program combining elements of the self-help, human potential, and holistic health movements in an effort to provide older adults with a personal growth experience. Offerings include exercise, group discussion, lectures and meditation. The program purports to influence a wide range of physical, psychological and social behaviors, although a recent extensive evaluation of some participants indicated that the program's effects, while positive, were not as widespread as claimed (Lieberman and Gourash, 1979).

Older adults may also seek fulfillment by working toward improving life for all other Americans. Some persons may take an active part in political action groups for older citizens, the largest being the National Council of Senior Citizens and the American Association of Retired Persons (Butler and Lewis, 1982). Such organizations work toward the advancement of the quality of life for older adults by lobbying for improvements in Social Security and Medicare benefits, housing, health care, and other services for older adults, as well as by providing their members with a variety of free or low-cost services, such as discounts on drugs, insurance and travel. The Gray Panthers, another such organization, also seek to improve the quality of life for older adults, although they have adopted a more activist strategy for change than the organizations already discussed. These and other such organizations for older adults provide them with opportunities for active involvement in helping their fellow older adults and those who will become older adults in the future. Participation in such organizations may promote feelings of self esteem productive achievement service and thereby serve to deter the development of mental health difficulties.

However, it must also be noted that the presumed established effects of such programs have not yet been reliably established in the literature. It is doubtful that active participation prevents all psychological problems, although it may well forestall more serious forms of mental disorders. Still very much needed are studies identifying the type of older adult who benefits most from such interventions and the type of disorders they are most effective in preventing or treating. It would be interesting to know, for example, if the persons volunteering and benefitting from such activities are those who have always been active in these pursuits, or whether the involvements represent new undertakings. Establishment of the latter would provide more convincing evidence for the efficacy of these preventive-type programs. Finally, little is presently known about the ages at which such programs have the most impact: whether the "young-old" and the "old-old" similarly benefit from such endeavors still needs to be determined.

Other Community Programs and Services

Community programs are also available for older adults with significant mental health needs. Rather than institutionalize such persons, day and respite care programs can provide maintenance care and permit relatives or friends to keep their loved ones at home. Day hospitals provide hospital treatment to older persons with mental health problems during the daytime hours. Such treatment is more intensive than outpatient treatment yet less intensive than hospitalization. Services provided in day hospitals usually include individual, group and family therapy, occupational therapy, recreational activities, drug therapy, medical care, and milieu therapy. These programs are particularly beneficial to persons returning to the community following hospitalization and to persons needing more intensive treatment than can be provided on an outpatient basis. Day care centers also offer daytime services to older adults with mental health needs, although such services are provided in a nonhospital setting. The focus of day care is on social and recreational activities rather than on psychological treatment (for example, individual, group, and family therapy). Medical assistance, while available, may be limited. These programs are most appropriate for individuals unable to stay at home alone without supervision and who can benefit from the stimulation provided by the activities.

Respite care provides a break for relatives and friends who are responsible for home care of older adults. This service allows the caregivers the opportunity to rest, vacation or be away from home for a period of time. Older adults may be cared for in their homes, or they may be transferred to residential facilities ("Information on Home Health Care," 1982). Such care may make the difference between older adults being maintained at home and being institutionalized, since most caregivers could not maintain their households, let alone their sanity, without having these periods of relief.

Examples of Home Mental Health Care for the Elderly

The following two cases illustrate the difficulties as well as the rewards of working with the elderly in home care settings. They illustrate the need for the nurse to be flexible in approach, to know limitations, and to be able to work as a member of a health care team to meet the complex health problems of the elderly.

CASE PRESENTATION: MRS. BALL

Mrs. Ball, a 76-year-old married black female, was referred to the Public Health Department in the community by her physician. Her doctor wanted the Health Department to monitor her physical and psychological health. Reportedly, Mrs. Ball had been mentally retarded since birth. While she had always required some supervision and guidance in her daily activities, her husband, age 75, had been able to provide the needed assistance. However, over the past ten years, Mrs. Ball's physical and mental health functioning had gradually declined, and her husband was having increasing difficulty in managing her care. In addition, Mr. Ball's own health was poor, limiting his ability to aid his wife.

She had poor vision. She had cataracts removed from both eyes and wore glasses with thick lenses. She also had impaired hearing and severe arthritis in both knees, limiting her mobility. While her low intelligence had always restricted her ability to function independently, in recent years her alertness had gradually deteriorated, her interest in living had declined, and her participation in household chores had decreased. The problems of Mr. and Mrs. Ball were compounded by their low income, lack of transportation, and minimal social supports.

Initially, the home health nurse focused her visits with the couple on establishing rapport and collecting information on their current health needs and health care goals. Mr. and Mrs. Ball enjoyed and appreciated the nurse's visit because of their desire for social contact and attention. They also appreciated the nurse's interest and efforts to improve their health status. After carefully assessing the couple, the nurse concluded that they would benefit from a home health aide who could help her bathe and provide some help with household chores. A volunteer could transport the couple to their doctor's appointments and to the grocery store. A mental health evaluation to assess Mrs. Ball's current mental functioning was also warranted.

Despite her retardation, Mrs. Ball had never been formally evaluated for intellectual functioning. On referral by the nurse, Mrs. Ball was assessed by a consulting psychologist at the local mental health center to determine her current intellectual and adaptive functioning. These data were then reported to the referring nurse who was able to use them in her care of Mrs. Ball. In addition, a written report on Mrs. Ball's mental functioning was prepared and filed in case documentation was needed for subsequent institutionalization.

By providing the couple with needed support services, the nurse was able to help the couple in their desire to remain in their home. Furthermore, by requesting an evaluation of Mrs. Ball's mental functioning, the nurse obtained needed and documented information on Mrs. Ball's current mental status.

CASE PRESENTATION: MRS. ABLE

Mrs. Able, a 75-year-old widowed white female, was referred to the community mental health center for a mental health assessment. In the months prior to the referral, Mrs. Able had demonstrated progressive deterioration in her physical and mental health status. Initially followed by the home health nurse because of hypertension and multiple social problems, Mrs. Able, with increasing frequency, refused to take her hypertensive medication, claiming that it was poisoned. In addition, she resisted going to bed at night, remaining in a lounge chair. At times, she verbalized a fear of turning black if she were to sleep in her bed. She also rejected most of her food, stating that it, too, was poisoned. On a number of occasions, she heard voices and talked to them but would not reveal their identities. Two months prior to her referral to the public health nurse, she experienced two significant losses—the death of a grandchild she had raised and the death of a favorite niece. When relatives attempted to help her mourn these losses, she refused to discuss them and became very hostile and verbally abusive. Mrs. Able's children, two of whom lived with her, were quite distressed by her behavior and sought the aid of the public health nurse. This was Mrs. Able's first known episode of mental disturbance.

After making several home visits, the home health nurse requested a consultation from the local community mental health center. She sought an evaluation of Mrs. Able's mental state and her need for psychiatric hospitalization. A psychologist and a psychiatrist visited Mrs. Able in her home after she failed to keep an appointment at the mental health center because of her refusal to leave the home.

Mrs. Able, a small, frail woman, was dressed in a bathrobe and slippers and sat in a lounge chair in her living room. When addressed by the mental health center staff, she did not acknowledge them nor did she respond appropriately to their questions. Throughout their visit, she alternated between sitting staring into space and talking animatedly to her voices. It was evident that her deteriorated physical condition, largely due to her poor intake and her refusal to take her hypertensive medication, posed a serious threat to her life and her depressed and paranoid mental state had isolated her from reality. The mental health center staff recommended to Mrs. Able's relatives, who had assembled for the review of the evaluation results, that Mrs. Able be hospitalized, in order to prevent further decline in her physical and mental health and to provide her with the opportunity for intensive treatment. The relatives, while desperate for assistance with Mrs. Able, resisted the notion of psychiatric hospitalization, particularly since they would have to commit Mrs. Able because she would undoubtedly refuse to sign herself into the hospital. Mrs. Able was not considered sufficiently severely disturbed to meet her state's rather rigid requirements for involuntary hospitalization by a non-relative. The relatives decided to postpone making a commitment decision at that time, and two days later called the mental health center to say that they had decided against hospitalization.

Subsequently, the home health nurse continued to provide care to Mrs. Able in her home, which was felt to be a less than ideal solution to Mrs. Able's problems. This case illustrates that external circumstances may force compromises in optimal health care given by home health nurses.

Summary

This chapter has provided an overview of issues important to delivering home mental health care to the elderly. It has demonstrated that psychological problems among the elderly are commonplace, and that even the medically oriented nurse must have a working knowledge of the various psychological disturbances commonly encountered in the aged. Three major mental health problems of older persons were reviewed in detail: depression and suicide; paranoid reactions; and organic brain syndromes. Each presents special issues of diagnosis and treatment. The chapter also presented an extensive review of the various treatment modalities which can be provided both in the home and the community to help maintain the older client at home. These treatment approaches are multiple, including in-home services such as psychological consultation and telephone reassurance programs, and community-based maintenance and preventive programs, such as day care and R.S.V.P. All can have substantial impact on the mental health of the elderly although more systematic evaluation and research are needed. Finally, two case examples were presented that illustrate the complexities of working with older persons in the community.

REFERENCES

Abrahams R B, Patterson R D: "Psychological distress among the community elderly: Prevalence, characteristics and implications for service." *Internat J Aging Human Develop*, Vol 9, No 1, 1978–79, pp 1–18

Bellak L, Karasu T B: *Geriatric Psychiatry*. Grune & Stratton, New York, 1976

Blake D R: "Psychosocial assessment of elderly clients," in Burnside I M (ed); *Psychosocial Nursing Care of the Aged*. 2nd ed. McGraw-Hill, New York, 1980

Brink T L: *Geriatric Psychotherapy*. Human Sciences Press, New York, 1979

Bruce M F: "Community resources for the elderly," in Hogstel M O (ed); *Nursing Care of the Older Adult*. John Wiley & Sons, Inc., New York, 1981

Burnside I M: "Organic brain syndrome." In Burnside I M (ed); *Nursing and the Aged*. 2nd ed. McGraw-Hill, New York, 1981

Busse E W, Pfeiffer E: *Mental Illness in Later Life*. American Psychiatric Association, Washington, D.C., 1973

Butler R N: "Psychotherapy in old age," in Arieti S (ed): *American Handbook of Psychiatry*. Vol. 5, 2nd ed. Basic Books, New York, 1975

Butler R N, Lewis M I: *Aging and Mental Health: Positive Psychosocial Approaches*. 3rd ed. C. V. Mosby Co., St. Louis, 1982

Cohen G D: *"Depression in the elderly."* N.I.M.H. Fact Sheet: Center for Studies of the Mental Health of the Aging. D.H.H.S. Pub. No. (ADM) 81–932, 1981

DSM-III: Diagnostic and Statistical Manual of Mental Disorders. 3rd ed. American Psychiatric Association, Committee on Nomenclature and Statistics, Washington, D.C., 1980

David R W, Klopfer W G: "Issues in psychotherapy with the aged." *Psychotherapy: Theory, Research and Practice,* Vol 14, 1977, pp 343–348

Eisdorfer C, Cohen D, Veith R: *The Psychopathology of Aging* (Current Concepts series). Upjohn, Kalamazoo, Michigan, 1981

Erikson E H: *Childhood and Society.* 2nd ed. Norton, New York, 1963

Gaitz C M: "Barriers to the delivery of psychiatric services to the elderly." *The Gerontol,* Vol 14, No 3, June 1974, pp. 210–214

Gallagher D: "Behavioral group therapy with elderly depressives: An experimental study," in Upper D, Ross S (eds): *Behavioral Group Therapy.* Research Press, Champaign, Illinois, 1981

Gallagher D, Thompson L W: *Elders' maintenance of treatment benefits following individual psychotherapy for depression: Results of a pilot study and preliminary data from an ongoing replication study.* Paper presented at the meeting of the American Psychological Association, Washington, D.C., August, 1982

Gallagher D, Thompson L W: "Assessment and treatment of depression in the elderly: A review" in Lewinsohnn P M, Teri L (eds): *Coping and Adaptation in the Elderly.* Pergamon Press, Ltd., London, In press

Gottsegen G B, Park P D (eds): *Psychotherapy: Theory, Research and Practice,* American Psychological Association, Washington, D.C., Vol 19, 1982

Havighurst R L: *Developmental Tasks and Education.* 3rd ed. David McKay Company, New York, 1974

Hayslip Jr. B: "Mental health and aging" in Ernst N S, Glazer-Waldman H R (eds): *The Aged Patient: A Sourcebook for the Allied Health Professional.* Yearbook Medical Publishers, Chicago, 1983

Hayslip Jr. B: "Treatment modalities," in Esberger K and Hughes S (eds): *Nursing Care of the Aged.* Brady, Bowie, Maryland, In press

Herman R: "Geriatric psychiatry is much enfeebled." *New York Sunday Times,* January 27, 1980

Information On Home Health Care Services: A Handbook About Care In the Home. American Association of Retired Persons, Washington, D.C.

Jones A: "Developmental tasks of later middle age and old age," in Hogstel M O (ed): *Nursing Care of the Older Adult.* John Wiley & Sons, Inc., New York, 1981

Kahn R L, Goldfarb A I, Pollack M, Peck A: "Brief objective measures for the determination of mental status in the aged." *Am J Psych,* Vol 117, Pt 1, October 1960, pp 326–328

Kastenbaum R: "The reluctant therapist," in Kastenbaum R (ed): *New Thoughts on Old Age.* Springer, New York, 1964

Kaufman G: *Shame: The Power of Caring.* Schenkman, Cambridge, Massachusetts, 1980

Kirkham A K: "Crime against the elderly," in Hogstel M O (ed): *Nursing Care of the Older Adult.* John Wiley & Sons, Inc., New York, 1981

Kramer M, Taube C A, Redick R W: "Patterns of use of psychiatric facilities by the aged: Past, present, and future," in Eisdorfer C, Lawton M P (eds): *The Psychology of Adult Development and Aging.* American Psychological Association, Washington, D.C., 1973

Lawton M P, Gottesman L E: "Psychological services to the elderly." *Am Psychol,* Vol 29, No 9, September 1974, pp 689–93

Lazarus L W, Weinberg J: "Treatment in ambulatory care setting," in Busse E W, Blazer D C (eds): *Handbook of Geriatric Psychiatry.* Von Nostrand, New York, 1980

Lieberman M A, Gourash N: "Evaluating the effects of change groups on the elderly." *Inter J Group Psychotherapy,* Vol 29, 1979, pp 283–304

Murray R, Huelskoetter M M, O'Driscoll D: *The Nursing Process in Later Maturity.* Prentice Hall, Inc., Englewood Cliffs, New Jersey, 1980

Peck R: "Psychological developments in the second half of life," in Neugarten B (ed): *Middle Age and Aging*. The University of Chicago Press, Chicago, 1968

Post F: "Paranoid schizophrenia-like and schizophrenic states in the aged," in Birren J E, Sloan R B (eds): *Handbook of Mental Health and Aging*. Prentice Hall, Inc., Englewood Cliffs, New Jersey, 1980

Ray D W K, Cooper A F, Garside R F, Roth M: "The differentiation of paranoia from affective psychoses by patients' premorbid personalities." *British Journal of Psychiatry*, Vol 129, 1976, p 207

Report to the President from the President's Commission on Mental Health (3 vols.) President's Commission on Mental Health, U.S. Government Printing Office, Washington, D.C., 1978

Sparacino J: "Individual psychotherapy with the aged: A selective review." *Internat J Aging Human Develop*, Vol 9, 1978–79, pp 197–220

Stenback A: "Depression and suicidal behavior in old age," in Birren J E, Sloane R B (eds): *Handbook of Mental Health and Aging*. Prentice Hall, Inc., Englewood Cliffs, New Jersey, 1980

The Aged and Community Mental Health: A Guide to Program Development. Group for the Advancement of Psychiatry, New York, Author, 1971

The Dementias: Hope Through Research. Pub. No. 81-2252, National Institute of Health, Washington, D.C., 1981

Welford A T: "Sensory, perceptual, and motor processes in older adults," in Birren J E, Sloane R B (eds): *Handbook of Mental Health and Aging*. Prentice-Hall, Englewood Cliffs, New Jersey, 1980

Whitehead J A: *Psychiatric Disorders in Old Age*. Springer, New York, 1974

Wolanin M P, Phillips L R F: *Confusion: Prevention and Care*. C. V. Mosby, St. Louis, 1981

BIBLIOGRAPHY

Herr J J, Weakland J H: *Counseling Elders and their Families: Practical Techniques for Applied Gerontology*. Springer, New York, 1979

Mace N L, Rabins P V: *The 36-Hour Day*. The Johns Hopkins University Press, Baltimore, 1981

Zarit S H: *Aging in Mental Disorders*. Free Press, New York, 1980

SAMPLE MASTER CARE PLAN FOR HOME CARE—

Nursing Diagnoses	Assessment	Planning
Depressed mood	• Degree of depression. • Suicidal risk (suicidal thoughts, plans). • Presence of a precipitant (death of a loved one). • Physical health status (acute and chronic health problems).	*Short-term goals* *Client will:* • elevate mood • reduce suicidal risk • have existing health problems treated • reduce level of stress
Withdrawal	• Frequency and quality of social interactions. • Social supports. • Number and frequency of activities outside the home (work and leisure). • Responsiveness to the nurse.	• increase the number of social interactions • increase the use of social supports • increase the number of activities outside the home
Physiological disequilibrium (sleep disturbance, decreased energy, lack of appetite)	• Daily sleep patterns at present (nighttime sleep and naps). • Food intake for the past two days (including alcohol consumption). • Physical appearance. • Physical health status, including nutritional status. • Current weight compared to usual weight. • Frequency and nature of daily activities.	• increase nighttime sleep and decrease naps • eat a healthy diet • increase physical activity. *Long-term goals* *Client will:* • obtain consultation if depression does not lift in six weeks • have a healthy life style (adequate diet, proper rest, regular physical exercise, minimal stress) • receive psychotherapy, medication and/or hospitalization if home management is ineffective.

DEPRESSION

Intervention: Nursing Orders	Intervention: Resources and Support Systems	Evaluation: Expected Outcomes
• Provide support. • Accept the client. • Listen to problems, concerns. • Encourage increased social interactions. • Encourage activities outside the home. • Encourage use of existing social supports. • Encourage expression of affect. • Suggest daily physical activity. • Teach healthy eating habits. • Suggest ways to improve sleep at night, e.g. daily exercise, warm milk before bed. • Discourage eating alone whenever possible. • Check on client often, either by phone or home visit. • Teach stress reduction techniques.	• Telephone Reassurance Program • Senior Center • Friendly Companion Program • Community Mental Health Center • Hospital-based Clinic • Area Agency on Aging • Retired Senior Volunteer Program • Gray Panthers	*Client has:* • elevated mood • increased social interactions • social support network • regular physical activity • healthy diet • adequate rest • increased number of activities outside the home • improved physical health status • medication, psychotherapy and/or hospitalization if necessary.

SAMPLE MASTER CARE PLAN FOR HOME CARE—

Nursing Diagnoses	Assessment	Planning
Suspiciousness and self-preoccupation	• Physical health status, especially hearing and vision. • Presence of recent losses (death of a loved one, loss of property, change of residence). • Duration of suspiciousness. • Disruptiveness of suspicious behavior to daily life. • Degree of threat to others. • Content of suspicions. • Mental status, especially thought processes.	*Short-term goals* *Client will:* • respond to reality–based precipitants • have existing health problems treated • increase social interactions • reduce stress • decrease the threat of aggression toward others *Long-term goals* *Client will:* • obtain consultation if thought disorder persists and disrupts daily living • receive psychotherapy, medication and/or hospitalization if home management is ineffective

PARANOIA

Intervention: Nursing Orders	Intervention: Resources and Support Systems	Evaluation: Expected Outcomes
• Accept the client. • Listen to problems, concerns • Approach client in a direct, honest, respectful manner • Provide explanations of all care given. • Make frequent but brief visits • Promote social interactions • Offer safe outlets for the expression of aggression • Teach the client ways of handling reality–based threats • Establish a long-term relationship with the client	• Trusted relatives, friends, neighbors • Community agencies and programs likely to be trusted by client • Trusted clergy • Health care providers accepted by the client	*Client has:* • decreased suspiciousness • reduced preoccupation with self • strengthened social support network • increased social interaction • medication, psychotherapy and hospitalization if necessary.

SAMPLE MASTER CARE PLAN FOR HOME CARE—

Nursing Diagnoses	Assessment	Planning
Confusion and disorientation	• Mental status including degree of confusion. • Physical health status, especially acute organic brain syndromes. • Home environment. • Daily routine including sleep, diet. • Degree of threat to self and others. • Physical activity. • Social supports. • Presence of precipitant (personal or environmental stress).	*Short-term goals* *Client will:* • reduce disorientation and confusion • have a consistent daily routine • have a safe home environment • have existing health problems treated • increase nighttime sleep and decrease daytime naps • reduce level of stress • remove any known precipitants • have regular physical activity • have social supports which are accepting and gentle
Physical aggression/ violence	• Degree of threat to self and others. • Daily routine. • Physical activity. • Presence of a precipitant. • Physical health status.	• reduce aggression/ violence • have safe outlets for the expression of aggressive feelings • have regular physical activity • have existing health problems treated • remove any known precipitants • reduce level of stress • have a consistent daily routine. *Long-term goals* *Client will:* • obtain help if problems persist • receive hospital care, medication or therapy if home management problems continue.

DEMENTIA

Intervention: Nursing Orders	Intervention: Resources and Support Systems	Evaluation: Expected Outcomes
• Provide orientation aids: e.g. watch, clocks, name band, calendar. • Maintain a stable home environment with furniture in fixed positions. • Raise window shades in the daytime and lower at night. • Introduce oneself and address the client by name. • Speak in simple language at a slow pace. • Notify friends and neighbors if client wanders or becomes aggressive. • Keep the outside doors locked at night. • Follow a consistent daily routine. • Accept the client's behavior. • Avoid overstimulation or understimulation.	• Friendly Companion program • Day care or day hospital programs • Home sitters • Physical activities programs • Home health aides • ADRDA (Alzheimer's Disease and Related Disorders Association) for information, home care tips, referrals for services, and support groups for caregivers.	*Client has:* • reduced disorientation and confusion • expression of aggression through safe outlets • medication, psychotherapy and/or institutionalization if necessary.

CHAPTER 11

METABOLIC DISORDERS

Monette Graves

Older aged individuals have fewer metabolic disturbances as a result of endocrine dysfunction than do young persons. Diabetes mellitus and thyroid abnormalities are the major metabolic disturbances in older people, with diabetes mellitus having a higher incidence than thyroid disturbances (Kart, Metress, and Metress, 1978, p. 160).

Diabetes Mellitus in the Elderly

The exact determination of the rate of diabetes in the older age population has never been made, but one source has estimated that 20% of all diabetic patients are 60 years of age or older (Kart, Metress, and Metress, 1978, p. 174). In the older age female population, non-white females develop diabetes twice as frequently as white females (Jones, 1982, p. 951). Diabetes is the seventh leading cause of death in the elderly (Eliopoulos, 1979, p. 185). The rate of diabetes is high in the elderly for several reasons. Since the discovery of insulin, more people who develop diabetes at a young age live to be old. One author (Gregerman, 1981, p. 1301) stated that certain cells show premature death or slower replacement of cells in the elderly. Some of the cells affected are the beta and alpha cells of the pancreas, the capillary endothelial cells, the cells of the retina, and the Swann cells. This can also account for the increasing incidence of diabetes in the older age group as well as some of the late complications of the disease.

Obesity in adulthood seems to carry a risk for the development of diabetes (Feldman, Sender, and Siegelaub, 1969, p. 478). In obesity, the fat cells enlarge and become less responsive to insulin. This condition necessitates the secretion of more insulin to allow glucose to enter the cells. Eventually the pancreas is unable to respond and diabetes occurs. Feldman et al. (1969, p. 478) stated that when fat is of the trunk and upper extremities as opposed to the hips and lower extremities, the risk of developing diabetes is greater for some yet unknown reason. Another reason there is a high risk of hyperglycemia in the elderly may be the number of medications taken by this age group that causes hyperglycemia, for example, furosemide (Lasix), cortisone or the thiazide diuretics.

Many older people who have diabetes have been diagnosed at a young age and require insulin for control. Others have maturity onset diabetes or non-insulin dependent diabetes and are controlled by an oral hypoglycemic agent and diet. Still others control the condition by diet alone. The older age person may be an undetected diabetic and begin to develop signs and symptoms of the disease at any time.

Clues to Undetected Diabetes

The older person may not have the usual and familiar signs and symptoms of diabetes such as polyphagia, polydipsia, and polyuria (Williams, 1979, p. 328). Fatigue may be the only symptom of the disease, or complaints may be caused by one of the complications of diabetes such as rapid changes in distance vision, sensory changes in the lower extremities, pruritis vulvae, impotence in the male, or inability to completely empty the bladder. Because of reduced glomerular filtration in the kidney of the older person, urine tests are often negative for sugar until blood sugar is elevated to 280-300 mgm per deciliter (Williams, 1979, p. 328). As the blood sugar rises, so does the osmolarity of the blood leading to severe dehydration and the possibility of hyperglycemic, hyperosmolar nonketotic coma (HHNK) (Luckmann, 1980, p. 1546). This type of coma is one of the life–threatening complications of non-insulin dependent diabetes. As many as 50% of the people who develop hyperglycemic, hyperosmolar nonketotic coma die from this complication. The older adult who is not under close supervision may develop this condition before being diagnosed as a diabetic (Kart, Metress, and Metress, 1978, p. 164).

Diagnosis of Diabetes in Elderly Clients

Many older people do not complain of the symptoms that would cause other family members to seek medical attention. All complaints deserve thorough assessment for a cause. Otherwise, diabetes may not be detected until severe complications are present. One elderly woman complained to her daughter that her vision was distorted and that she was unable to keep up with her usual activities because of severe fatigue. Her daughter, fortunately, was a nurse and recognized that her symptoms could indicate diabetes and requested that she call her physician to schedule a glucose tolerance test. Her blood sugar, two hours after a glucose load, was 900 mgm %. She was placed on an oral hypoglycemic agent, a strict 1000 calorie diet, and assured that her symptoms would clear with time, but she received no explanation about why she had the symptoms. She later received an explanation of why the symptoms were present and the length of time required for them to clear. She stated she felt much better after a brief explanation of what was occurring and why.

When diabetes is suspected, an oral glucose tolerance test is the usual means of determining whether diabetes is present. For this test to be accurate, the individual should receive a moderately high carbohydrate diet for three days prior to the test. In elderly persons, the fasting blood sugar level is usually normal, but the blood sugar two hours after administration of the glucose load is approximately 10 mgm percent higher for each decade of life (Hayter, 1981, p. 33). Tobin and Andres, in Pomerantz (1982, p. 315) have developed a normogram categorizing in percentile ranks those who show a certain blood glucose level two hours after the loading dose. It is suggested that older people whose glucose level is in the top seventh percentile on the normograph be diagnosed as diabetics. Williams (1979, p. 328) suggested that the use of the normogram for the glucose tolerance test, or a two–hour post–prandial blood glucose level that is repeatedly 250 mgm %, and/or the presence of any of the complications of diabetes be used to determine whether the elderly person has diabetes. Medications that will raise blood sugar are nictonic acid, estrogen, furosemide (Lasix) and the thiazide diuretics. These drugs will need to be withheld for an accurate glucose tolerance test result. Drugs that lower blood sugar and should be withheld are propranolol (Inderal) and high doses of aspirin (Eliopoulos, 1979, p. 185).

When an individual is ill, the fasting blood sugar will be elevated due to the increased secretion of cortisone and possibly epinephrine, both of which elevate blood sugar levels. Therefore, persons who have no overt signs of diabetes should be retested after recovery from acute illness.

Many older adults are often determined to have diabetes during a routine office visit for other symptoms (Moss, 1976, p. 52). One elderly woman had none of the classical symptoms of diabetes, but on a routine visit to the physician for follow-up care after a myocardial infarction, her urine was positive for glucose. The initial test for blood sugar level found it to be excessive and subsequent post–prandial blood sugar level was approximately 300 mgm %. Diabetes was first diagnosed in this instance at the age of 70.

Treatment of Diabetes in the Older Client

The goal of treatment of the person with diabetes is control of the disease because there is no cure at present. The primary goal is the same, whether the person is insulin dependent or non-insulin dependent. It is becoming more evident that blood sugar should be as well–controlled as possible in order to slow the development of long-term complications. In one long-term study of diabetics, the incidence of the three major complications of diabetes (neuropathy, nephropathy, and retinopathy) was correlated highly with the level of hyperglycemia (Hayter, 1981, p. 32). A relatively new laboratory test has been developed to detect the degree of hyperglycemia over a long period. The test is for glycosylated hemoglobin (Hgb A_{lc}) (Hayter, 1981, p. 33). This test shows the amount of glucose bound to hemoglobin and is determined by the level of blood glucose over a period of time. It is used to determine the degree of control. Once the glucose is bound to the hemoglobin, it remains bound for the remainder of the life of the red cell (Hayter, 1981, p. 53).

Insulin Dependent Diabetes in Elderly Clients

In older age diabetics who have had the disease since their younger years, treatment will remain similar to the treatment the client is accustomed to having. However, as aging progresses, the person must be observed carefully for signs of either too much or too little insulin administration. As muscle mass decreases with age, body metabolic needs also will decrease. As physical activity slowly decreases or when other chronic illnesses occur such as congestive heart failure or arthritis, there will be a significant decline in physical activity. Therefore, total calories will need to be reduced to prevent obesity. Any decrease in activity can mean the person will need an increase in exogenous insulin to assist in the utilization of calories ingested, or a decrease in calories. The need for protein, vitamins and minerals will remain the same so the caloric reduction will be in carbohydrate or fats (Shuman, 1971, p. 75). Caloric needs are increased by fever or by extremely hot or cold temperatures due to increased body metabolism. The very old individual may not be able to increase body metabolism in extremely cold environments, however. If the elderly individual decides to begin an exercise regimen, adjustments in insulin and/or calories will need to be made because treatment is based on a balance of insulin, diet and exercise.

Treatment of the Older Client with Insulin

Insulin or oral hypoglycemic agents are not usually necessary when diabetes occurs in older persons. During acute illness or hyperglycemic, hyperosmolar nonketotic coma, insulin will be required in small amounts. Some physicians recommend insulin when diet alone does not control hyperglycemia or if glycosuria and weight loss occur (Shuman, 1976, p. 75). Shuman recommends an intermediate insulin be used and that the dose begin with 10-20 units daily. It is very important that treatment not produce a rapid fall in blood glucose and the resultant hypoglycemia. If the older person has persistent episodes of hypoglycemia, the dose can be divided and given two-thirds in the morning and one-third before the evening meal, or the total dose lowered slightly (Shuman, 1976, p. 75). If too much insulin is administered, blood sugar falls causing glucagon to be secreted by the pancreas and a rise in blood sugar resulting in rebound hyperglycemia. This is known as the Somogyi effect. The client should be questioned for the presence of weakness, hunger, sweating or irritability at the time the insulin would have its peak effect to determine whether mild hypoglycemia has occurred. The treatment is to reduce the insulin given.

Insulin dependent diabetic persons who exercise sporadically will have problems with hypoglycemia unless they are taught to eat a snack before exercising and to carry a rapidly absorbed substance at all times for use if hypoglycemia should occur. Some responsible person who will be with the client during exercise must know that the client is a diabetic and the action to take if a hypoglycemic episode occurs. If consiousness is lost, honey or syrup coated over the buccal surfaces will be absorbed. When consciousness returns, the client should eat 10-20 grams of rapidly absorbed carbohydrate, such as hard candy, or a small amount of a cola–type (not diet) drink.

Monitoring Blood Glucose at Home

For better control of the insulin–dependent diabetic, many clients are beginning to monitor blood glucose at home by means of a finger stick. There are a number of blood glucose monitoring systems available. Each has advantages and disadvantages. The Dextrostix must have the drop of blood rinsed off the stick after 60 seconds and the color change determined at once because the color fades rapidly. With Chemstrip bG, one drop of blood is placed on the reagent and wiped off after sixty seconds. The colors on these strips are such that the older person may have difficulty seeing them. The Dextrostix can be interpreted by a machine, but the machine currently costs about $300 (Stevens, 1981, p. 2026). There is no doubt the home monitoring of blood glucose will increase in an effort to maintain a steady blood glucose level. Researchers think that the long-term complications of diabetes will be delayed by better control of blood sugar. If they are correct, fewer older persons who are insulin dependent diabetics should have the devastating complications seen so often after 10-15 years of diabetes (Hayter, 1981, p. 32).

Non-insulin Dependent Diabetes in Elderly Clients

For non-insulin dependent diabetics, the diet may need revision as activity declines to prevent obesity or to correct obesity. Obesity leads to a need for more insulin which the pancreas cannot supply. Activity remains important in the control of diabetes in the elderly just as in the young diabetic. Exercise is known to increase muscle uptake of glucose without insulin (Luckmann, 1980, p. 1564). Dietary management is the preferred treatment for the maturity onset older age person with diabetes. If diet alone is found not to be successful after a reasonable period of time, the oral hypoglycemic agents may be added to the treatment program. The oral medication should be given cautiously because of the danger of hypoglycemia (Williams, 1979, p. 328).

Oral Hypoglycemic Agents in the Treatment of Diabetes

When diet, exercise and weight control have not been successful in reducing hyperglycemia in the older person, one of the oral hypoglycemic agents is sometimes added to the medical regimen. In patients who have maturity onset, or non-insulin dependent diabetes, some insulin is secreted but it is insufficient to meet the needs of the person. The oral hypoglycemic agents stimulate the pancreas to release the preformed insulin. Sulfonylurea is also thought to increase the peripheral utilization of insulin (Todd, 1981, p. 291). The sulfonylureas are the only oral hypoglycemics available today since the Food and Drug Administration has banned the use of the biguanide drug in America. Clients who have previously been allergic to sulfonamide drugs should not take sulfonylurea (Todd, 1981, p. 291). The most commonly used oral hypoglycemic agents are summarized in Table 11.1.

Because the renal function of older people is reduced, the use of oral hypo-glycemic agents necessitates observing the person very closely for hypoglycemia induced by failure to excrete the drug. Intolerance to alcohol is present when individuals take the sulfonylurea drugs. Together the two produce an antabuse-like reaction. Symptoms are a sensation of warmth, flushing of the face, redness of the conjunctiva, headache, nausea, tachycardia and dizziness (Nickerson, 1977, p. 103).

Drugs that enhance the effect of oral hypoglycemia agents include alcohol, aspirin in large doses, coumarin, phenylbutazone (Butazolidin), probenecid and pro-pranolol (Inderal). Drugs that increase blood glucose and cause need for more insulin include corticosteroids, epinephrine, lithium, thiazide diuretics, birth con-trol pills, and thyroid hormone (Todd, 1981, p. 294).

TABLE 11.1
Oral Hypoglycemic Agents

Drug	Usual Dose	Half-life	Duration of action	Metabolism & Excretion
tolbutamide (Orinase)	500 mgm	4-5 hrs	12 hrs.	Metabolized by liver, ex-creted by urine as inert substance
tolazamide (Tolinase)	100 mgm	4-6 hrs	12-24 hrs.	Metabolized by liver, ex-creted in urine
chlorpropamide (Diabinese)	100 mgm	34-36 hrs.	60 hrs.	Excreted unchanged in urine
acetohexamide (Dymelor)	250 mgm	6-8 hrs.	12-24 hrs.	Metabolized by liver Metabolite is the active ingredient excreted in urine

Sources:
1. Todd, Betsy. "Drugs and the Elderly, When the Patient is taking a Sulfonylurea." *Geriatric Nursing*, July/Aug. 1981, p. 291.
2. Askew, Gail. "Oral Agents, Combating Convenience." Chapter 4, pages 35-48 in "Managing Diabetes Properly," *Nursing Skill Book*, Skillbook 77. 1977 Intermed Communications, Horsham, Pa.
3. Nickerson, Donna. "Oral Hypoglycemic Agents." Chapter 10, Gutherie and Gutherie, *Nursing Management and Diabetes Mellitus*, 1974, 1974, C.V. Mosby Co.

Hypoglycemia is a serious risk for the older adult who is taking sulfonylurea to control diabetes. As pointed out earlier, hypoglycemia has been known to cause other complications such as stroke, myocardial infarction, or retinal hemorrhages (Moss, 1976, p. 57). Symptoms and treatment of hypoglycemia will be discussed under nursing implications.

Treatment by Diet

When diabetes is diagnosed, the physician will determine the diet prescription based on the needs of the individual patient. If a client is overweight, the total calories will be planned for slow weight reduction. Calories are determined for weight loss, weight maintenance, or weight gain, and with consideration of the physical activity of the particular client. If the client is receiving insulin, the diet will provide for mid-afternoon and bedtime snacks to prevent nighttime hypoglycemic episodes. After the diet prescription is written by the physician, either a nutritionist or the nurse will explain the diet to the patient. The particular diet will be developed around the client's ethnic, cultural or religious needs, as well as particular life style. If these factors are not considered, it is very unlikely that the diet will be adhered to very well. The American Diabetes Association and the American Dietetic Association have jointly prepared a list of foods with equivalent grams of carbohydrate, protein and fat per serving. The foods are arranged as exchanges of servings, and the client is assisted to plan a number of daily menus in order that the diet can be continued at home. The total calories for the day are distributed as 50% carbohydrate, 20% protein, and 30% fat, and further divided into three meals and snacks if the client is receiving insulin. These percentages may vary, particularly when the client has a very high level of serum cholesterol or fatty acids. In that case, fats may be reduced and complex carbohydrates increased as total percent of calories for the day. Various well–known clinics vary the distribution of calories in other ways (Kaufman, 1977, p. 29).

Studies have shown that people in underdeveloped countries have a much lower incidence of diabetes and a much higher amount of fiber in their diets. The total calories consumed are probably less. Also, a high–fiber diet means a more rapid transit through the intestinal tract and possibly less absorption. Much of the fiber is complex and non–digestible, therefore it is not absorbed and does not affect the blood sugar (Luckman, 1980, p. 1551). Some authors recommend a diet high in fiber for non-insulin dependent diabetics and have found that even with a higher percent of very complex carbohydrate, the glucose tolerance of the person is improved (Luckmann, 1980, p. 1551). This high–fiber diet includes low–fat dietary intake. Because many older people have diverticulitis, this diet would not be appropriate and is not currently recommended by the American Diabetes Association.

The client, and affected family members, need much support in learning to manage the prescribed diet when diabetes is diagnosed. The first step in helping the client adjust to the diet is to determine customary dietary habits and preferences and conform to them as much as possible. The dietary habits of most elderly people are well established and not easily changed. The diet plan should be prepared to meet the individual needs and be written. A copy of the American Diabetes Association exchange list should be explained and presented to the client. It will be helpful to the older person who has just been diagnosed as having diabetes if some arrangement is made for having questions answered as they arise during the time the person is learning to use the exchange list. Since so many older persons take some of their meals at a Senior Center or fast food restaurant, copies of most usual food items and the exchange equivalents have been prepared by many of the fast food chains and are available for clients (Kloster, 1982, p. 184). If the client is a vegetarian, the diet is planned so that high protein vegetables that complement each other's amino acids are used in the same meal to provide complete protein. Information on vegetarian diets and food at fast food restaurants is given at the end of this chapter. (Cook, 1979, p. 72).

Regardless of whether diet and insulin, diet and oral hypoglycemic agents, or diet alone is used to treat diabetes in older individuals, the treatment should lead to a slow decline in blood sugar. Overly vigorous treatment can lead to hypoglycemia which can cause cerebral vascular accidents, retinal hemorrhages, or myocardial infarction (Moss, 1976, p. 57).

Exercise in Treatment of Diabetes in the Elderly Client

Exercise is an important component of therapy in diabetes. Exercise promotes insulin secretion and utilization of glucose by muscles (Kart, Metress, and Metress, 1979, p. 165). The elderly person with diabetes should be encouraged to walk or take some other form of exercise daily. Walking is considered to be one of the best forms of exercise for older people. In many cities, shopping centers open their doors early and have special markings or colored stripes in the halls that allow persons to tell approximately how far they have walked. At some shopping centers, the same persons walk daily and form friendships among their fellow walkers. Within the mall, the walking surface is smooth, well–lighted, warm in winter, cool in summer, and provides for socializing as well as exercise. At one mall in the Midwest, one of the coffee shops open early so the walkers can rest temporarily during the walk.

In one study, subjects who participated in rather vigorous exercise such as walking, swimming or tennis had one-third the risk of heart disease as those clients who did not participate in any exercises (Ganda, 1980, p. 935). The same study showed that in mild non-insulin dependent diabetes, physical conditioning improved the plasma lipids and glucose levels. Physical activity or exercise leads to an increase in the level of high density lipoprotein (HDL) as opposed to low density lipoprotein, and therefore less atherosclerosis. The benefits of exercise are reduction in obesity, less need for insulin or oral hypoglycemic agents, slowed development of atherosclerosis, and increased socialization.

Older persons who cannot take part in vigorous exercise or walking can be taught muscle setting and range-of-motion exercises. They should be encouraged and/or supervised in the daily performance of the activity as a means of improving their health status.

Nursing Implications

Anyone giving or supervising care of the older person in the home needs to be alert to the possibility of the development of an overt diabetic state or the development of long–term complications of diabetes, in either insulin dependent or non-insulin dependent diabetics or in the person who has not been diagnosed as a diabetic.

Older persons who have insulin–dependent diabetes will probably have had the disease many years, therefore multiple complications are probable. People who have had diabetes 15 years or longer are especially prone to develop retinopathy as well as neuropathy and nephropathy (Morse, 1976, p. 59). However, many older adults who have never been diagnosed as having diabetes develop symptoms of long-term complications, such as peripheral neuropathy, autonomic neuropathy, or visual or renal symptoms of microvascular disease. Nurses who have clients in the home should be alert for the early manifestations of diabetes or its complications in their assessment of each elderly client.

Assessment

Assessment of the elderly client should include careful history taking to detect subtle changes, such as disturbance in distance vision. As blood glucose rises, the lenses absorb glucose or sorbitol, causing fluid retention and distortion of vision. Careful ophthalmological examination can reveal signs of microaneurysms, hermorrhage or cotton wool spots of the retina which indicate long standing hypoglycemia and the need for medical attention. Narrow-angle glaucoma is another visual problem more common in diabetic clients due to neovascular tissue formation of the iris or the chamber angle. Glaucoma can be detected early and treated adequately. Symptoms that occur are pain in the eye, headache, redness of the conjunctiva, and blurred vision (Morse, 1976, p. 59; Jones, 1982, p. 775).

When distant vision is altered along with weakness or lethargy, the nurse refers the client to his or her physician to determine whether diabetes may be the cause. As hyperglycemia decreases with treatment, vision will gradually be restored, but it may take several weeks. One older person had recently been diagnosed as a diabetic. Her primary fear was that of blindness because of her visual changes. After the cause was explained and reassurance given that the problem would clear within four to five weeks, she was less fearful and thanked the nurse several times for listening and providing her with information.

Assessment for Neuropathy

Neuropathy of diabetic origin should be suspected when the older client complains of burning or aching pain of the lower extremities. The pain may be worse at night with rest rather than with activity. On examination, one may find the achilles reflex is absent, loss of ability to feel painful stimuli, or the presence of injury to the feet. The feet of all elderly diabetics should be inspected at each home visit. Pedal and popliteal pulses should be palpated. Atherosclerosis decreases circulation to the feet and the development of atherosclerosis is twice as rapid in the diabetic client as in the non-diabetic individual (Moss, 1976, p. 59). When neuropathy of diabetes occurs, foot care is essential to prevent an infection that may fail to heal. Neurotrophic ulcers of the feet are most often found on the pressure points on the ball of the foot. These ulcers are painless and may fail to heal resulting in eventual amputation.

If ulcers or infections are present on the feet of the elderly diabetic individual, the client and the caregiver are taught the principles of handwashing prior to wound care, the use of asepsis with wound care, to warm any solution used on the feet, and to maintain a warm environment during care of the lesions. When any abrasion or cut occurs, it should be cleansed with a sterile dressing applied immediately. If foot soaks are to be used when lesions are present, the water needs to be boiled for 10 minutes and allowed to cool before use. The foot to be soaked should be cleansed with soap and water prior to placing in the foot soak solution so that bacteria on the foot will not contaminate the wound (Schaefer, 1982, p. 183).

Elderly people often do not see well enough to trim their own nails. As nails thicken with age, the danger of improperly trimmed nails increases. Amputation is a major threat to any elderly diabetic because of the rapid development of atherosclerosis, the increased tendency to develop infections which do not heal, and the presence of neuropathy so that pain is not felt (Moss, 1976, p. 56).

In addition to the neuropathy of the lower extremities, neuropathy may also affect the autonomic nervous system. Diplopia may occur due to damage of the fourth and sixth cranial nerves. Cranial nerve damage is assessed by checking the extra occular eye movements in all six directions and by questioning the client regarding acuity of vision (Bates, 1974, p. 22).

More frequently noted is an atonic bladder with incomplete emptying and often overflow incontinence. A distended bladder often results in an infection and pyelonephritis. When a client has been diagnosed as having a neurogenic bladder, the client must be taught to empty the bladder frequently and to use the Credè method if necessary. Family members or the diabetic client, or both as appropriate, can be taught to palpate the bladder to be certain it is empty after voiding. Chronic urinary retention and neuropathy lead to a relaxed detrussor muscle and make palpation of the bladder difficult. If the bladder cannot be palpated, percussion just above the symphysis pubis may aid in the detection of a full relaxed bladder. Palpation of the bladder may result in incontinence, if the bladder is full (Caird, 1977, p. 45). The relationship of chronic urinary retention to the development of pyelonephritis and ultimately to renal failure is explained to the client and/or caregiver. Renal failure may be the ultimate crisis for older diabetic clients whose kidneys are already compromised by the aging process and possibly by nephropathy of diabetes. Autonomic nervous system dysfunction can also manifest itself in gastric atony with a feeling of fullness, failure to eat the prescribed diet, and a lack of diabetic control. The client with these complaints will need smaller, more frequent meals to prevent weight loss and malnutrition.

Impotence is a complaint of elderly male diabetics. Many authors believe that with good control of hyperglycemia the impotence may be relieved. If not, the client needs careful evaluation to determine whether some other factor is causing the problem. The silastic penile implant can be helpful if the client desires this type of prosthesis (Gutherie, 1977, p. 59).

Assessment of nephropathy. Diabetic nephropathy is one consequence of microvascular disease resulting in thickening of the basement membrane of the glomerular tuft and eventual destruction of the glomerulus. This condition results in further reduction of renal functioning in addition to what advanced age has already produced. According to Williams (1978, p. 330), physicians should annually assess renal functioning in diabetic clients. Nurses who have contact with older diabetic clients in the home can encourage them and their caregivers to ensure that this evaluation is carried out in order to detect and treat early stages of renal disease and try to prevent uremia. Hemodialysis has not been very successful in very aged diabetic clients because their blood vessels show advanced atherosclerosis, causing problems attaining and maintaining access for dialysis.

Assessment for hyperglycemia. During each visit to the home of the older diabetic client, the nurse will review the results of the urine tests since the last visit. Since urine tests are negative for sugar in most older diabetics until blood sugar reaches 300 mg %, the nurse will assess for other indications that hyperglycemia is present. The urine should be checked for acetone periodically to detect for ketosis if the client is an insulin–dependent diabetic. The client is observed for lethargy, weakness or new visual disturbances. If the older person is a non-insulin dependent diabetic, assessment will be directed toward detection of hyperglycemia prior to development of hyperosmolar coma. Skin turgor is assessed as well as dry tongue and lips, rapid pulse, and low blood pressure. The client is questioned concerning the volume of urinary output. When neuropathy is present, the parasympathetic nervous system can be affected and heart rate will not be able to speed up even with dehydration (Moss, 1976, p. 55). If hyperglycemia is severe, urine sugar will be present, but acetone will be negative since some insulin is being secreted and prevents lipolysis and the resulting ketone bodies.

The nurse should observe the feet carefully for the presence of any infection since any stress will increase the need for insulin but the pancreas cannot respond to the need. The client will be questioned regarding the presence of urgency or burning upon urination, either of which can indicate a urinary tract infection and increased stress.

Assessment for hypoglycemia. Assessment of the older person who has insulin–dependent diabetes or who is receiving an oral hypoglycemia drug will include questions to determine whether symptoms of hypoglycemia have occurred and have not been recognized. Nocturnal hypoglycemia is sometimes the cause of restlessness during sleep. If long-acting insulin or oral agents are used, the early autonomic nervous system symptoms of hunger, nervousness and tachycardia are often not detected and the symptoms of severe hypoglycemia develop. The symptoms that family members are often able to relate are irritability, personality changes, slurred speech, or combativeness (Jones, 1982, p. 769). Too often family members and medical personnel consider these symptoms a result of the aging process and fail to recognize the real cause. When the above symptoms are elicited during assessment, the physician should be notified. The nurse can help determine what precipitated the hypoglycemia. For instance, is the client not eating all the food allowed? Is the client exercising more than usual, or has the insulin or oral medication not been taken as prescribed? Has the client's vision deteriorated to the point that there is a problem with insulin measurement?

Teaching the Older Diabetic Client

Teaching elderly people who have had diabetes for many years can be a real challenge. Clients often think they know all about diabetes and have been administering insulin and regulating their diet for a long time. The nurse should assess their knowledge and share new information that was not available when they developed diabetes. By approaching clients in this manner, the nurse will get them interested in learning. The client should also see the nurse as a knowledgeable person. Any successful teaching program or session demands client participation. Assessment of the clients' understanding of diabetes and the relationship of insulin, diet and exercise to the control of diabetes is an initial step in teaching. By allowing clients to share what they know, the nurse can help fill in the gaps and correct any misconceptions. The decision concerning what needs to be taught, the timing of specific segments of information, and methods chosen for presentation must be based on the client's needs. Because restrictions are so often emphasized, the positive approach is preferred.

When the elderly client has recently been diagnosed as having diabetes, the nurse may detect a high degree of anxiety that prevents learning. By allowing the individual to discuss what diabetes means, the nurse can help reduce the anxiety and allow some learning to occur. Teaching is best received when carried out in short segments with the information that has meaning for the client.

Insulin administration and complications. A demonstration by the client or caregiver of the procedure used to prepare and administer insulin will reveal any aspect of insulin administration that needs to be explained, clarified and/or changed. Since U 100 insulin is now used by most diabetics, there is less likelihood that a U 40 syringe will be used to prepare and give U 80 insulin. But if Iletin (regular) insulin is mixed with long-acting insulin, the nurse needs to determine that the insulins are drawn into the syringe in the same sequence each time. For instance, if the long-acting insulin is usually drawn into the syringe first followed by the regular insulin, this sequence needs to be used at all times. Otherwise, the dose of regular insulin may be greater if it is drawn into the syringe first due to the dead space in the syringe and the needle. The newer insulin syringes have a very small dead space and a short needle, so the medication error will not be as great as with the older syringes and longer needles. The client should be taught to cleanse the tops of both vials of insulin with alcohol and inject the correct amount of air, determined by the insulin dose, into each vial. Authors vary in their recommendations of which insulin to draw up into the syringe first. Wolfe (1977, p. 53) recommended withdrawing the long-acting insulin into the syringe first and then the regular insulin, being careful that no long-acting insulin enters the regular insulin vial. Burke (1977, p. 92) recommended withdrawing the regular insulin into the syringe first, then the long-acting insulin. The author prefers the latter procedure because it prevents modified insulin from entering the regular insulin vial.

The client is taught to rotate the vial between his or her hands to mix the medication thoroughly. If the vial is shaken, air bubbles form in the insulin and the dose will not be accurate. If insulin is refrigerated, the prepared dose is allowed to warm to room temperature prior to administration in order to reduce the incidence of lipodystrophy, either atrophy or hypertrophy. Atrophy occurs more often in women than men and ranges from a mild dimple to severe loss of tissue. Hypertrophy occurs more often in young males and occurs on the anterior and lateral thigh. Both atrophy and hypertrophy have little blood supply so insulin injected into the area is absorbed very slowly (Jones, 1982, p. 767). When the client has been using the hypertrophic area for insulin injection and the site is changed, the insulin will be absorbed more quickly and can cause signs of hypoglycemia. Other causes of lipodystrophy are failure to rotate sites of insulin injection so that repeat injections are given in the same site day after day, and failure to inject the insulin between the subcutaneous fat and the muscle. The actual injection should be observed in order to ensure the correct placement of the insulin. With the short needles on the new insulin syringes, it is sometimes difficult to penetrate the fatty layer in an obese client. Standard texts on medical nursing will have pictures demonstrating the best means of assuring the correct injection angle and depth (Luckman, 1980, p. 1550).

The older person who is visually impaired or blind will need assistive devices to enable the withdrawal of the correct dose of insulin. Some clients will depend upon the nurse to prepare a week's supply of insulin in the syringes and leave them refrigerated to be used daily. Insulin will adhere to glass or plastic syringes so the dose may vary slightly when prepared and left for the client to use. The assistive devices depend upon hearing and touch rather than vision. Boyles (1977, p. 1456) has described seven different assistive devices and gives the advantage and disadvantage of each.

In teaching the client about the administration of insulin, nurses should emphasize the following points:

- correct measurement of the prescribed dose;
- aseptic technique in preparation and administration of insulin;
- rotation of sites according to a chart prepared with the client so that each day of the month is shown on a stick man figure (assures adequate rotation of sites used);
- injection of insulin between the fat and muscle layers;
- the vial of insulin currently being used need not be refrigerated, but the bottle purchased and kept available is refrigerated until ready for use;
- when insulin is necessary for control of diabetes, the diet prescription should be adhered to regarding calories and timing of meals, so that hypoglycemia does not occur;
- 5 or 6 small hard candies should be carried in case hypoglycemia occurs;
- an identification card or a Medi-Alert bracelet should be worn stating the client is a diabetic and takes insulin. (The card will have the name of the person's attending physician and the type and amount of insulin taken.)

Teaching needs related to oral hypoglycemic drugs. Occasionally an elderly client taking one of the sulfonylurea medications will develop an intolerance and have a rash when exposed to sunlight. Clients need to contact their physician if this occurs. Older adults taking chlorpropamide (Diabinese) must be cautioned against the use of alcohol. This drug is most likely of all the sulfonylureas to produce the antabuse-like reaction when alcohol is ingested. The symptoms of this reaction occur very shortly after ingesting alcohol and include a vasomotor response with flushing of the face, redness of the conjunctiva, a feeling of warmth, nausea and vomiting, shortness of breath, and tachycardia. The symptoms usually last no more than one hour but could be very frightening. Many over-the-counter medications contain alcohol, so the client should be warned to check all medications for alcohol content (Nickerson, 1977, p. 104). Oral hypoglycemic agents also produce hypoglycemia in some individuals. When the elderly overweight person has oral hypoglycemic agents prescribed, it is important the client be taught to return for repeat blood sugar evaluations at the time intervals stated by the physician. As the person loses weight, the need for the oral hypoglycemic drugs may decrease causing hypoglycemia. After the passage of time or the development of nephropathy, and the older person's renal function decreases, the drug will not be excreted as quickly as previously, leading to an overdose and hypoglycemia. The signs and symptoms of hypoglycemia from the oral preparations are those of central nervous system origin, such as irritability, personality changes, slurred speech, or combativeness (Luckman, 1980, p. 569; Kayne, 1981, p. 359).

Elderly clients on oral medications and a family member need to know the symptoms of hypoglycemia. Many times family members will be aware of the altered behavior but attribute it to senile dementia or other causes. The client may fail to recognize the symptoms. As soon as the symptoms are noticed, a small amount of available glucose should be taken. Ten to 12 Gms of available glucose is usually sufficient. This represents two teaspoons of sugar, syrup, or honey, four ounces of orange juice, or five or six life savers. The rapidly available glucose is followed by a food with complex carbohydrate such as a slice of bread or a small glass of milk. Caution should be used not to overtreat and result in hyperglycemia.

Teaching elderly diabetics to maintain dietary restrictions. The nutritional goals for any client who is a diabetic are to achieve optimum weight, to maintain blood sugar levels without wide variations, to avoid concentrated carbohydrate, and to maintain normal serum fatty acid levels. The diabetic diet also provides for a balanced diet.

The diet of the older person should be altered as little as necessary to control diabetes. In many older persons the taste buds have changed so that the perception of sweet is less, leading to a desire for very sweet foods (Hayter, 1981, p. 36). If dentures are worn, they also cover taste buds on the upper palate and mask the taste of food. Older persons can be helped to enjoy food by using lemon juice, herbs, and spices to enhance the taste of food, especially meat and vegetables, without adding salt and sugar. The diabetic diet is usually first explained by a dietitian, but often the nurse, who visits in the home of the client will need to answer questions regarding dietary modifications. By being in the home, the nurse can evaluate the availability of shopping centers to purchase food, transportation for shopping, as well as facilities for storing and cooking food.

The dietitian will provide the client with a list of food exchanges, the number of servings from each exchange for the meals of the day, and midafternoon and evening snacks, if insulin is required. The nurse can assist the elderly client or caregiver to choose foods that are available and will be eaten by the client. The client's preferences are considered; therefore the diet regimen will more likely be followed. If the ethnic food preferences are not listed on the exchange sheet, most dietitians have copies of this information available. The client is instructed not to use sugar, jelly or honey since these are simple sugars and elevate the blood sugar immediately. Caffeinated drinks cause the blood sugar to rise and should be limited. If the elderly client insists on having alcoholic beverages, caution is recommended. Alcohol is high in calories, reacts adversely when oral hypoglycemics are taken, and prevents the liver from converting glycogen, protein, or fat into glucose if hypoglycemia occurs. With the physician's approval, small amounts of alcoholic drinks can be included in the menu. Insulin–dependent diabetics or those taking sulfonylurea need their meals on a regular schedule. If a meal must be delayed, a glass of milk should be taken at the regular meal time to prevent hypoglycemia. The calories in the milk are subtracted from the meal when it is eaten (Luckman and Sorensen, 1980, p. 1555). When meals are eaten in restaurants, the client should order foods without sauces or gravy, no fried foods, and food with little fat. A broiled steak, a small baked potato, without sour cream, and a salad will usually meet the requirements for a meal. If eating in a fast foods restaurant, foods should be chosen that have the calories allowed for the meal such as a small hamburger and a salad instead of french fries (Kloster, 1982, p. 184).

Elderly diabetics should be taught that exercise will increase caloric utilization and food should be taken prior to exercise, or where applicable, the dose of insulin can be reduced by a few units with the physician's approval. One important fact that should be emphasized is that the diabetic menu provides the basis for family meals also. Non-diabetic members of the family can add foods in addition to the diabetic menu or have larger portions of food. Foods from the various exchange lists can be used in combination during preparation and a portion served to conform to the exchanges for that meal for the diabetic client.

Teaching the older person who is a diabetic what to do when ill. Illness, no matter how mild, causes some degree of stress which results in increased metabolism, increased gluconeogenesis, and elevated blood sugar. Minor illnesses such as diarrhea or a gastrointestinal upset can be a crisis for older persons who are diabetic. The older individual with diabetes will be taught some specifics that help prevent serious consequences if a short term illness of less than 72 hours in duration occurs. The insulin–dependent diabetic should not omit insulin. Instructions should be obtained from the physician concerning his or her preference for insulin administration when illness occurs. Some physicians will have the client take regular insulin according to the results of the urine tests. Other physicians will have the client take a portion of the usual insulin dose and supplement that with regular insulin according to the results of the urine test (Garofano, 1977, p. 84). If the client is taking oral hypoglycemic agents and cannot eat, the drug is omitted. Vomiting and diarrhea will need to be controlled to prevent fluid and electrolyte problems.

The ill diabetic client should remain in bed and keep warm. Someone will need to remain with the individual in case a hypoglycemic reaction occurs or the illness progresses. Urine should be tested for sugar and acetone every four hours for all elderly diabetics, whether insulin–dependent or not. The illness may result in a temporary need for insulin.

The client should be encouraged to take oral fluids each hour. The fluids should replace some of the lost electrolytes as well as the water. Broth is a good liquid to take if the client will drink it. Some fluids should contain carbohydrates which is better tolerated than protein or fat. Ginger ale is a good source of carbohydrate and is usually well tolerated. If the client is not able to eat after two or three meals, the physician should be notified (Petrokas, 1977, p. 84).

Teaching care of the feet to elderly diabetic clients. Elderly clients who are diabetic have a high risk of decreased circulation to the feet and legs. Because of the decreased circulation and the excess glucose in tissues, the danger of infection of the feet increases. Hygienic measures designed to protect the feet and legs of elderly diabetic clients should include the following instructions:

1. Wash the feet daily in warm water using mild soap. Dry the feet thoroughly, especially between the toes. Avoid vigorous rubbing because this could injure the skin.
2. Use a mild lotion on the feet, but not between the toes, after the feet are dry.

3. If the older person or caregiver is able, trim the toenails straight across. Do not cut the corners of the toenails. Always soak the feet in warm water 10 minutes before trimming the toenails.
4. If toenails are thick or tend to split, visit the podiatrist every 2-3 months to have the toenails trimmed.
5. Keep the feet warm.
6. Wear clean socks and change daily.
7. Wear proper-fitting supportive shoes with room for the toes and no pressure on bony prominences. Wear shoes at all times to protect the feet.
8. Inspect the feet daily for skin breaks, ulcers or blisters.
9. Do not use a heating pad or hot water bottle on feet.
10. Do not cut corns or calluses.
11. Refrain from tobacco because it constricts blood vessels and reduces circulation.
12. Any lesion, cut or ulcer demands medical attention because healing is delayed.
13. If an injury of the foot occurs, wash the area and cover with a sterile gauze.
14. Do not wear garters or hose that constrict and reduce circulation.
15. See the physician concerning any lesion that does not heal promptly.

The above measures can help protect the feet from injury and infection which could turn gangrenous and result in amputation (Smiler, 1982, p. 178).

Teaching the insulin–dependent diabetic to travel safely. Whenever the older age insulin–dependent client wishes to travel, here are some suggestions that make travel easier and safer:

1. Obtain a prescription for insulin and syringes and carry the prescription while traveling.
2. Carry an extra supply of insulin and syringes on the trip. If traveling by plane, wrap the insulin in a towel and put it in a carry-on bag to protect from extremes of heat or cold in the baggage area.
3. Protect insulin from heat. Do not place insulin in the trunk of the car or the glove compartment where heat is intense.
4. If traveling outside the country, discuss with the physician whether insulin can be purchased in other countries and used.
5. If traveling by car, plan to eat smaller meals and eat about 10 grams of a carbohydrate food each hour. Stop frequently and walk around.
6. Carry rapid-acting carbohydrates in case of hypoglycemia. Also carry some longer lasting carbohydrate food in case there is a delay between meals. Peanut butter or cheese crackers and fruit are good choices.
7. If traveling across time zones, consult the physician about adjusting diet and insulin dose.
8. The same fundamentals apply when the person is taking sulfonylurea agents.
9. Always wear a Medi-alert bracelet and carry a card stating you are a diabetic, with the type and amount of insulin taken (Garofano, 1977, p. 91).

Diseases of the Thyroid in the Elderly Population

The thyroid gland gradually decreases in size with age and shows some changes in cell structure. However, these changes do not indicate a disease process. There is a decrease in the serum concentration of triiodothyronine (T3) in the elderly individual, but no significant decrease in thyroxine (T4) (Asch and Greenblatt, 1978, p. 316). Some physicians who care for elderly patients recommend that thyroid function be evaluated in older age persons who come in for diagnosis (Kart, Metress, and Metress, 1978, p. 161). Both hypothyroidism and hyperthyroidism occur in the older age population, but the signs and symptoms are different than in the younger age group (Pomerantz, 1982, p. 314). Kart, Metress, and Metress (1978, p. 161) stated that pathology of the thyroid occurs frequently in the elderly population, but the symptoms of disease are diminished or different than symptoms seen in young adults.

Hypothyroidism

Hypothyroidism in the elderly person may not be detected because physicians and nurses are not alert to the possibility of this disease. The symptoms occur slowly, mimic the aging process, atherosclerosis, or nutritional deficiencies, and so hypothyroidism is not suspected (Asch and Greenblatt, 1978, p. 161). Symptoms of hypothyroidism in the elderly client may range from mental depression to chronic joint pain. The person may be more sensitive to cold, have gradually increasing lethargy, depression, a puffy face, forgetfulness, a hoarse voice, and severe constipation. The elderly person may also have a slow pulse, low blood pressure, and a temperature too low to register on the usual clinical thermometer. Severe myxedema is seen less frequently in the elderly than is thyrotoxicosis. However, some researchers believe that mild hypothyroidism may be present in as many as 40% of the population (Galton, 1975, p. 97). Primary hypothyroidism is seen frequently in the individual who has diabetes and when it occurs, a decrease in the dosage of insulin may be required (Kozak and Cooper, 1982, p. 347). Myxedema occurs more often in women than in men and is seen most commonly in women over 60 years of age (Luckman and Sorenson, 1980, p. 1585). With hypothyroidism, there is an increase in the development of atherosclerosis leading to ischemic heart disease and angina pectoris (Kart, Metress, and Metress, 1980, p. 162). When thyroid production is decreased, there is an increase in circulating cholesterol, phospholipids, and triglycerides which results in accelerated atherosclerosis (Guyton, 1966, p. 1073).

Diagnosis

The diagnosis of hypothyroidism is made by testing the serum levels of T3 and T4. The cholesterol level and triglyceride levels are usually elevated also (Fischback, 1980, p. 493).

Treatment

Treatment of hypothyroidism in elderly clients is initiated very gradually with low doses of thyroid hormone. The most usual medications used today are synthetic thyroxine (Synthroid) or triiodothyronine (Cytomel). If hypothyroidism is severe, the person should be observed carefully for any signs of cardiac abnormalities or adrenal crisis (Asch and Greenblatt, 1978, p. 317). When the thyroid gland fails to secrete thyroid hormone, there is an increased secretion of thyrotropin by the pituitary gland and a decrease in the amount of corticotropin secreted. Consequently, if rapid thyroid replacement occurs, the level of thyrotropin decreases but the corticotropin may not increase as rapidly, resulting in a deficiency of cortisone and lead to adrenal crisis (Guyton, 1966, p. 1060).

Nursing Implications

Nurses supervising care of elderly clients in the home should be alert for the possibility of inadequate thyroid function and assess for this deficit, rather than assume that progressive symptoms are because of the aging process or atherosclerosis. Documentation of signs and symptoms typical of lack or insufficient thyroid function can be made, and requests for tests of thyroid function are more likely to be honored. Assessment of signs other than decreased mental function that may lead to the suspicion that there is a lack of thyroid hormone can save the client from being institutionalized because of paranoia or psychosis due to hypothyroidism (Pomerantz, 1982, p. 314).

If treatment is begun with replacement thyroid, nursing assessment will include observations of improvement of mental and physical functioning, lessening of the edema noted by decreasing puffiness of the face, and weight loss. Intake and output should be evaluated since the fluid trapped in the interstitial spaces will be gradually mobilized and excreted. Blood pressure and pulse rate, volume and regularity are evaluated frequently so that if the replacement of the thyroid hormone is too rapid and signs of cardiac problems develop, they will be detected early. Angina pectoris, myocardial infarction, or cardiac irregularities are likely to occur if the body metabolism is speeded up too suddenly. Any major change in pulse or the occurrence of angina should be reported to the physician at once and the thyroid medication withheld until the client is seen. If dyspnea occurs, the client should be observed carefully for signs of congestive heart failure. Cardiac function may not be adequate to meet the increased demands made by thyroid hormone and the resulting metabolism.

Persons who suffer from significant hypothyroidism are very sensitive to narcotics and barbiturates, therefore when analgesics or sedatives are given the dosage should be only one third to one half the usual dose. After administering the medication, the nurse should observe for respiratory depression (Luckmann and Sorenson, 1980, p. 587).

As the thyroid replacement begins to take effect, the client will need less clothing or covering. The temperature will begin to increase as the body metabolism rises and the peripheral areas become warmer.

With the administration of thyroid hormone, mental acuity and physical strength will improve. The client will need encouragement to be more active, to take part in household activities, and be more responsible for self care. Caloric restrictions are sometimes needed if much weight has been gained prior to diagnosis. Weight will need to be checked accurately to help determine whether the replacement hormone dose is adequate or too high. There is frequently a rapid weight loss when therapy is initiated due to the mobilization and excretion of retained fluid. The puffiness around the eyes and face should decrease as the extra fluid is lost from the tissues. Constipation will usually resolve itself as activity levels increase and as intestinal motility returns to normal. The elderly client still needs to be encouraged to drink at least eight to ten glasses of fluid each day to prevent constipation and dehydration. A stool softener is sometimes needed to prevent straining with constipation.

After the thyroid hormone is started, frequent laboratory measurements of thyroxine levels are recommended until the correct maintenance dose has been reached (Asch and Greenblatt, 1978, p. 317). Nursing personnel will help the elderly client and/or the caregiver realize that once the maintenance dose of thyroid hormone has been achieved, the medication will be needed for the remainder of the individual's life. Emphasis will be placed on the fact that the body is no longer producing the thyroid hormone; therefore, it must be replaced daily to maintain normal metabolism.

Specific teaching needs of the elderly client who has hypothyroidism. The nurse should teach the client and/or the family the following:

1. Use layers of clothing or covers to protect oneself from cold.
2. Thyroid medication will be needed each day for the remainder of his or her life, unless symptoms of overdose occur. If there is suspicion of an overdose, blood levels of T3 and T4 will likely be determined in order to adjust the dosage of medication.
3. Signs and symptoms of overdose of medication are weight loss, tachycardia, fatigue, confusion, angina pectoris, or atrial fibrillation. When symptoms suggest overdosage, the physician should be notified so that tests can be made to determine whether the dose needs to be revised or whether something else is causing the symptoms.
4. The client should avoid sedatives or narcotics until the replacement hormone has become effective. If the client must take these medicines, the caregiver will observe carefully for signs of respiratory depression.
5. As the client's energy level increases, encourage more activity and greater responsibility for self care.
6. If weight gain has been a problem, a calorie–restricted diet will be needed until ideal weight is accomplished. As the thyroid hormone reaches normal levels,

calories will need to be increased slightly to prevent too rapid a weight loss and increasing fatigue.

Hyperthyroidism

Hyperthyroidism is not as common in the elderly population as it is in the young adult (Kart, Metress, and Metress, 1978, p. 161). Approximately 10 to 15% of persons who have hyperthyroidism are in the older age group (Asch and Greenblatt, 1978, p. 317). Symptoms of hyperthyroidism in the elderly are very different from those seen in the 20-year-old person. Symptoms of hyperthyroidism in the elderly are more often related to congestive heart failure, atrial fibrillation, angina pectoris, or myopathic weakness (Locke and Galaburda, 1978, p. 135). These conditions are often accompanied by confusion, weight loss, weakness and fatigue. Since this group of symptoms is frequently seen in elderly people, the thyroid state is often not considered as a cause. Polydipsia is frequently present in the elderly client with hyperthyroidism, probably because of increased blood flow to the kidney and increased fluid excretion by kidneys unable to conserve fluid as readily as in the young person (Asch and Greenblatt, 1978, p. 317).

Diagnosis

One researcher suggested that thyroid function should be routinely tested in all elderly persons because the disease produces different symptoms in the elderly than in young individuals. The same laboratory tests used to diagnosis hypothyroid states are used to diagnose hyperthyroidism. Both triiodothyronine (T3) and thyroxine (T4) levels are increased. The radioiodine uptake test (RAI) shows a very rapid concentration of the iodine in the thyroid gland (Pomerantz, 1982, p. 314).

Treatment

Elderly clients are more sensitive than younger individuals to drugs, so treatment protocols take this fact into consideration. The antithyoid drugs and radioactive iodine are the therapies most often used. Radioactive iodine is recommended for elderly patients (Locke and Galaburda, 1978, p. 135). This drug can be given in small doses and the client can be observed at home. As the radioactive iodine is absorbed by the thyroid, some of the functioning cells are gradually destroyed and the secretion of thyroid hormone diminishes. Several weeks may be necessary for symptoms of hyperthyroidism to subside. A second small dose of the radioactive iodine is sometimes necessary to control the production of thyroxine. This therapy eliminates the necessity of continued drug administration for long periods (Asch and Greenblatt, 1978, p. 317). The client will need to have the function of the thyroid gland checked after symptoms are relieved to determine whether or not hyperthyroidism has occurred from the medication.

Anti-thyroid drugs. Anti-thyroid drugs are sometimes used to control hyperthyroidism. Both proplythiouracil and methimazole (Tapazole) act by inhibiting the synthesis of the thyroid hormone. Both drugs, when given over a long period of time, sometimes cause toxic effects. The most serious toxic effect is agranulocytosis. Another possible side effect is a rash. A baseline white blood cell count should be performed before either of these drugs are started, and periodically during therapy (Luckmann and Sorenson, 1980, pp. 1589-1590). The client and/or caregiver should be taught to report signs of sore throat, fever or rash to the physician and withhold the drug until the physician gives approval to resume taking the drug. In the elderly client, either of these drugs should be started at a very low dose and gradually increased until a maintenance dose is reached. Adrenergic blocking agents, especially propanolol (Inderal) may be needed to control the cardiac symptoms such as atrial fibrillation, tachycardia, or tremors, until the anti-thyroid drugs have reduced the production of thyroid hormone (Asch and Greenblatt, 1978, p. 317).

Nursing Implications

When supervising care of elderly clients in the home, the nurse should be alert for signs of hyperthroidism. If atrial fibrillation has not been diagnosed previously, but a rapid irregular pulse is detected, the nurse should assess further for symptoms of cardiac and non-cardiac origin. If apathy, confusion, fatigue, muscle weakness, and weight loss are present, one needs to suspect hyperthyroidism as a cause. Exophthalmos is seldom seen in the elderly person. The client and his or her family will be questioned concerning the client's complaints, such as being hot or wearing less clothing than previously. The temperature will be higher than the base line for this client. Hyperthyroidism rarely occurs in persons over 70, but there has been an apparent increase recently. It is not known whether the increase is because of better diagnosis or increasing longevity (Kart, Metress, and Metress, 1978, p. 161).

Once a diagnosis of hyperthyroidism has been made and treatment begun, the elderly client and his or her family will need a careful explanation of the regimen. Diet should be adequate to meet the additional caloric needs until weight has been stabilized. Rest is necessary to conserve energy and spare the heart extra work. An explanation of the treatment ordered and the length of time needed to relieve the symptoms will be necessary. It usually requires four to eight weeks for manifestations of hyperthyroidism to be corrected. If the anti-thyroid drugs are used, one to two years of therapy may be necessary to completely control the condition (Kart, Metress, and Metress, 1978, p. 160). If radioactive iodine is given, the client and family should be assured that there is no danger from the small dose utilized. A cool environment will aid in providing comfort for the individual. The client and family members should be told that confusion and fatigue will begin to clear as the physical condition improves with treatment. Information regarding times to administer the anti-thyroid drugs, if ordered, is important. The client and/or caregiver needs to be provided with information to reinforce knowledge of toxic symptoms of the medication. The client should be encouraged to keep medical appointments for follow-up care. At each visit the nurse will assess the status of the cardiac system by listening to heart sounds and by observing carefully for new or different sounds such as an S3 or gallop rhythm. These heart sounds often indicate early congestive heart failure. Since atrial fibrillation often occurs when the elderly person has hyperthyroidism, an apical pulse should be checked on each visit and any change in rate or rhythm noted and/or reported to the physician. During assessment, the nurse should observe for the presence of a rash or sore throat. If either one is present, a report is made to the physician and the anti-thyroid drug withheld until the doctor has been consulted.

Specific Teaching Needs for the Elderly Client with Hyperthyroidism

1. If radioactive iodine is given, the dose is so small there is no danger to the client or others from radioactivity.
2. If an anti-thyroid drug is ordered, a schedule is made to help remind the client when to take the medication, and the dosage.
3. A careful explanation of possible drug reaction is necessary. Reinforce the fact that only a few people have any toxic side effects. The side effects that are observed are a rash or the presence of a sore throat and fever (Luckmann and Sorenson, 1980, p. 1590).
4. Family members or caregivers are cautioned to continue to observe for dyspnea, angina or altered rhythm of the pulse, because cardiac complications can occur before the medication has become effective (Asch and Greenblatt, 1978, p. 317).
5. Reinforce that frequent follow-up visits to the physician are essential to determine whether adequate amounts of the drug are being administered or whether the dose is too great or too small. When anti-thyroid medications are given for long periods, hyperthyroidism can occur. Early signs and symptoms of hyperthyroidism in the elderly person should be explained to family members or the caregiver.

Summary

Endocrine diseases in general are more prevalent in young persons than in the elderly. When endocrine diseases occur in older persons, the symptoms are often nonspecific and different than the signs and symptoms the same disorders cause in younger people. Therefore, the nurse caring for clients in the home should assess the client carefully and be aware of the possible implications of endocrine disease when nonspecific complaints are voiced. Many complaints of the older person who is developing an endocrine disorder are similar to problems encountered with the aging process. Early detection and adequate treatment will prevent many complications of endocrine disorders in elderly clients. The nurse in the home has the opportunity to listen and evaluate each complaint of the older person for all possible causes and to initiate appropriate action. Teaching the older diabetic client is a very rewarding activity for the nurse with the patience to persevere.

REFERENCES

Asch R H, Greenblatt R: "Geriatric endocrinology," in Reichel W (Ed): *Clinical Aspects of Aging*. Williams and Wilkins Co., Baltimore, 1978, pp 315–26

Blainey C: "Diabetes mellitus," in Carnevali D, Patrick, M: *Nursing Management for the Elderly*. J.B. Lippincott, Philadelphia, 1979, pp 295–309

Blake D R: "Physical assessment of the aged: differentiating normal and abnormal change," in Burnside I M: *Nursing and the Aged*. 2nd Ed. McGraw-Hill Book Co., New York, 1981, Chapter 29

Boyles V: "Injection aids for blind diabetics." *Am J Nurs*, Vol 77, No 9, September 1977, pp 1456–1458

Burke E: "Insulin," in Gutherie D, Gutherie R: *Nursing Management of Diabetes Mellitus*. C.V. Mosby, St. Louis, 1977, pp 86–101

Cahil G F: "Diabetes mellitus," in Wyngarden J, Lloyd Smith C: *Textbook of Medicine*. 16th Ed. W.B. Saunders, Philadelphia, 1982, pp 1045–1053

Cook K A: "Diabetics can be vegetarians." *Nursing 79*, Vol 9, No 10, October 1979, pp 70–73

Eliopoulos C: *Gerontological Nursing*. Harper and Row, New York, 1979, pp 185–194

Eliopoulos C E: "Foot care for diabetics." *Am J Nurs*, Vol 78, No 5, May 1978, pp 884–88

Feldman R A, Sender J, Siegelaub A B: "Difference in diabetic and non diabetic fat distribution patterns by skin fold measurements." *Diabetes*, July 1969, pp 478–486

Fischback F T: *A Manual of Laboratory Diagnostic Tests*. J.B. Lippincott Co., Philadelphia, 1980, pp 493–495

Galton L: "Don't Give Up on an Aging Parent." Crown Publishers, New York, 1975, p 97

Ganda O P: "Pathogenesis of macrovascular disease in human diabetes." *Diabetes 29*, Vol 29, No 11, November 1980, pp 931–939

Garofano C: "Advising the peripatetic diabetic," in *Managing Diabetes Properly*. Horsham, Philadelphia, 1977, pp 89–95

Gregerman R L, Bierman E: "Diabetes mellitus and aging," in Williams R: *Textbook of Endocrinology*. 6th Ed. W.B. Saunders, Philadelphia, 1981, pp 1201–1225

Gutherie D, Gutherie R: *Nursing Management of Diabetes Mellitus*. C.V. Mosby St. Louis, 1977, pp 52–61

Hayter J: "Diabetes and the older person." *Geriat Nurs*, Vol 2, No 1, January-Feburary 1981, pp 33–36

Kozak G, Cooper R: "Diabetes mellitus and other endocrine diseases," in Kozak G: *Clinical Diabetes Mellitus*. W.B. Saunders Co., Philadelphia, 1982, pp 342–352

Kaufman S: "Diet: Enforcing the sine que non," in Chaney P S: *Managing Diabetes Properly*. Horsham, Philadelphia, 1977, pp 27–34

Kayne R: "Drugs and the aged," in Burnside I M: *Nursing and the Aged*. 2nd Ed. McGraw-Hill Book, Co., New York, 1981, pp 349–359

Kart D S, Metress E S, Metress J F: *Health and Aging*. Addison Wesley Publishing Co., Menlo Park, 1978, pp 160–174

Kloster P: "Nutrition—fast food, is it junk?" *Geriat Nurs*, Vol 3, No 3, May/June 1982, pp 184–185

Locke S, Galaburda A: "Neurological disorders of the elderly," in Reichel W: *Clinical Aspects of Aging*. Williams and Wilkins Co., Baltimore, 1978, p 135

Luckmann J, Sorensen K C: *Medical Surgical Nursing: A Psychophysiological Approach*. 2nd Ed. W.B. Saunders Co., Philadelphia, 1980, pp 1542–1598

Lundin D V: "Reporting urine test-results: switch from + to %." *Am J Nurs*, Vol 78, No 5, May 1978, pp 878–879

McCarthy J A: "Diabetic nephropathy." *Am J Nurs*, Vol 81, No 11, 1981, pp 2030–2033

Moss J: "Pitfalls to avoid in diagnosing diabetes." *Geriatrics*, Vol 31, No 10, October 1979, pp 52–100

Morse P H: "Ocular signs and symptoms of diabetes." *Geriatrics*, Vol 31, No 10, October 1976, pp 59–66

Petrokas J: "Explaining axioms of sick days," in Chaney P S (Ed): *Managing Diabetes Properly.* Horsham, Philadelphia, 1977, pp 83–88

Plasse N J: "Monitoring blood glucose at home: A comparison of three products." *Am J Nurs,* Vol 81, No 11, November 1981, pp 2028–2029

Pomerantz R: "Considerations in the physician's approach." *Geriat Nurs,* Vol 3, No 5, Sept/Oct 1982, pp 311–315

Porte D, Halter J B: "The endocrine pancreas," in William R: *Textbook of Endocrinology.* 6th Ed. W.B. Saunders, Philadelphia, 1981, pp 758–837

Schaefer A M: "Common concern: Nursing measures to maintain foot health." *Geriat Nurs,* Vol 3, 1982, pp 182–183

Schultz J, Williams M: "Blind diabetics, breeding independence," in Chaney P S: *Managing Diabetes Properly.* Horsham, Philadelphia, 1977, pp 175–181

Schumann D: "Disturbances in glucose metabolism," in Jones, D A, Dunbar C F, Jiroyec M: *Medical Surgical Nursing.* New York, 1982, pp 745–782

Shuman C, Owen O E: "When and how to use insulin in the elderly diabetic." *Geriatrics,* Vol 31, No 10, October 1976, pp 75–82

Smiler I: "Common concern: Foot problems of elderly diabetics." *Geriat Nurs,* Vol 3, No 3, May/June 1982, pp 177–181

Stevens A D: "Monitoring blood glucose at home: Who should do it and how." *Am J Nurs,* Vol 81, No 11. November 1981, pp 2026–2027

Todd B: "Drugs and the elderly, when the patient is taking a sulfonylurea." *Geriat Nurs,* Vol 2, No 4, July/August 1981, pp 291–294

Todd B: "Drugs and the elderly—for arthritis—plain aspirin or an aspirin substitute." *Geriat Nurs,* Vol 3, No 3, May/June 1982, pp 191–194

Welk D S: "Preventing insulin induced lipodystrophy." *Nursing 79,* Vol 9, No 12, December 1979, pp 42–45

Williams T F: "Diabetes mellitus in older people," in Reichel W: *Clinical Aspects of Aging.* Williams and Watkins Co., Baltimore, 1979, pp 327–330

Wolfe L W: "Insulin: Easing the dialy routine," in Chaney P S: *Managing Diabetes Properly.* Horsham, Philadelphia, 1977, pp 49–55

BIBLIOGRAPHY

Bonar, J R: *Diabetes.* 2nd Ed. Medical Examiners Publishing Co., New York, 1980

Duncan T G: "Teaching commonsense health care habits to diabetic patients." *Geriatrics,* Vol 31, No 10, October 1976, p 93

Durgin, S J: "The pharmacist's evaluation." *Geriat Nurs,* Vol 3, No 1, Jan/Feb 1982, pp 31–33

Forbes K, Stokes S A: "Saving the diabetic foot." *Am J Nurs,* Vol 84, No 7, July 1984, pp 884–88

Fredhold N Z: "The insulin pump: New method of insulin delivery." *Am J Nurs,* Vol 81, No 11, November 1981, pp 2024–2025

Graham S, Morley M: "What 'foot care' really means." *Am J Nurs,* Vol 84, No 7, July 1984, pp 889–91

Griffin, A: "How to prepare and inject insulin with one hand." *Geriat Nurs,* Vol 1, No 2, July/August 1980, pp 111–113

Jones D, Dunbar CF, Jirovec M: *Medical Surgical Nursing: A Conceptual Approach.* 2nd Ed. McGraw-Hill Book Co., New York, 1982

McCarthy J: "Somogyi effect." *Nursing 79,* Vol 9, No 2, February 1979, pp 39–41

Metzger M J: "A new test for blood sugar." *Am J Nurs,* Vol 83, No 5, May 1983, pp 763–64

Williams R: *Textbook of Endocrinology.* 6th Ed. W.B. Saunders Co., Philadelphia, 1981

Wyngarden J B, Lloyd Smith C: *Textbook of Medicine.* 16th Ed. W.B. Saunders Co., Philadelphia, 1982

Information on Meal Planning for the Diabetic

Exchange Lists for Meal Planning from American Diabetes Association, 600 Fifth Avenue, New York, N.Y. 10020. 1976

The Effective Application of Exchange Lists for Meal Planning, American Diabetes Association, 600 Fifth Avenue, New York, N.Y. 10020.

The American Diabetes Association/American Dietetic Association Cookbook (Prentice-Hall), Published 1980.

Fast Food Facts by Diabetic Education Center, 4959 Excelsior Boulevard, Minneapolis, Minnesota 55436.

Franz, Marion: "Fast Foods," Diabetes Forecast, Vol. 36, No. 1 (January/February), 1983, pp 16–20.

Vegetarian Entree Recipes for Diabetic Diets, Loma Linda Company, Loma Linda University Medical Center, Loma Linda, California.

Nutrient Information for Commercial Vegetarian Products:

1. Morningside Farm Products, Miles Laboratory, Inc., Grocery Products Division, 7123 West 65th Street, Chicago, Illinois 60638.
2. Loma Linda Foods, 11503 Pierce Street, Riverside, California 92505.

Information for Clients:

Diabetes and Aging, US Department of Health and Welfare, U.S. Government Printing Office, 1978, 720-295/4089-31.

"What is Diabetes?" Ely Lily and Co., Indianapolis, Indiana 46206.

Foot Health and Aging, American Podiatry Association, 20 Chevy Chase Circle, N.W., Washington, D.C. 20015.

Foot Care for the Diabetic Patient, U.S. Department of Health, Education and Welfare, Public Health Service, Diabetes and Arthritis Program, Washington, D.C. 20201.

SAMPLE MASTER CARE PLAN FOR HOME CARE—

Nursing Diagnoses	Assessment	Planning
I. Nutrition alteration in ability to utilize carbohydrate, protein and fat, due to diabetes mellitus resulting in possible hyperglycemia, ketoacidosis, or hypoglycemia. A. Hyperglycemia	● Assess for weakness, visual changes, dehydration. ● Observe record of urine testing since last visit. ● Assess dietary intake for consistency with diet plan. ● Assess amount and frequency of exercise or strenuous activity. ● Assess insulin dosage taken and the time of administration in relation to meals. ● Assess for presence of acetone on the breath or in urine when tested. ● Assess results of home glucose monitoring, if used.	*Short-term goals* ● Blood glucose will be within normal limits on next examination. ● Urine glucose will be negative. *Long-term goals* ● Blood sugar will remain within normal limits with minimal high or low swings. ● Long-term complications will be delayed, prevented or, detected early.

DIABETES MELLITUS, insulin dependent

Intervention: Nursing Orders	Intervention: Resources and Support Systems	Evaluation: Expected Outcomes
• Teach client how to prepare and administer the type and amount of insulin prescribed. • Teach client to check the blood glucose with Dextrostix (or other material) as prescribed. • Assess client's interpretation of the blood glucose test. • Observe client test urine with method used. Ask client to interpret results. • Review client's dietary plan, meal plans, and total daily calories including between meal and bedtime snacks, as ordered. • Review with client the usual exercise or activity pattern. • Determine the usual regimen of client when minor illness occurs.	• American Diabetes Association, local affiliate. • "Diabetes Forecast." ADA magazine for members. • Local hospital education department classes for diabetics. • Nutritionist from home health agency.	• Client can successfully prepare and administer the prescribed dose of insulin. • Insulin is administered between the subcutaneous fat and muscle. • Client can document the site used and use site rotation. • No lipodystrophy occurs. • Client varies the menu while maintaining the ratio of carbohydrate, protein, and fat, as well as total daily calories. • Client tests the urine accurately and interprets the results correctly. • Client knows when to notify the physician of possible problems of control. • Client can use the materials to test blood glucose.

SAMPLE MASTER CARE PLAN FOR HOME CARE—

Nursing Diagnoses	Assessment	Planning
B. Ketoacidosis, potential	• Assess for nausea, vomiting, pain in the abdomen, excessive thirst, excessive urination, deep difficult respiration, odor of acetone on the breath, drowsiness, flushed face or loss of consciousness. • Assess for the presence of any undetected illness, such as flu, infection of the extremities. • Assess whether the client has taken the prescribed insulin. • Check the blood sugar, if the client uses a home testing method. • Test the urine for acetone.	*Short-term goals* • Ketoacidosis will not occur or will be detected and treated early. *Client will:* • know and state why ketoacidosis might occur when insulin is omitted or when too many calories are consumed • be able to state why fluids with minerals are essential when ill and unable to eat • be able to state why bouillon or Gatoraide are good fluids to drink when ill. *Long-term goal* • Ketoacidosis will be prevented.

DIABETES MELLITUS, insulin dependent (continued)

Intervention: Nursing Orders	Intervention: Resources and Support Systems	Evaluation: Expected Outcomes
• Teach the client to contact the physician for insulin orders when blood sugar is 240 mg. % or higher or to administer the dosage of regular insulin recommended by the physician. • Administer oral fluids, if client is conscious. Encourage client to take a glass of fluid each hour if the blood sugar is over 240 mg. %, or if urination is frequent and in large amounts. • Treat and report all illnesses to the physician early. • Arrange for someone to stay with the client until recovery occurs or the client is hospitalized, if illness occurs. • Notify the physician if nausea and vomiting continue or if Kussmaul breathing occurs. • Test urine every 4 hours or more often if indicated for acetone.	• American Diabetes Association, local affiliate • Physician • Family members • Neighbors • Live-in help, if needed	• Ketoacidosis will not occur *Client:* • can state how illness increases the need for insulin • recognizes when the potential for ketoacidosis occurs • can state the early signs of potential ketoacidosis • takes regular insulin by reaction or according to blood glucose, when illness occurs • can state the relationship of skipping insulin dose to the development of ketoacidosis. • drinks fluids with calories and minerals when ill and unable to eat.

SAMPLE MASTER CARE PLAN FOR HOME CARE—

Nursing Diagnoses	Assessment	Planning
C. Hypoglycemia, potential	• Assess for undetected hypoglycemic events. • Assess for tremulousness, hunger, personality changes, nighttime perspiration or restlessness. • If above symptoms have occurred, assess for alteration in diet, insulin administration, or exercise as possible causes. • Determine whether appropriate site rotation is used for insulin administration. • Observe for the presence of atrophy or hypertrophy at injection sites. • Determine any over-the-counter drugs the client has taken that may alter the action of insulin.	*Short-term goals* *Client will:* • be able to state the symptoms of hypoglycemia that have been experienced. • be able to state the actions to take when the above symptoms occur. • help determine what might have led to the hypoglycemia. *Long-term goals* • Blood glucose will remain within normal limits with minimal variation. • Client will be able to state the relationship of diet, exercise, and insulin to hypoglycemia.

DIABETES MELLITUS, insulin dependent *(continued)*

Intervention: Nursing Orders	Intervention: Resources and Support Systems	Evaluation: Expected Outcomes
• Observe the client pre-pare and administer the ordered type and amount of insulin. • Observe for accuracy of measurement, sterile technique and admin-istration technique. • Plan for site rotation with client. Encourage client to maintain a rec-ord of daily injection sites that provide the longest time period be-tween reuse of sites. • Observe for lipodystro-phy at injection sites. • Determine whether al-tered vision prevents the client from measur-ing insulin accurately. • Ask the client what the usual mid-afternoon and bedtime snack consists of and determine whether sufficient com-plex carbohydrate is in-cluded.	• American Diabetes As-sociation, local affiliate. • Family members. • Friends, neighbors. • Ophthalmologist.	• Client states the symp-toms of hypoglycemia experienced. • Client takes 4 oz. of or-ange juice or 6-8 life savers at the first sign of hypoglycemia. • Client can, in retrospect, state what probably causes hypoglycemia. • Client relates excessive exercise or too little food to hypoglycemic attacks. • Client's blood glucose is within normal limits on each visit to the physi-cian's office.

SAMPLE MASTER CARE PLAN FOR HOME CARE—

Nursing Diagnoses	Assessment	Planning
2. Skin integrity, impairment of, potential. Lesions of feet or legs	• Assess the circulation to the extremities with each visit. • Assess the state of toenails and skin of feet and legs. • Assess for the presence of numbness, tingling or pain in the lower extremities. • Observe the feet for any break in skin integrity. • Assess the client's ability to trim nails correctly.	*Short-term goals* • Nails will be trimmed straight across and even with end of toes. • Skin on feet and legs will remain intact. • No numbness, tingling or pain will occur in feet or legs. • Pedal pulses will be present at each visit. • Client will demonstrate self inspection of skin integrity. *Long-term goal* • No lesions will occur on the lower extremities.

SAMPLE MASTER CARE PLAN FOR HOME CARE—

Nursing Diagnoses	Assessment	Planning
Nutrition, alteration in utilization due to hypothyroidism.	• Observe for puffy face, croaky voice, slowed mental and physical response. • Assess for cold intolerance, constipation and angina pectoris.	*Short-term goals* • Client will be able to carry out Activities of Daily Living. • Signs and symptoms will decrease after treatment. *Long-term goal* • Metabolic equilibrium will be restored.

DIABETES MELLITUS, insulin dependent (continued)

Intervention: Nursing Orders	Intervention: Resources and Support Systems	Evaluation: Expected Outcomes
• Teach client to inspect feet and legs each day for any break in the skin. • Teach client to wear clean socks. • Teach client to wear well-fitted shoes to protect the feet from injury. • Teach the client to cut nails straight across, even with the end of the toes, only after a ten–minute soak in *warm* water. • Encourage the client to test bath water and foot soak water temperature by using the forearm or elbow rather than the hand. • Inspect the lower extremities for any break in skin, or for a corn or callus that is injured or infected.	• Podiatrist. • Family member to help with trimming nails.	*Client:* • wears correctly fitted shoes and clean socks at all times • visits the podiatrist every 2-3 months if unable to trim own toenails • notifies physician of any injury to the feet and legs.

HYPOTHYROIDISM

Intervention: Nursing Orders	Intervention: Resources and Support Systems	Evaluation: Expected Outcomes
• Document signs and simptoms that might indicate hypothyroidism. • Assess for hyperthyroidism at each visit. • Prevent client from harming self until treatment is effective. • Weigh weekly until metabolism is normal. • Explain to client and family relationship of inadequate thyroid hormone and symptoms. • Explain the need for continued treatment.	• Family members • Friends • Home health nurse.	• Client excretes the retained tissue fluid gradually. • Mental and physical activity is normal for client. • Client's weight returns to normal.

SAMPLE MASTER CARE PLAN FOR HOME CARE—

Nursing Diagnosis	Assessment	Planning
Nutrition, alteration in need for nutrients due to hyper-thyroidism.	• Assess for the presence of an S3 heart sound, pedal edema, and abnormal lung sounds. • Assess the cardiac rhythm for atrial fibrillation (rapid, irregular irregularity). • Determine whether polydipsia is present. • Assess for apathy or confusion, muscle weakness and fatigue. • Assess for weight loss.	*Short-term goals* • Weight will increase 1 to 2 lbs. weekly. • Lung sounds will gradually return to normal range and will be regular. • Pulse rate will be within normal range and will be regular. • Depression and apathy will gradually resolve. • Muscle strength will improve weekly. *Long-term goals* Body metabolism will return to normal within 6 months.

HYPERTHYROIDISM

Intervention: Nursing Orders	Intervention: Resources and Support Systems	Evaluation: Expected Outcomes
• Teach client and/or family member how the medication is to be taken. • Weigh each week. • Listen to heart and lungs each visit; document changes and notify the physician if indicated. • Assess for mental ability each visit. • Assess for increased muscle strength each visit.	• Family members • Friends • Home health nurse	• Client states the name of the medication taken and how and when to take it. • Client keeps physician appointments as recommended. • Weight increases 1-2 lb. each week. • Heart and lung sounds gradually return to normal. • Mental ability shows improvement each visit. • Muscle strength shows slight improvement each visit.

CHAPTER 12

PULMONARY PROBLEMS

Davida Michaels and Carol Stephenson

Chronic lung disease is a leading cause of disability affecting both the client and the family. It strains personal, family and community resources because the client must adjust to a complex medical regimen at a time when there are decreased physical, financial, psychological and social resources. Chronic lung disease affects multiple body systems: cardiovascular, respiratory, renal, neurological and musculoskeletal. Common treatment modalities often include medications such as bronchodilators which can cause added tremors and nervousness in addition to problems caused by acidosis and the aging process. When prescribed, steroids may affect mental status, causing confusion, irritability and irrational behavior in clients who, because of hypoxemia and hypercapnia, may have an already compromised mental status. Additionally, the presence of dyspnea often causes anxiety which, in turn, increases the sensation of dyspnea. All of these situations make it difficult for the client to master the necessary technical procedures and adhere to medication schedules.

Clients with chronic lung disease can better cope with their condition through an effective, comprehensive pulmonary home care program. Nursing is a major component of such a program.

Pulmonary Changes Related to Aging

Planning intelligently for the care of elderly clients with pulmonary problems requires that the nurse recall the effect of the aging process on the respiratory system as well as the pathophysiological changes caused by any disease which is present. Table 12.1 summarizes the pulmonary changes which occur during the aging process.

TABLE 12.1
Pulmonary Changes in Aging

Structural Change	Implications for Client Care

A. Structure and tissue changes
  1. Chest wall stiffens somewhat.
  2. Reduced respiratory muscle strength.
  3. Reduced alveolar—capillary diffusion surface.
  4. Alveolar enlargement.
  5. Increased airway closure.
  6. Possible kyphosis.
	1. ↓ ability to cough effectively.
	  a. Instruct patient in proper cough techniques.
	  b. Position patient carefully to avoid restricted chest movement and decreased ventilation
	2. ↓ excerise capacity.
	  a. Instruct in energy conservation, work simplification and ADL's "how to do more with less."

Altered neurologic control	

1. Less precise neurological control of respiration.
2. Blunting of chemoreceptor responses to hypoxemia and hypercapnia.
3. Defense mechanisms.
4. Reduced immune defense mechanisms.
5. Reduced mucociliary clearance.
	1. ↓ reserve; patient tolerates stress poorly.
	  a. Caution with administration of sedatives and tranquilizers
	  b. Instruct patient in prevention of infection, early recognition, and prompt seeking of medical attention.

The respiratory changes of aging are usually minimal in the healthy person. Clinical evidence of these changes may not be clear. However, if the client becomes ill or has other risk factors, such as disease or smoking, he or she is much more susceptible to respiratory problems than a younger person. Older people are also more susceptible to the hazards of drug therapy, such as respiratory depression, and are less able to adjust ventilation to extreme demands of exercise or stress.

Pulmonary Problems Requiring Home Care

Chronic lung disease includes obstructive conditions such as asthma, emphysema, and chronic bronchitis as well as restrictive conditions such as interstitial lung disease.

Obstructive Diseases

Obstructive lung diseases are a group of diseases characterized by expiratory airway obstruction and resistance to airflow. According to West (1982, pp. 59–60), three major conditions cause airway obstruction:

• Conditions inside the lumen of the conducting airways such as secretions and foreign bodies.

- Conditions affecting the wall of the airway. These include hypertrophy of the mucous glands, smooth muscle contraction (bronchospasm), or inflammation and edema of the mucosa.
- Conditions outside the airway affect the caliber or size of the airway. There may be destruction of lung tissue surrounding the airway which causes a loss of airway support. Imagine the airway held open by springs around it; if the spring is weak or destroyed, the airway will collapse, most noticeably on expiration. This condition happens in emphysema. Pressure on the airway due to such conditions or tumors may compress the airway with direct pressure.

Obstruction is usually more of a problem on expiration because the airway normally widens on inspiration because of the "pull" of the lungs as they expand. On expiration, the airways normally narrow. If there is an obstruction inside the airway, outside the airway, or loss of the spring-like traction, the airway may collapse and prevent air from being exhaled.

Chronic Obstructive Pulmonary Disease (C.O.P.D.)

C.O.P.D. is a collective term applied to a group of chronic, frequently progressive, respiratory disorders which appear to be related but with no single etiology. The category of C.O.P.D. generally includes emphysema and chronic bronchitis. Asthma is also included although asthma is considered to be a reversible disorder. Clients with C.O.P.D. experience a slow but progressive shortness of breath, cough, decreased exercise tolerance, and impaired gas exchange. They are much more prone to respiratory infection than persons not affected.

Cigarette smoking has been shown to be a major etiological factor in the development of emphysema and chronic bronchitis. There is a definite relationship between "pack years" of smoking (packs smoked per day times number of years) and development of C.O.P.D. Other less–important factors implicated in the etiology of C.O.P.D. are air pollution, occupation, repeated infections, and genetic factors such as alpha/antitrypsin deficiency.

Emphysema

Emphysema is a pathologic diagnosis more than a clinical one. In emphysema, the alveoli are distended and/or destroyed. This condition leads to loss of gas exchange capability, loss of lung elasticity, and decreased elastic recoil. Without the alveolar and bronchilar support, the airways tend to collapse on expiration causing air trapping. The pulmonary capillary bed is partially destroyed along with the alveoli which results in decreased perfusion and diffusion.

Chronic Bronchitis

Chronic bronchitis is defined by its clinical symptoms. A person who has a chronic cough and sputum production for three months of the year for at least two consecutive years has chronic bronchitis. There is chronic inflammation of the bronchial walls along with mucosal edema, increase in size and number of the mucous glands, and excessive mucus production. Degenerative changes occur in the bronchi with loss of cilia, scarring and mucus obstruction. As a result, the airways are narrowed on expiration, causing air trapping and ventilation-perfusion imbalance. Emphysema and chronic bronchitis rarely occur in isolation, although a given client may have a primary pathology of one disease or the other. Asthma may occur in combination as well.

Clinical presentation. Emphysema and chronic bronchitis are progressive diseases. Although their clinical presentation varies somewhat according to which disease predominates and by the severity of the disease, they are more alike than different. The clinical presentations of emphysema and chronic bronchitis are compared in Table 12-2.

Clients seldom seek attention until late in the course of C.O.P.D. when they are extremely short of breath and there is significant deterioration of pulmonary function. Clients with C.O.P.D. demonstrate a predictable progression of airway obstruction with a mean rate of decline of 75–80 ml. of tidal volume per year (Burrows, 1978, p. 26.) Table 12-3 presents a guide for estimating respiratory impairment and the resultant effect on the patient's ability to perform activities of daily living.

Asthma

Asthma is a condition in which three pathological changes occur: 1) bronchospasm, or narrowing of the airway by spasm of its muscles; 2) mucosal inflammation, causing edema of the airway mucosa and subsequent narrowing from within; and 3) increased sputum production, leading to plugging of the airway by sputum.

Asthma may occur in adults as well as children and may occur alone or in combination with emphysema or chronic bronchitis. The combination of chronic bronchitis and asthma is called asthmatic bronchitis. Asthma is an episodic condition, with attacks being caused by such stressors as allergy, infection, exercise and emotional stress. None of them will cause an asthma attack, however, unless the potential for asthma pathology is present in the client's airways. Theoretically, the airways return to normal between attacks, although this is not true for many adults.

Symptoms of an asthma attack usually occur first at night, with dyspnea, coughing, orthopnea and wheezing while the client is lying down. If untreated, the attack progresses in a few days to the same symptoms while sitting up, along with chest tightness due to air trapping, anxiety, tachycardia and reduced exercise tolerance.

Bronchiectasis

Another less–common obstructive pulmonary disease is bronchiectasis. Bronchiectasis refers to a permanent, focal dilatation of the bronchi. These dilated areas commonly contain purulent secretions. Repeated infection is commonly believed to be the cause of the bronchial wall damage. Other factors that may

TABLE 12.2
Clinical Hallmarks:
Predominant Bronchitis Versus Predominant Emphysema

	Predominant bronchitis	Predominant emphysema
General appearance	Mesomorphic; overweight; dusky with suffused conjunctivae; warm extremities	Thin, often emaciated; pursed-lip breathing; anxious, prominent use of accessory muscles; normal or cool extremities
Age, years	40–45	50–75
Onset	Cough	Dyspnea
Cyanosis	Marked	Slight to none
Dyspnea	Moderate	Disabling
Cough	More evident than dyspnea	Less evident than dyspnea
Sputum	Copious	Scanty
Upper respiratory infections	Common	Occasional
Breath sounds	Moderately diminished	Markedly diminished
Cor pulmonale and right-sided heart failure	Common	Only during bout of respiratory infection, and terminally
Radiograph	Normal diaphragm position; cardiomegaly; lungs normal or with increased bronchovascular markings	Small, pendulous heart; low, flat diaphragms; areas of increased radiolucency
Course	Ambulatory but constantly on verge of right-sided heart failure and coma	Incapacitating breathlessness punctuated by life-threatening bouts of upper respiratory infections; prolonged course, culminating in right-sided heart failure and coma

Reprinted with permission from Fishman, Alfred P., *Pulmonary Diseases and Disorders*, McGraw-Hill Book Co., 1980, p. 459, Table 35-1.

predispose the patient to the development of bronchiectasis include inhalation of foreign bodies, aspiration pneumonia, immune deficiency states, and cystic fibrosis. Many clients can date their symptoms from the development of childhood respiratory illnesses. These symptoms include a chronic, productive cough, recurrent chest infection, and intermittent hemoptysis. The sputum is characteristically

TABLE 12.3
Guide for Estimating Permament Respiratory Impairment

Estimate to Nearest 5%	None	Slight 10–25%	Moderate 30–50%	Marked 55–75%	Severe 80–90%
Dyspnea	Grade I: patient's breath is as good as that of other individuals of same age and build at work, on walking, and on climbing hills and stairs.	Grade II: patient is able to walk with normal persons of same age and build on the level but is unable to keep up on hills or stairs.	Grade III: patient is unable to keep up with normal persons on the level but is able to walk a mile or so at own speed.	Grade IV: patient is unable to walk more than 100 yards on the level without a rest.	Grade V: patient is breathless on walking or talking or is unable to leave the house because of breathlessness.
Estimated work capacity	Unrestricted.	Can perform moderate activities.	Can do light work not involving hurrying, climbing or heavy lifting.	At most, can do sedentary work.	Completely disabled.
Activities of daily living (ADL)	No significant restriction of normal activities.	Not dyspneic during essential activities; some restriction in other activities.	Dyspneic during showering or dressing; can manage with assistance.	Depends on others for some essential ADL, such as bathing or dressing.	Dependent on help for most needs.
SaO₂(%)*	95–94	93–92	91–89	88–85	<85
Pa_o2(mm Hg)**	80–75	74–70	69–60	59–50	<50
Pa_co2(mm Hg)***	44–46	47–49	50–59	60–65	>65

*SaO₂ - Oxygen saturation. The ratio of amount of oxygen each hemoglobin molecule is carrying in relation to how much oxygen it is able to carry.
**PaO₂ - Patrial pressure of oxygen in arterial blood.
***PaCO₂ - Partial pressure of carbon dioxide in arterial blood.

Adapted with permission from: Fullager, Leonard D. "Basic Information About Pulmonary Procedures" in Michaels, Davida, *Diagnostic Procedures The Patient and the Health Care Team*, John Wiley & Sons, 1983, p. 357, Table 22.2

foul smelling and mucopurulent. In advanced cases, it separates into three layers with a foamy top layer, a serous intermediate layer, and a bottom layer with yellow-green pus and debris. The affected bronchial mucosa show loss of ciliated epithelium, squamous metaplasia, and infiltration with inflammatory cells (West, 1982, p. 182). Bronchiectasis is often accompanied by chronic bronchitis and areas of localized emphysema. There may also be chronic paranasal sinusitis associated with the bronchiectasis.

In addition to the productive, often disabling cough and recurrent infections, the client often develops chronic malnutrition, weakness and fatigue. Complications include lung abscess, chronic respiratory insufficiency, and cor pulmonale. Metastatic brain abscess may occur, although this complication is rare today. Hemoptysis occurs in the majority of clients.

Although bronchiectasis is rarely life threatening, it is a frightening occurrence for the client. Life style may be altered considerably due to the social implications of constantly producing large amounts of foul-smelling sputum.

Successful control of bronchiectasis depends on prompt recognition and treatment of infection, usually with a broad spectrum antibiotic. Septra DS or Bactrim DS (sulfamethoxazole and trimethoprim) is useful in reducing volume of sputum and eliminating pathogens and is frequently used on a long-term outpatient basis (Davis, 1980, p. 1217). Other useful drugs are tetracyline and amoxicillin. Other care includes frequent postural drainage and the same measures as are used for the other obstructive pulmonary conditions. Early recognition and treatment of infection is of special importance.

Restrictive Disorders

According to West (1982, p. 92),* "restrictive diseases are those in which expansion of the lung is restricted either because of alterations in the lung parenchyma or because of disease of the pleura, chest wall or neuromuscular apparatus . . . These diseases are . . . very different from the obstructive diseases in their pure form, although mixed restrictive and obstructive conditions may occur."

Restrictive diseases can best be described as stiff lung syndromes. This means that although the client cannot take as deep a breath as normal, there is no actual resistance to airflow in the airways. Obstructive and restrictive disorders are compared in Table 12.4

Interstitial lung diseases

One category of restrictive plumonary diseases is interstitial lung disease. Interstitial lung diseases comprise a group of disorders characterized by injury to the lung parenchyma, inflammatory response, and alveolitis. There are a wide variety

---

* Reprinted with permission from West, John B., *Pulmonary Pathophysiology*, Baltimore: Williams and Wilkins Publishers, 1982, p. 92.

TABLE 12.4
Comparison of Obstructive and Restrictive Disorders

Obstructive	Restrictive
Definition Difficulty getting air out. Lungs very compliant, like a "floppy balloon," easy to inflate but due to loss of elasticity, difficult to deflate.	*Definition* Difficulty getting air in. Lungs not complaint, like a "stiff balloon," difficult to inflate but empty easily.
Breathing Pattern Long exhalation phase; air trapping	*Breathing Pattern* Rapid, shallow

Medical Treatment
1. Treat cause; reverse that which is reversible.
2. Relieve obstruction
   a. Loosen and remove secretions.
Humidity, hydration, cough, suction, postural drainage.
   b. Treat infection
   c. Decrease swelling
     Steroids
   d. Relieve spasm
     Bronchodilator
     Avoid known irritants
3. Teach breathing control
Pursed lip breathing, abdominal diaphragmatic.
	Medical Treatment
	1. Treat cause; reverse that which is reversible.
	2. Prevent further damage.
	   a. Remove from source of irritants.
	   b. Decrease inflammatory response.
	     Steroids
	3. Assist patient to get air in;
	   I.P.P.B.
	   Incentive Spirometry (preventive measure).

of etiological agents that cause interstitial lung disease. Some interstitial lung diseases that might be seen in the home care of the older client include pulmonary fibrosis, collagen diseases such as scleroderma, lupus erythematosus, asbestosis, silicosis, and sarcoidosis.

These diseases progress very slowly. Often the initial exposure to the causative agent began as much as 20 years prior to the onset of pulmonary fibrosis symptoms. Such chronic exposure can affect firemen, asbestos workers, glass workers, and farmers for example.

If the causative agent is not removed early and the disease progresses, there will be pulmonary cellular and connective tissue alterations. As healing takes place, fibrous tissue replaces normal lung tissue. This distorts the architecture of the alveoli and airways, stiffens the lung, and increases the distance through which respiratory gases must diffuse.

Clinical Signs and Symptoms. Diffuse interstitial lung disease begins insidiously. Clients usually complain of progressive shortness of breath, first during activity and ultimately at rest. The client is usually tachypneic, weakened and fatigued as the illness progresses. Weight loss is common. The clinical picture may resemble neoplasia or chronic hypoxemia. Characteristically there is the presence of fine, end inspiratory crackles (velcro rales) at the lung bases. There may be a dry cough; sputum production is uncommon unless there is infection superimposed on the interstitial lung disease.

Early in chronic interstitial lung disease oxygenation is usually normal; later the client develops hypoxemia. The client is unable to adapt ventilation to the demands of exercise, so exercise worsens hypoxemia. As the disease continues to advance and the lungs progressively stiffen, work of breathing continues to increase and exercise tolerance decreases. Complications include infection, cor pulmonale or right-sided heart failure, hypercapnia, or carbon dioxide retention, and finally respiratory failure.

The major goals of therapy and management of the client with interstitial lung disease are very similar to those of C.O.P.D. In addition to the usual management of C.O.P.D., steroids are considered important therapy for many clients. They are not effective in all cases, however. The steroids would then be tapered and discontinued after an unsuccessful clinical trial.

Effects and Complications of Lung Diseases

Hypoxemia

Both C.O.P.D. and interstitial lung disease result in hypoxemia, or a reduced amount of oxygen dissolved in the blood. Besides the actual lung pathology, factors which contribute to hypoxemia are hypoventilation, secretions, mucosal edema, and bronchospasm. The chronically ill client can tolerate a more severe level of hypoxemia than can a person who suddenly becomes hypoxemic, as from a chest injury. In chronic lung diseases, a pO_2 in the low 60's is considered adequate.

Hypoxia (below 60 mm Hg) affects the nervous system, the circulatory system, the musculoskeletal system, the digestive system, and the respiratory system, among others. The circulatory effects of hypoxia are the result of sympathetic nervous system stimulation. The heart works harder to supply blood to the body tissues. The heart rate increases and the blood pressure rises as a result of this effort. Later, as the heart becomes more hypoxic, cardiac irritability and subsequent arrhythmias may occur. The heart ultimately fails, and consequently, blood pressure and heart rate fall as well. Cyanosis is a late and unreliable sign of hypoxemia. It is affected as much by skin color and hemoglobin level as it is by circulatory status. The falling cardiac output is reflected in lowered urinary output as less blood is moved to the kidneys for filtration. Hypoxemia, if chronic and severe, can also lead to pulmonary hypertension and cor pulmonale, which will be discussed separately.

The respiratory response to hypoxemia is to attempt to increase the respiratory rate as much as possible. There may be an accompanying sensation of dyspnea as the work of breathing increases. Respiratory failure occurs when the work of breathing uses more oxygen and generates more carbon dioxide than the client can move.

The brain is very sensitive to reduced oxygenation. Hypoxemia, therefore, can result in a variety of changes in mental functioning. Anxiety and restlessness are considered classic signs of respiratory distress. Other mental changes which may occur in any combination include confusion; disorientation; impaired judgment, memory, and coordination; irritability; paranoia; or delirium. There may also be impaired visual perception. Ultimately, if the hypoxemia continues unchecked, the client may progress to stupor and coma.

The musculoskeletal system responds to hypoxemia with reduced exercise tolerance because the muscles are not properly oxygenated. As the client exercises less, this compounds the problem because disconditioned muscles require more oxygen to support a given activity than do conditioned muscles. Digestion also requires a great deal of oxygen and may be impaired in the hypoxic client.

The hypoxic client has no reserve and therefore, little tolerance to stressors such as breath holding, activity, emotional upset, infection or other pathologic processes. Even a mild stressor may be enough to move the client from chronic respiratory insufficiency to acute respiratory failure.

Hypercapnia

Hypercapnia, or carbon dioxide retention, does not occur in all clients with C.O.P.D. or interstitial lung disease. Carbon dioxide retention is important, not only for the symptoms it causes, but also for its effect on the respiratory drive.

In the normal individual, respiration is stimulated by the effect of carbon dioxide (CO_2) accumulation. When CO_2 accumulates to a certain point, the respiratory center is stimulated, and the person takes a breath.

If a person chronically retains CO_2 so that the CO_2 level is always above normal, the respiratory center loses its sensitivity to CO_2. Therefore, CO_2 accumulation no longer provides a stimulus to take a breath. Instead, the body switches to a hypoxic respiratory drive. That is, when the person's oxygenation (pO_2) falls to a certain level, peripheral chemoreceptors take note of this and cause him or her to take a breath. If enough oxygen is given to this person to raise the pO_2 above what is normal for this client (usually in the 60's or low 70's), the individual loses the stimulus to breathe and indeed does not breathe until the pO_2 falls below what it was before the oxygen was given. This phenomenon is called CO_2 narcosis. It can, in its most severe form, cause respiratory arrest. This not infrequently occurs in the home setting where someone increases the liter flow of the home oxygen supply as a way of dealing with respiratory distress. CO_2 retention is not a contraindication for oxygen therapy. Oxygen should be administered at low liter flows (1–2 min.) and started by nasal cannula.

In chronic CO_2 retention with cor pulmonale there is often sodium and water retention with resultant edema. The kidneys retain bicarbonate to compensate for the hypercapnia and buffer the blood pH. Clients who have a slow, gradual rise in CO_2, with time for kidneys to compensate, may tolerate very high levels of CO_2.

Carbon dioxide is a vasodilator which leads to many of the clinical symptoms of hypercapnia: flushing, reduced mentation, and severe basal headaches which occur most often during sleep. The headaches occur most while asleep because everyone breathes less efficiently when asleep. If the client is barely managing adequate air exchange when awake, it is not surprising that the person may hypoventilate and accumulate CO_2 when asleep. The headaches which awaken the person are precursors of cor pulmonale and are indicators for oxygen therapy while asleep.

Cor pulmonale

Cor pulmonale, or right–sided heart failure, is a common complication of C.O.P.D. and interstitial lung disease. Chronic hypoxemia causes pulmonary hypertension which, in turn, increases the work load of the right side of the heart as it attempts to pump blood into the pulmonary vessels. The right ventricle is not built for this workload and fails, that is, cor pulmonale occurs.

The symptoms of cor pulmonale are those of right-sided heart failure: insidious onset, jugular venous distention (JVD), weight gain, dependent edema, and if severe, liver enlargement. There may or may not be basal headaches at night. The assessment of dependent edema is important to the nurse; whether or not the person is up walking or sitting in a chair, whether legs and feet are dependent and the site of edema formation. If, however, the client is constantly in bed, the sacrum is the most dependent area and should be checked for edema. Clients with chronic lung disease should be taught to weigh themselves once or twice weekly and report sudden weight gain because it is an early symptom of cor pulmonale.

Management of cor pulmonale consists of improving ventilation and oxygenation, reducing fluid load (often with salt restriction and diuretics), steroids to reduce inflammation, treating infection, if it is present, and other management as indicated for the chronic lung disease and any complications which may arise.

Digitalis preparations are usually reserved for clients with left ventricular failure. If it is used in the presence of hypoxia, it increases cardiac irritability, already a problem for the hypoxic heart. Clients with chronic lung disease may also tend to be sensitive to the effects of digitalis because of hypercapnia, electrolyte imbalance, or acid-base imbalance as well as the cardiac effects of their medications, such as Xanthimes and sympathomimetic agents (Fishman, 1980, p. 859), used to relieve bronchospasm. If such failure exists and digitalis is necessary, the client should be maintained on the lowest dosage possible. Digitalis toxicity is always a possibility for which the client should be carefully assessed at each home visit.

Retained Secretions

Increased secretion production, impairment of mucociliary clearance, decreased ability to cough, and impairment of the function of the aveolar macrophages may result in retained secretions. Ciliary movement may be impaired by the lung pathology, airway irritants (allergens, pollution), infection, hypersecretion of mucus, and medications that dry secretions. Coughing may be impaired because of very thick secretions, or the inability to take a deep breath and generate sufficient expiratory flow rates to move secretions. Retained pulmonary secretions lead to inflammation and infection of airways, and partial or total airway plugging with resultant increased resistance and work of breathing.

Infection

Pulmonary infection occurs commonly in clients with C.O.P.D. In fact, it is the most common cause of acute respiratory failure. The most common organisms involved are *Hemophilus influenzae* and *Streptococcus pneumonia*. Less common are *Klebsiella pneumoniae* and *Psuedomonas*. It is vital that efforts are aimed at prevention and early recognition and treatment of infection. The client must take an active part in this aspect of care. Infection is discussed further in the section on management of care.

Acute Respiratory Failure

Other causes of acute respiratory failure in these clients include pulmonary embolism, heart failure, use of sedatives, acute episodes of bronchospasm, bronchial plugging, and misuse of oxygen. Infection is the most common cause of acute respiratory failure, hospitalization, and cor pulmonale in these clients. Many chronic pulmonary clients overlook the early signs of respiratory infection or other respiratory problems even after thorough instruction. The nurse, therefore, must be very astute in observing the homebound respiratory client for changes or problems, and should look for changes in sleep habits due to dyspnea, orthopnea, wheezing or coughing, reduced exercise tolerance, increased dyspnea, thickening or color change of the sputum, and mental changes. Teaching of the client should be done repeatedly and at the client's level of understanding. Table 12.5 provides a guide to aid the client in deciding when to call the physician.

An important assessment factor in the client who has bronchospasm or asthma is wheezing. Early in the attack, auscultation will reveal expiratory wheezing because the airways normally close more in expiration than inspiration. Excess narrowing due to bronchospasm, therefore, will first be apparent on expiration. As the attack progresses, auscultation reveals both inspiratory and expiratory wheezing. If the client is not treated by this point in the attack and the nurse examines the client a day or two later, no wheezing at all may be heard. The nurse should then listen very carefully for breath sounds. The most notable cause of this lack of wheezing is that the airways are so closed that the client is not even moving enough air to wheeze. This client, who has greatly diminished breath sounds and has stopped wheezing, needs immediate treatment if acute respiratory failure is to be avoided.

TABLE 12.5
Client Guide for When to Call the Doctor

Call your doctor when:

1. There is any change in your level of shortness of breath, wheezing, coughing, or if you have chest pain.
2. You are having difficulty sleeping because of wheezing, coughing, or shortness of breath.
3. You think you are having side effects from your medicines.
4. There is a change in your sputum, such as from white to yellow, green, gray, or bloody, or your sputum is thicker and more difficult to cough up.
5. You have fever or chills.
6. You notice weight gain or swelling of your feet or legs.
7. You need a prescription refilled.
8. Planning to take any drug prescribed by another physician or any over-the-counter medicine.

Management of Chronic Lung Disease and Interstitial Lung Disease

Management of these conditions is aimed at reversing that which is reversible, providing symptomatic relief, preventing complications, and assisting the clients and their families to live with their condition. Both acute care and home care attempt to achieve the same goals and utilize the same types of activities. Along with the care by the health team, it is vitally important that the client be educated so that he or she becomes a full participant in his or her care. The client needs to understand every aspect of the disease and its care. An outline for client education may be seen in Table 12.6. Written materials and visual aids should be liberally incorporated into the teaching process.

The management of chronic lung disease is detailed below and in the sample master care plan at the end of the chapter.

Improve Ventilation

The first management goal is to *improve ventilation*. The client can be assisted to move air more effectively in several ways:

- Liquify sputum. When sputum is thin, it is easier to expectorate and thus clear the airway.
- Aid in removal of secretions. This may be done by chest physiotherapy and coughing techniques. Occasionally, suctioning is necessary.
- Open the airway using bronchodilating and steroid drugs.
- Promote effective breathing pattern by teaching breathing techniques and their use and with the use of relaxation and conditioning techniques.
- Avoid respiratory suppressants.

TABLE 12.6
Client/Family Education Plan for Chronic Lung Diseases

Assess client and family knowledge, beliefs, practices.

Normal lung structure and function.

Basic disease process
- Definition, pathophysiology, effect on lung function
- Relate pathology to symptoms

Drug therapy
- Why taken, when taken, adverse effects
- Relate drug actions to symptoms and pathology

Daily living and coping
- Relaxation techniques
- Conditioning
  - Gradual, planned exercise program
  - Breathing exercises, breathing control, respiratory and abdominal muscle strengthening
- Nutrition
- Pulmonary hygiene
  - Hydration, cough, chest physiotherapy
  - Equipment—operation, assembly, cleaning
  - Emergency care in power failure
- Oxygen
  - How much and when to use
  - Equipment
- Self-care activities
  - Work simplification and energy conservation
- Avoiding airway irritants and hazards
- Monitoring, decision making
  - Prevention and recognition of infection
  - Deciding when to call the doctor
- Community Resources
  - American Lung Association, Better Breathing Club, Transportation

Hydration

Liquification of sputum can be accomplished in a variety of ways. The most important is a high fluid intake. The adult client should routinely drink at least eight to ten eight-oz. glasses of fluid a day, excluding milk and milk products. Milk may tend to thicken secretions, so it should be used only in very limited amounts. If the client notices secretions thickening, he or she should increase fluid intake to even higher levels. If fluid retention is a problem, diuretics should be used to balance the fluid load, but fluid intake should not be restricted. If water intoxication becomes a problem, more balanced fluids such as juices may be substituted for free water intake.

Aerosol Therapy

Aerosol therapy is particularly helpful for clients with thick secretions, such as those with chronic bronchitis and bronchiectasis. An aerosol is a suspension of particles in a gas. Aerosols are usually produced by a device such as a nebulizer which break water or saline into tiny droplets for delivery to the pulmonary mucosa. Clincially, the penetration and deposition of aerosols in the airway is affected by the clients' ventilatory pattern. The preferred pattern is a slow, deep breathing one with a slight end inspiratory breath hold (Shapiro, 1979, p. 172.)

The technique is easier to master than Intermittent Positive Pressure Breathing (I.P.P.B.) and the equipment less expensive and simpler to maintain.

Aerosol therapy is useful in the breaking up of retained dry secretions and in promoting sputum mobilization and cough. During the administration of therapy, the client should sit up, if possible, with the body in proper alignment and breathe through the mouth with slow, deep breaths using diaphragmatic breathing. Coughing should be encouraged several times during the treatment. If too much sputum is mobilized, suction may be necessary to avoid airway obstruction. The nurse should check the clients' ability to clean the equipment. Some manufacturers have devised fancy equipment with tiny holes which are easily plugged and difficult to clean by clients with decreased vision and peripheral muscular tremors.

Methods of Administration

Heated mist. Heated mist or nebulizers are capable of delivering an aerosol of moderate density. The mist is delivered, by means of wide-bore tubing, to either a face mask or face tent. Heated mist is usually given as an individual treatment two to four times a day for 15 to 20 minutes after bronchodilator therapy.

Ultrasonic nebulizer. The ultrasonic nebulizer delivers a high volume of aerosol. Particle size is very small, which aids deposition in the smaller bronchioles. Wide-bore tubing must be used to deliver the mist. Therapy may be given two to four times a day, up to every four hours, for 20 to 30 minutes following bronchodilator therapy.

Hazards of aerosol therapy. Shapiro (1979, pp. 181–2), has identified several hazards of aerosol therapy, especially ultrasonic nebulization, that should be remembered in caring for the client in the home care setting.

Swelling of dried, retained secretions. The dried secretions may swell and completely occlude an already partially occluded airway. If this occurs, the client will experience increased shortness of breath and respiratory distress. The client should be taught to stop the treatment in such a case. Suction equipment should be available when it is a major problem to prevent or minimize this hazard; a bronchodilator should be administered before the aerosol treatment.

Precipitation of bronchospasm. The aerosol droplets, as foreign bodies, may precipitate bronchospasm. The secretions themselves, as they move along the airway, may also cause spasm. Bronchodilator administration prior to nebulization helps to prevent bronchospasm.

Contamination of equipment is also a hazard. The tubing should be cleaned every 24 hours using the proper technique.

Fluid overload. Although Shapiro does not believe that overload is a concern in the adult client, it may become a concern in fluid sensitive adults such as those with cardiac or renal failure.

Aerosols may increase airway resistance, especially in clients with hyperreactive airways.

Chest physical therapy (postural drainage)

Chest physical therapy includes postural drainage with or without percussion or vibration. Postural drainage aids in the mobilization of secretions by the use of gravity. Secretions are forced from the periphery of the lung toward the trachea where they are removed by coughing. Some conditions involving actual or potential retained secretions in which postural drainage may be of benefit are chronic bronchitis, bronchiectasis, pneumonia, atelectasis, and lung abscess.

There are 12 basic postural drainage positions to drain specific areas of the lung. It is neither necessary nor practical to utilize all of these in the chronic pulmonary client. The physician, nurse, client and therapist should work together to choose the appropriate combination of positions to drain the affected lung areas while being maximally tolerated by the client. The elderly pulmonary client probably will not tolerate the extreme tilt of the Trendelenburg position that is described in most texts on postural drainage.

In addition, there may be other problems such as arthritis or back pain as well as a compromised cardiovascular system. Additionally, adjustments must be made for the home setting if the client does not have a hospital-type bed. Pillows and foam wedges may be utilized in propping the client in the required position. The semi-prone, side position seems to be the best tolerated by the elderly client. This position can be accomplished with the client lying on one side on a bed or sofa with two or three pillows under the hips. (See Figure 12.1) Upper lobes should be drained with the client sitting up (See Figure 12.2) before being placed in a position to drain the lower lobes in order to avoid redeposition of secretions. Often individual adjustments have to be made in choosing the optimal positions for each client. When therapeutically draining a client with disease of one lung, the

FIGURE 12.1
Modified Position for Postural Drainage with Chest Percussion of Lower Lobes and Lateral Areas

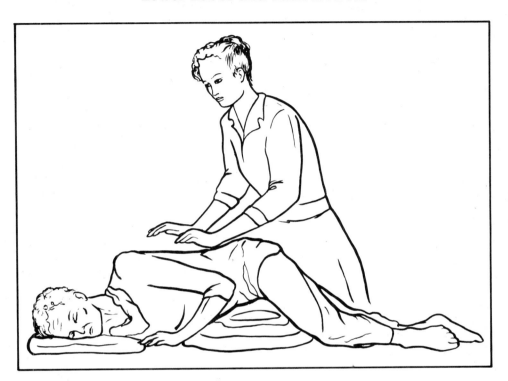

contralateral lung should also be drained in order to decrease the spread of disease.

Postural drainage is intended to augment the client's cough mechanism. It is, therefore, important to reinforce cough technique with the client before and during the treatment. The client should cough several times during the treatment, even in the absence of the natural desire to do so, to aid movement of the secretions. Although the client may feel the urge to sit up and cough, this should be discouraged because this position allows the mucus to run back down the airway. If there is increased shortness of breath during drainage and coughing, the client should be encouraged to cough against pursed lips rather than use a forceful or hacking cough. Many clients do not produce secretions during the procedure but will cough productively several hours afterwards, particularily if they are active.

How long should the client maintain each drainage position? This is an individual matter and depends on patient tolerance, amount of sputum produced, and time

FIGURE 12.2
Position for Postural Drainage with Chest Percussion of Upper Lobes

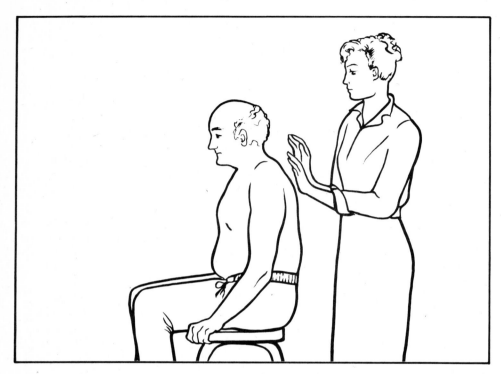

available. Usually the client should remain in each position for 15 minutes in order to allow the tenacious secretions time to mobilize. Treatments should be scheduled at least one hour prior to or two hours after mealtime to prevent regurgitation.

The frequency of chest physiotherapy will vary according to client needs. Clients who have emphysema, asthma, and interstitial lung disease need it only when they are producing secretions (during an infection or an asthma attack). They do not need it on a regular daily basis.

Clients who produce sputum on a daily basis, such as those with chronic bronchitis, can benefit from daily chest physiotherapy. It is unrealistic to expect that the client who is doing relatively well will spend the time and energy required to do chest physiotherapy four to six times daily.

It is, therefore, best to teach the client *plan A and plan B*. Plan A is the plan that the client will use during the times when he or she is relatively stable. The nurse should ask the client to select a time of day when secretions are particularly troublesome, and do chest physiotherapy at that time. Often, by the nurse's next visit, the client has found the treatment so helpful that he or she has selected a second time of day to use it as well.

Plan B is the plan the client should switch to at the first sign of increased or thickened secretions, increased respiratory distress, or other problems. In this plan, the client increases hydration and does chest physiotherapy four to six times a day in an effort to prevent a crisis episode. Along with these activities, the client should confer with the physician and be placed on an appropriate program of drug therapy.

The technique of chest physiotherapy or postural drainage involves percussion and vibration. Percussion, or cupping, is the technique of using cupped shaped hands to clap the chest wall. Percussion is performed continuously for three to five minutes at the start of the drainage period and may be repeated in the middle of the drainage period. When properly performed, there should be no discomfort or pain. When performing percussion, hands are maintained in a cupped shape to trap air between the hand and the chest wall. This produces an energy wave which is transmitted to the lung tissue and shakes the secretions loose. The sound produced should be hollow, not flat; a flat sound indicates slapping rather than cupping. When percussing the client, the scapula, clavicles and spine should be avoided as should the kidneys and female breast tissue. Semi-soft rubber caps are available that help the partially disabled or arthritic spouse perform this technique at home without injury or pain.

Vibration is a technique of producing a vibratory motion in the air while compressing the chest wall. The hands are flattened and placed over the affected area of the chest. The wrists and arms are held stiffly and a vibratory motion is produced by the shoulder muscles as the client exhales. This procedure is repeated for four or five exhalations. It is a gentle technique, usually well tolerated by the client. Some clients may own or rent a vibrator which may enable them to perform the procedure themselves or make the technique easier for another person to accomplish. If a mechanical vibrator is used, it is applied for two to three minutes at the start of the drainage period and may be used for another two to three minutes in the middle of the drainage procedure.

Precautions and contradictions. Clients with compromised cardiovascular systems may tolerate position changes poorly. The head–down position may interfere with venous return and is contraindicated in clients with increased intracranial pressure or cardiac disease. Clients with rib fractures, major heart disease, osteoporosis, or lung cancer should not have chest physical therapy.

Cough Technique

Clients with C.O.P.D. should not force their cough as this tends to close the airway prematurely and may cause airway spasm. They should be taught a controlled cough technique. The object of a controlled cough is to work the mucus slowly up the airway and out without precipitating airway closure or spasm.

Controlled or cascade cough. The client takes a slow, deep breath using diaphragmatic breathing. The breath is held a few seconds; then the client coughs several times during the same exhalation with the mouth slightly open. It helps to lean forward slightly when coughing. After several short coughs, the client should pause, even if no secretions are produced, and inhale by sniffing to avoid pushing the secretions further down the airway. The procedure is then repeated until the secretions are removed. Coughing is one of the most effective ways to clean the airway in the case of respiratory distress. It is even more effective if done after the administration of a topical bronchodilator. Medicines to suppress the cough or dry the secretions should be avoided in the client with lung disease.

Bronchodilators

Bronchospasm is often associated with chronic pulmonary disease. It results in symptoms such as wheezing, shortness of breath, reduced exercise tolerance, tachycardia, and orthopnea. As previously described, other pulmonary conditions involve airway closure on expiration. With the exception of wheezing, the symptoms of these conditions are similar to those of bronchospasm.

Bronchodilators are useful in preventing or reversing bronchospasm and widening the airway to decrease airflow obstruction. The base for all bronchodilator therapy is aminophylline, which comes in a variety of preparations and brand names. It may be administered orally or intravenously. There is a rectal suppository, but its absorption is erratic and unpredictable so it should not be used. It takes several hours to attain a blood level of the drug when it is given orally so this is not a drug of choice for relief of respiratory symptoms. Instead, it should be taken on a regular basis to maintain a blood level of the drug.

Because theophyllin is supplied in many names, the nurse should check the client's drugs to be sure that he or she is taking only one theophylline preparation. The client should be instructed to take it regularly and with food.

Because aminophylline is individually metabolized, dosage adjustment is sometimes a problem. This may be monitored by doing aminophylline blood levels. The level should be drawn one hour before a scheduled dose of the drug in order to ascertain the *trough* or lowest point of the drug's blood level. Therapeutic range is 11-20 mg. %.

A common sign of aminophylline toxicity is nausea and vomiting. If the client develops this, the nurse should obtain a thorough description of the circumstances. If the nausea or vomiting developed soon after taking the drug on an empty stomach, the problem is probably gastric irritation and can be remedied by taking the drug with food. If the problem develops several hours after taking the drug, it is probably toxicity. The client's next dose should be held and the aminophylline level checked.

A variety of drugs are available that combine small amounts of aminophylline with ephedrine (a poor bronchodilator) and phenobarbital to counteract the stimulation of the ephedrine. These are much less effective than an adequate dose of aminophylline. In addition, they are dangerous, not only because of their stimulating effects but because ephedrine can cause urinary retention in elderly men.

Adrenergic drugs such as epinephrine are sometimes used as bronchodilators. These are the major components of most over-the-counter bronchodilators. They are short acting and have dangerous cardiac effects. They are inappropriate as therapy for elderly patients with pulmonary diseases.

Terbutaline (Brethine, Bricanyl) is another very useful bronchodilator. Chemically different from aminophylline, its action is synergistic with the theophyllines. It may be administered either orally or subcutaneously and should be given on a regular rather than on an as needed schedule. The drug may cause tremors, especially at first, but these subside somewhat after a few weeks on the drug. If the tremors continue to be a problem, the dose may need to be adjusted.

Other useful bronchodilators include isoetharine (Bronkosol), albuterol (Proventil), and metaproterenol (Alupent). Of these, Proventil and Alupent are supplied both as metered-dose (cartridge) inhalers and as oral drugs. Bronkosol is supplied as a liquid to be used in a nebulizer or I.P.P.B. machine. Proventil and Alupent are both effective bronchodilators which may be used along with the theophyllines on a regular basis. Any one of the three drugs is appropriate for topical use, both on a regular and an as–needed basis. For "as needed" use, the client should be taught to use the drug at the onset of symptoms, but no more often than prescribed (four hours for Alupent and Bronkosol and six hours for Albuterol). It is also helpful to use the topical drug prior to activities that usually cause wheezing or dyspnea (such as exercise or housework). Anticholinergics are being experimentally used as an adjunct to potentiate the effects of the bronchodilators by stabilizing the airways. There is a danger of dried retained secretions and airway obstruction.

Use of the metered dose device (inhaler). Hand–held pressurized cartridges are frequently prescribed to deliver aerosolized medications. They are quick and easy to use, but may be easily abused (overused) by clients seeking quick relief of symptoms. To be effective, the client must be instructed in their proper use. First, emphasis must be placed on the fact that the device delivers potent medicine and should be used only as prescribed. The cartridge should be shaken well and turned upside down. The client should take a deep breath, exhale fully, then place the inhaler just inside the mouth. As the client inhales slowly through the nose and mouth, the cartridge is pressed and the medication released. The breath is held to a count of three and then slowly released. The breath hold allows maximum deposition and distribution of the medication. If the physician orders two "whiffs" or puffs, the patient should wait five to ten minutes between puffs.

Some authorities (Bushnell and Brooks, 1979, p. 137) have suggested that the client hold the device an inch away from the mouth to prevent deposition in the oropharynx. Other physicians attach a short piece of flex tubing and a mouth piece to the inhaler to trap large particles before they get to the mouth to decrease systemic side effects (Miller and Geumei, 1978, p. 72). If the client is to receive a bronchodilator such as albuterol (Proventil, Ventolin), metaproterenol (Alupent), or isoetharine (Bronkosol) and a steroid, beclomethasone (Vanceril), the bronchodilator should be given before the steroid for maximum effectiveness and to prevent bronchospasm. The client should wait at least 15 minutes between bronchodilator and steroid for maximum effectiveness. The mouth should be rinsed after the steroid is administered.

Delivery of unassisted bronchodilator. Bronchodilators may be administered by means of an air compressor attached to a small reservoir jet nebulizer (aerosol), as described earlier in this chapter.

Intermittent Positive Pressure Breathing (I.P.P.B.). I.P.P.B. therapy consists of the application of positive pressure to the airway during inspiration. It has been prescribed for use at home in clients with chronic lung disease to decrease the work of breathing, improve gas exchange, and administer medications. Controversy surrounds I.P.P.B. because it is expensive and hazardous. Many clients who are short of breath have used I.P.P.B. to relieve their dyspnea by taking a few puffs on the machine at frequent intervals. If the client can be taught to use proper breathing control, the shortness of breath can be relieved without relying on the machine. As one client observed after having undergone an extensive rehabilitation program, he used to be afraid to go out of the house away from his machine. Breathing control not only worked for him, it was much more portable.

Although the work of breathing may be decreased during the treatment, it only lasts for the time of the treatment. In many cases, work of breathing actually increases during the treatment. The use of proper breathing control will provide a lasting decrease in the work of breathing. As to drug delivery, there is no evidence to demonstrate that bronchodilators are more effectively administered by I.P.P.B. than by inhalers or compressor–driven nebulizers.

Problems associated with the use of I.P.P.B. are expense, infection, CO_2 narcosis, hyperventilation, decreased cardiac output, pneumothorax, and psychological dependence. Improper cleaning of the I.P.P.B. machine may result in frequent infections. If the client has I.P.P.B. equipment, he or she must be taught to clean the machine properly. The client should be taught to care for the machine and should be given written directions so that the nurse can use these periodically to check the client's technique of machine care. One method is described in Figure 12-3.

Occasionally, clients will hyperventilate with the I.P.P.B. machine and become dizzy or faint. If they commonly retain carbon dioxide, they may develop CO_2 narcosis during an I.P.P.B. treatment as described in the section on hypercapnia.

It is all too common for some clients to rapidly cycle the machine and receive a large volume resulting in hyperventilation and decreased $PaCO_2$ causing dizziness and faintness. It is also possible to have a significant decrease in venous return to the heart resulting in a decreased cardiac output, tachycardia, dyspnea, and a frightened, anxious patient. Clients with C.O.P.D. may also suffer a pneumothorax secondary to the rupture of a bleb (a bubble-like area on the lung periphery). According to Shapiro and others (1979, p. 191), it is not the I.P.P.B. itself that

FIGURE 12.3
Cleaning Your Breathing Equipment

EVERY DAY: CLEAN ALL TUBING (except small, narrow tubes)

EQUIPMENT NEEDED

1 Basin (or 2 if you have them)
Liquid detergent—Joy, Ivory, etc.
Long-handled bottle brush
Toothbrush
White vinegar

HOW TO CLEAN
1. Take equipment apart
2. Wash in warm, soapy water in basin
3. Clean all small parts with toothbrush
4. Clean wide tubing with the bottle brush
5. Rinse well
6. Make vinegar solution (1 part vinegar to 3 parts water)
7. Soak in vinegar for 20 minutes. (Use basin)
8. You do not have to rinse vinegar off
   Some prefer to rinse the mouthpiece so that there is no vinegar taste
9. Let drain over night
   Put the wide tubing over a hanger OR hang by a clothes pin from the hanger
   Put the small pieces on a clean cloth towel or paper toweling
10. Reassemble equipment and use

AFTER EACH TREATMENT
Clean the mouthpiece and nebulizer in warm water and soap and rinse.

Do not let medicine stand in nebulizer from one treatment to the next.

ruptures the bleb because pressures at the mouth of 20 cm H_2O generate alveolar pressures of 10 cm H_2O, insufficient to rupture blebs. More air may enter the bleb which then may rupture secondarily to cough at high bleb pressure. If the I.P.P.B. treatment is continued with a pneumothorax, the result is a tension pneumothorax. Complaints of sharp chest pain and increased difficulty breathing must be investigated promptly.

Many clients develop a psychological dependence on their I.P.P.B. machines. Much of their life is spent assembling, cleaning their equipment, preparing their medications, and taking treatments. Travel is difficult because they become afraid to leave their homes and machines. If it is prescribed, I.P.P.B. should be administered correctly for maximum effectiveness. The client or family member should periodically be observed preparing the medication, performing the treatment, and cleaning the equipment.

To receive a proper I.P.P.B. treatment, the client should sit upright in proper body alignment, place the mouthpiece between the teeth, and make a tight seal with the lips. All breathing should be through the mouth. There must be a leak proof system or the unit will cycle off. The client should start to breathe in normally with just a slight inspiratory effort which will initiate the machine's cycle. When the preset pressure is reached, the machine will cycle off. The client should exhale completely through the mouthpiece. In some clients who have difficulty with air trapping, a device with a small diameter orifice is placed in the expiratory opening to slow exhalation. This acts in the same manner as pursed lip breathing to keep the small airways open longer. The client may need to stop and cough at intervals and should not cough into the mouthpiece.

Steroid Medications

Inflammation is a major component of chronic bronchitis at all times and of the other diseases during acute exacerbations. When the inflamed respiratory mucosa swells, it occupies what would otherwise be open space in the airway and thus contributes to airway obstruction.

At home, steroid medications may be either given as oral or inhaled drugs. The oral drugs most commonly used are prednisone and prednisolone. If possible, these should be used only during acute illnesses, after the client is off the intravenous steroids. If given for short periods, their hazards are minimal, including increased gastric acid secretion (contributing to peptic ulcers), increased appetite, and increased feeling of well-being.

As the client improves, the steroids are tapered both in dose and frequency until, at hospital discharge, those who are still on steroids are receiving a low dose once daily or every other day. It is important that this single dose be taken upon arising in the morning and that it be tapered rather than being abruptly stopped. To abruptly discontinue steroids is to almost guarantee an acute exacerbation of the condition.

A variety of systematic effects can occur if the client is on oral steroids long-term. The steroids may impair thought processes that are already affected by hypoxemia, arteriosclerosis, or other problems. As a result, there may be decreased understanding or retention of information. Instructions should be given simply, with much repetition. Written reinforcement is essential. Many clients are labeled as "noncomplaint regarding medications" because a nurse or physician did not provide a written list of medications. In the case of the confused older adult, education should be aimed at the caregiver responsible for the client.

Steroid psychosis is another fairly common problem. It causes some difficulty in care because, although removing the steroids can reduce the psychosis, it also can exacerbate the pulmonary status. Most physicians, however, tend to taper the steroids in this case and treat the pulmonary problem more vigorously with other drugs, chiefly bronchodilators.

Other long-term effects of steroids include adrenal suppression, abnormal fat deposits and water retention, osteoporosis, hypertension, peptic ulcer, cataracts, electrolyte imbalances, easy bruising, increased appetite and feeling of well-being. The client has lower resistance to infection, but the early signs of infection may be masked by the steroid. It is more difficult to control diabetes in the steroid-dependent client. If the steroid–dependent client is ill or stressed, the physician will need to increase the steroid dose. Also, the client's medic-alert should include the information that he or she is steroid-dependent.

If a client is to be started on long-term steroids he or she should have a P.P.D. skin test before the drugs are begun. Long-term steroid use can lead to release of walled–off tuberculosis organisms and an active case of the disease. If the client's skin test is positive, he or she usually receives a year of prophylactic I.N.H. (Isoniazid) along with the steroids.

A topical steroid (Beclomethasone, Vanceril) is a useful alternative to oral steroids for the maintenance of many clients. It is supplied in a cartridge inhaler to be used after using a topical bronchodilator. Like oral steroids, suddenly stopping its use can lead to pulmonary exacerbations. Unlike oral steroids, Vanceril does not cause systemic body effects, so it is much safer for long-term use. Vanceril is not effective during an acute exacerbation, however. During these episodes, the client needs short-term intravenous and oral steroids. In order to prevent opportunistic infections (Candida) of the mouth, the client should rinse the mouth well after every dose of Vanceril. The nurse should periodically check the client's mouth for the telltale white patches of Candida, or thrush, and report these to the physician if they occur.

Keeping the airways open and non-irritated also involves the avoidance of irritants. Of course, the most important of these irritants is cigarette smoke. It is essential that pulmonary clients avoid being around smoking or stop smoking. They will not get better if they do not do so. Excellent programs to assist in this effort are available through the American Lung Association and the American Cancer Society.

Other irritants and allergens should be avoided. These include pollens to which the client is sensitive, dusts, chemicals such as outdoor sprays, indoor cleaning fluids, and the like. Even brief exposure can cause extreme distress and respiratory failure in some clients. Industrial dusts and pollutants should also be avoided if possible. If this is not possible, the client should wear a mask when in the industrial area.

Promote Effective Breathing Patterns

The sensation of dyspnea is a subjective one. It is especially important that the client understand that a moderate amount of dyspnea is acceptable and can be tolerated. For example, all persons become dyspneic on exertion. If a young man plays tennis and becomes dyspneic, he does not panic but accepts it as normal and rests until his dyspnea subsides. In contrast, a man with C.O.P.D. may become dyspneic during his morning walk. This creates a great deal of anxiety so that he panics and attempts to hyperventilate. This increases his hypoxemia and thus makes him more dyspneic—a vicious cycle. If he can learn to relax and breathe in an appropriate pattern until the dyspnea subsides, he can often gain control of his breathing within one minute.

Relaxation techniques may be taught by the nurse or as a part of biofeedback therapy. The client may be referred to a biofeedback center for instruction in relaxation and/or decreasing tension, or very simple progressive relaxation techniques may be taught by the nurse. Relaxation reduces the muscle tension which many dyspneic clients experience because of their respiratory efforts. It reduces their oxygen need and aids them in gaining control of their breathing.

Pursed lip breathing is a very effective method of prolonging exhalation and gaining respiratory control. To accomplish pursed lip breathing, the client should inhale through the nose and exhale through pursed lips, taking longer to exhale than inhale. A suggested pattern is twice as long to exhale as inhale: breathe in for a mental count of 1, 2 and exhale to a mental count of 1, 2, 3, 4. It is helpful to tell clients not to force expiration because this causes airway closure. They should be cautioned against taking an excessively deep breath which many of them do instinctively. Clients need help to develop a positive attitude and belief that they can control their breathing; their breathing does not have to control them.

Pursed lip breathing should be taught at a time when the client is comfortable and not in distress. The client should practice often until able to master the technique, thus being able to use it to gain control in times of respiratory distress. The client should not be expected to use the technique at all times. Pursed lip breathing should be used when the client is short of breath or in distress.

Pursed lip breathing can also be used to advantage during exercise and activity. The client should plan to do the activity on pursed lip exhalation and then rest to inhale. For example, in stair climbing, the client should climb 2 steps on exhalation, and then rest to inhale. To tie the shoes, inhale, bend over and tie one shoe on exhalation, sit up to inhale, and tie the other shoe on exhalation. Shaving is often a problem for men due to instinctive breath holding. Using the pursed lip technique while shaving prevents the breath hold and enables the client to accomplish the task.

While these techniques may sound simple, they require a good explanation on the part of the nurse and practice on part of the client. It may take weeks for the client to feel comfortable with the breathing techniques. Every effort should be expended to encourage clients to continue to practice these techniques because many of them have found these techniques helpful in relieving dyspnea and increasing exercise tolerance.

Clients with C.O.P.D. often breathe in a rapid, shallow, uncoordinated and ineffective manner. This is partly due to air trapping and decreased diaphragmatic excursion. Abdominal diaphragmatic breathing seeks to correct this problem by teaching the client to use abdominal muscles to increase diaphragmatic excursion.

Abdominal diaphragmatic breathing should be done along with pursed lip breathing. The client is taught to place one hand on the upper thoracic rib cage to monitor its movement while placing the other hand on the abdomen just below the xiphoid to monitor abdominal movement. The client should inhale while letting the abdomen gently balloon out as far as possible and exhale, through pursed lips, while the hand pushes the abdomen inward and upward. A book or small weight may be used to exert additional pressure on the abdomen. While walking, the client should be taught to use abdominal breathing combined with pursed lip breathing. A suggested rhythm is to inhale while walking one to three steps and exhale while walking two to six steps.

Postural Techniques

General postural techniques can augment these techniques to gain control in times of respiratory distress. When an attack of breathlessness occurs, the client should assume one of the following positions and perform pursed lip diaphragmatic breathing to relieve the attack:

High side lying. Lie on one side slightly rolled forward with a slope of four pillows to raise the shoulders and an extra pillow placed between the body and underlying arm to fill the gap between the waist and armpit to maintain a straight spine. The knees are slightly bent and the top leg is placed in front of the lower one.

Forward lean sitting. Two or three pillows are placed on a table. Relax the upper chest and head resting against the pillows. Maintain a straight spine since too much forward bending at waist can inhibit diaphragmatic movement.

Relaxed sitting. Sit leaning forward with a straight back, with the forearms resting on the thighs, and the wrists relaxed.

Forward lean standing. Stand leaning forward from the hips with the forearms resting on an object of suitable height (e.g. stair rails, window ledge, mailbox, wall).

Relaxed standing. Lean back against the wall with the feet approximately twelve inches from the wall. The shoulders should be relaxed with arms hanging loosely at the sides.

The body's muscles are stronger, function more effectively, and require less oxygen per unit of work when they are well conditioned. Therefore, the client should participate in an ongoing general conditioning program of gentle conditioning exercises and regular progressive walking, stair climbing, or bicycling. The client should perform all exercises utilizing pursed lip breathing and use the postural exercises as necessary to gain respiratory control. The program should be systematically graduated by increasing repetitions of the exercises, or increasing distance. An individualized home exercise program should be planned by the physician, the client, and the other health care professionals. The physician should prescribe the exercise target rate and the client taught to monitor pulse and other symptoms as a guide to deciding if the exercise should be terminated (see Table 12-7).

TABLE 12.7
Client Guide to Exercise Termination Points

My target pulse rate is: _____

I should stop exercising and rest if any of the following occur:

1. SEVERE shortness of breath (some shortness of breath is acceptable).
2. Chest pain, suggestive of angina.
3. Extreme fatigue
4. Dizziness or faintness
5. Lack of coordination, mental confusion, marked apprehension
6. Sudden onset of perspiration or cyanosis
7. Increase or decrease in my heart rate of more than 15 beats per minute
8. Pulse rate over my target pulse rate

Avoid Respiratory Depressants

It is critical that the client who has chronic pulmonary disease avoid both prescribed and over-the-counter respiratory depressants. Even a small dose of such drugs as Valium or sleeping aids can depress the ventilation significantly.

Improve Oxygenation

The second management goal is to *improve oxygenation*. Although long-term oxygen therapy greatly improves the quality of life, it does not alter lung function nor does it prolong life. Benefits cited for long-term outpatient oxygen therapy are reduced pulmonary artery pressure, reduction of red cell mass, increased mental function and well-being, reduction in hospitalization and, in many clients, increased activity and return to work. While oxygen supplements may increase well-being, some clients, especially men, are reluctant to start oxygen in the home. It is sometimes perceived as a step "down hill" and a threat to independence rather than an aid to activity and independence. The home use of oxygen also identifies the user as "ill" or different.

Indications for home oxygen therapy are arterial oxygen tension of 55 mmHg or less, cor pulmonale, hematocrit above 55 secondary to polycythemia, exercise induced hypoxemia with limitation of activity, and sleep disturbances related to hypoxemia. In clients with advanced lung disease, studies have demonstrated that continuous (24 hr/day) oxygen therapy is more beneficial than intermittent therapy of 12 or 15 hours per day (Petty, 1982, p. 85).

Oxygen may be delivered by a variety of devices including masks and nasal cannula. In the home, the most convenient method is the two pronged nasal cannula which can be worn 24 hours a day and interferes very little with activities of daily living. The nose, naso and oropharynx act as an anatomic reservoir containing

normal–sized meal often results in a "too full" feeling which causes increased difficulty breathing.

Many clients have abdominal distention because of a tendency to swallow air during aerosol therapy. Gas further increases abdominal distention and respiratory distress. Lack of energy results in decreased ability to prepare a well-balanced diet. Lack of activity and a balanced diet also contribute to a common complaint of the elderly—constipation—which increases pressure in the diaphragm and leads to straining and breath holding.

Moser et al. (1980, pp. 67–9), offered suggestions for clients to deal with dietary difficulties.

- Eat six small meals. Since digesting food requires energy, eating smaller meals requires less energy at a given time.
- Avoid gas–forming foods such as members of the cabbage family, melons, carbonated beverages, onions, and radishes.
- Eat slowly and leisurely. Share mealtime with a friend.
- Avoid fatty or fried foods which take longer to leave the stomach.
- Eat high protein foods. Protein content may be increased by additing nonfat dry milk to sauces, casseroles and puddings. Protein supplements may be helpful.
- Take medications with food, if appropriate, to decrease nausea.
- Vary the menu and use garnishes to brighten the plate.
- To save energy, prepare one-dish meals or prepare a recipe in a large quantity and freeze some.

Meals-on-Wheels may be helpful to some elderly clients who cannot provide for their own nutritional needs.

Many clients with chronic lung disease are on low–sodium diets and need to be instructed in foods high and low in sodium. Clients on diuretics or steroids may suffer potassium depletion, so potassium supplements may be ordered. Instruction should cover foods high in potassium such as bananas, oranges, raisins, prunes, spinach, decaffeinated coffee, and meats.

Energy Conservation and Work Simplification

Another goal is maximizing the client's ability to carry on the activities of daily living. One way to help achieve this is with *energy conservation and work simplification.* Clients with chronic hypoxemia who are often weak and fatigued benefit from referral to an occupational therapist for instruction in energy conservation and work simplification. Much energy can be saved by planning and organizing activities around rest periods. Rest periods should be short and frequent, for example, 15 minutes every hour rather than one hour of rest after four hours' work. If possible, the client should sit for as many activities as possible.

Proper body mechanics and breathing control should be used with all activities. Exhalation should take place during the strenuous part of any activity such as pushing, pulling, bending, or lifting, or with activity requiring motion toward the body. Rushing should be avoided because it will only increase discomfort. Likewise, the client should use slow, rhythmic movements while working.

Psychosocial Aspects of Living With Chronic Lung Disease

Another major goal is to help the client and family learn to live with chronic lung disease. Emotional states that imply an action orientation require increased oxygen consumption as the result of increased work of breathing, increased muscular tension, and increased cardiac output. Clients with chronic lung disease are often unable to meet these increased demands required for social interaction, which leads to the use of defense mechanisms and changes in their social life. Dudley (1973, pp. 389–393), found that their clients used denial, isolation and repression. Many clients, when dyspnea and anxiety increase, withdraw gradually and cut off social interaction thus isolating themselves from potential emotionally laden events. Some clients use denial very actively to prevent anxiety. One client informed the nurse during a visit to her home that the nurse was not allowed to mention "sickness" because she insisted she was not sick; she just could not breathe. Her overusage of her I.P.P.B. and inhaler could not be discussed, nor her need to continue the activity program agreed upon in the hospital rehabilitation program which she had just completed. Any mention of these topics resulted in her throwing herself back on the bed crying: "I can't breathe!"

Clients may also utilize regression as a coping mechanism. Regression may be adaptive in an acute illness; not so in chronic illness where clients must be active partners in management of their care. The client who overutilizes regression may become an over–dependent, demanding person who completely regresses to a childlike state and completely gives up adult responsibilities. Such a state is counter-productive in the home care setting.

As the client's losses increase—loss of bodily function, loss of social contacts, loss of job (disability, retirement)—and there are role changes at home, depression is likely to result with feelings of hopelessness, helplessness and sadness. Irritability and anger are common among clients with chronic lung disease, partly because of hypoxemia and hypercapnia and partly because of grief and loss. The client may lash out in frustration at the helping people in the environment, both professional, personnel and family members, often pushing away those most necessary and wanted.

Depression may decrease ventilation resulting in decreasing PaO_2 and increasing $PaCO_2$ thus intensifying the client's complaint of dyspnea and further increasing anxiety.

The attitude of the nurse, as well as the client's family, physician and other health care providers significantly affects the client's course. Abrams (1972, p. 262) identified several negative caregiver attitudes toward clients with pulmonary disease.

These negative attitudes included:

- Overconcern and overinvolvement. Nurses should be aware of their motives in their relationships with clients. If there is a great desire to cure, then the client who does not get well may represent an affront to the nurse's ability. Families may become over-protective of the client who remains ill.
- Anger and rejection. If the client does not adhere to the medical-nursing regimen, the nurse may react with anger and rejection. The client is then labeled "noncompliant" and "uncooperative." The family may also reject the client for such behavior.
- Lack of sensitivity. The nurse should make every effort to understand the meaning of the illness to the client. If there is decreased sensitivity to psychological issues, care will be hampered.

The above attitudes are human responses. In order to develop a therapeutic relationship, the nurse must be aware of his or her feelings and motivations in each relationship. In the development of a therapeutic relationship, the nurse should recall that the client reacts for a reason. The client with respiratory problems is often avoided. This may, in part, be related to the sometimes adverse coping mechanisms utilized by these clients. In addition, it may be related to the uneasiness of dealing with the client who is extremely dyspneic.

In caring for clients with chronic lung disease, it is helpful to maintain a realistic approach. The client should be expected to behave within societal norms. Dependency on the nurse should be minimized. From the initial interview, the relationship is facilitated by an attitude of concern. Active listening is helpful to identify the client's perceptions of his or her illness and goals. Interventions should be goal directed. To be effective, the goals must be mutually set between the client, family and the nurse.

Clients with chronic lung disease do not do well in either individual or group psychotherapy which is focused on the exploration of affect, interpersonal conflict, or any threat to the defense mechanisms necessary for their survival. They tend to be more comfortable when discussing the disease and physical methods to control anxiety and shortness of breath such as breathing contol.

Social support has the ability to protect against the health consequences of life stress (Cobb, 1976, p. 300). Mastery of new tasks takes place best under supportive conditions. While the nurse is part of the clients' support system, this relationship must, of necessity, be temporary if the goal is self sufficiency. The client needs family or friends who can form a supportive network. The client may find mutual support in a group of peers such as that offered by the American Lung Association and its Better Breathers' Club. Even the homebound client can find support in receiving their newsletter and participating in a telephone network. These groups offer the person with chronic lung disease a chance to explore areas of mutual concern, such as coping with shortness of breath, community resources, and death and dying.

Summary

Chronic lung diseases are a group of conditions which have a slow, insidious onset. They are a leading cause of disability affecting a largely elderly client population. Chronic lung disease strains personal, family and community resources. People with chronic lung disease require knowledgeable, concerned nursing care as well as the support of a comprehensive pulmonary home care program.

Treatment of chronic lung diseases is generally aimed at reversing that which is reversible, providing for symptom relief, preventing and treating of complications, and assisting the client and family to live with the condition and adhere to the medical regimen.

Treatment modalities include medications such as bronchodilators to decrease airway spasm, steroids to decrease airway spasm and inflammation, and antibiotics for infection. Efforts are aimed at removal of retained secretions which are causing increased hypoxemia and infection. Secretions are liquified by systemic hydration measures and aerosol therapy. Postural drainage is useful in selected clients to aid removal of secretions. Supplemental oxygen may be prescribed to increase tissue oxygenation and improve mental and physical functioning. Breathing control techniques such as pursed lip breathing and abdominal diaphragmatic breathing are taught to clients in order to reverse the ineffective breathing pattern.

Clients with chronic lung disease have many problems in common. Among these are anxiety, nervousness, weakness, fatigue with decreased exercise tolerance, and decreased ability to perform activities of daily living. There is often poor nutrition. The client is often irritable and has decreased self-esteem. As the disease progresses and energies diminish, there may be increasing depression. Many clients become socially isolated as a means of conserving energy which results in further depression. Clients are often difficult to care for because of dyspnea, hypoxemia, hypercapnia, and accompanying irritability and poor judgment. Family relationships and resources are often strained under the physical and financial burden.

Care of the client requires that the nurse not only be skilled and knowledgeable in the care of clients with respiratory problems, but also that he or she have a positive attitude of care and concern for these clients. A team approach to pulmonary home care is recommended to maximally assist the client and family to increase self sufficiency, decrease hospitalization, and improve the quality of life.

REFERENCES

Abram H S: "Psychology of chronic illness." *J Chronic Dis,* Vol 25, No XX, 1972, pp. 659–64
Burrows B: "Course and prognosis in advanced disease" in Petty T L (ed): *Chronic Obstructive Pulmonary Disease.* Marcel Dekker, Inc., New York, 1978, p 26
Bushnell S S, Brooks R A: "Humidification and aerosol therapy," in Morrison M (ed): *Respiratory Intensive Care Nursing.* Little Brown Publishers, Boston, 1979, p 137

Cobb S: "Social support as a moderator of life stress." *Psychosomatic Medicine,* Vol 38, No 5, September-October 1976, pp. 300–312

Davis A L: "Bronchiectasis," in Fishman A P: *Pulmonary Diseases and Disorders.* McGraw-Hill Book Co., New York, 1980, p 1217

Dudley D, Wermuth C, Hague W: "Psychosocial aspects of care in the chronic obstructive pulmonary disease patient." *Heart and Lung,* Vol 2, No 3, May-June 1973, pp 389–93

Miller W F, Geumei A M: "Respiratory and pharmacologic therapy in COPD" in Petty T L (ed): *Chronic Obstructive Pulmonary Disease.* Marcel Dekker, New York, 1978, p 72

Moser K M et al.: *Better Living and Breathing: A Manual for Patients.* C.V. Mosby Co., St. Louis, 1980, pp 67–9

Petty T L: *Intensive and Rehabilitative Respiratory Care.* 3rd ed. Lea and Febiger, Philadelphia, 1982, p 85

West J B: *Pulmonary Pathophysiology: The Essentials.* 2nd ed. Williams and Wilkins, Baltimore, 1982, pp 59–60

BIBLIOGRAPHY

Ciuca R: "Cor Pulmonale." *Nursing '78,* Vol 8, No 12, December 1978, pp 46–49

Dudley D: "Coping with chronic COPD: Therapeutic options." *Geriatrics,* Vol 36, No 11, November 1981, pp 69–74

Fuhs F, Stein A M: "Better ways to cope with COPD." *Nursing '76,* Vol 6, No 2, February 1976, pp 28–38

Hudgel W, Madsen L A: "Acute and chronic asthma: A guide to intervention." *Am J Nur,* Vol 80, No 10, October 1980, pp 1791–95

Kaufman J S, Woody J W: "For patients with COPD: Better living . . . through teaching." *Nursing '80,* Vol 10, No 3, March 1980, pp 57–61

Kirilloff L H, Tibbals S C: "Drugs for asthma: A complete guide." *Am J Nurs,* Vol 83, No 1, January 1983, pp 55–61

Mathers J A L, Cooper K, Galuser F: "Office management of COPD." *Geriatrics,* Vol 36, No 1, January 1981, pp 103–110

Mizuki J A: "There's no place like home." *Am J Nurs,* Vol 84, No 5, May 1984, pp 646–48

Pierson, J: "Asthma in the elderly: special challenge." *Geriatrics,* Vol 37, No 4, April 1982, pp 87–95

Sexton D L: "The supporting cast-wives of COPD patients." *Am J Nurs,* Vol 10, no 2, February 1984, pp 82–85

Stanley L: "You really can teach COPD patients to breathe better." *RN,* Vol 41, No 4, April 1978, pp 43–49

Materials for Client Education

Moser K M et al: *Better Living and Breathing: A Manual for Patients.* 2nd ed. The C.V. Mosby Co., St. Louis, 1980

Chronic Obstructive Pulmonary Disease—A Guide for Teaching Patients. Chicago Lung Association, 1440 W. Washington Blvd., Chicago, Illinois, 60607, N.D.

Help Yourself to Better Breathing, American Lung Association, Vermont Lung Association, 1980

SAMPLE MASTER CARE PLAN FOR HOME CARE—

Nursing Diagnoses	Assessment	Planning
I. Respiratory Impairment: (Difficulty breathing) related to:	• Auscultate lungs each visit. • Vital signs each visit. • Check respiratory rate, rhythm, excursion. • Observe for hypoxemia: restlessness, mental confusion, irritability, altered blood pressure or pulse. • Observe for hypercapnia: headache, flushed cheeks, palms, tremors, confusion, hypertension.	*Short-term goals* • Client will exhibit decreased to absent s/s hypoxemia, hypercapnia, dyspnea. • Client's respiratory pattern will be normal. • Client will be able to state, in own terms, lung changes related to disease. • Client able to state and demonstrate coping mechanisms to be used when short of breath. *Long-term goals* *Client will maintain adequate:* • tissue oxygenation. • ventilation (PaCO$_2$) • acid-base balance (pH).
a. Bronchospasm (wheezing)	• Auscultate all lobes for wheezes. • Client complains of "tight chest" dyspnea, orthopnea, reduced breath sounds or heart sounds.	*Short-term goals* • Client will have decreased to absent wheezes. • Client statements will reflect relief of chest tightness. • Client able to state name of bronchodilator, dose, why taken, when taken side effects.
	Long-term goals • Client adheres to medication regimen. • Side effects absent or, if present, medication adjustment made.	• Client demonstrates correct administration of MDD or inhaler. • Client able to state precautions related to use of steroids and side effects.

CHRONIC LUNG DISEASE

Intervention: Nursing Orders	Intervention: Resources and Support Systems	Evaluation: Expected Outcomes
• Inform physician of change in client status. Arterial blood gases if ordered. • Supplemental oxygen as ordered (Usually 1-2 L/nasal cannula). • Instruct client in structure and function of lung, disease process, symptomatology and what to do to cope with symptoms. • If client smokes, urge to stop smoking.	• Medical supply company: cylinder, liquid system or concentrator. • Refer to American Lung Association • Better Breathing Club • A-V Aids, Patient Education References: • Flip chart: *Chronic Lung Disease* The Robert Brady Co. Author: Hilary D. Sigmon RN, MSN. • Book: Moser, Kenneth et al. *Better Living and Breathing*, (St. Louis, C.V. Mosby) 1980	• Client has improved mental function, absent restlessness, normal vital signs. • ABG's: pH 7.35-7.45, PaO_2 above 55mmHg, $PaCO_2$ 35-45 (if elevated, pt. will have compensated) • Client states lung changes related to disease in own terms. • Client utilizes proper breathing control when short of breath.
• Teach and monitor compliance with medical regimen. • Bronchodilator medications • Steroids: Teach proper use and precautions.	• MedicAlert bracelet or other warning system re medications (steroids) and medical condition.	• Decreased to absent wheezes or dyspnea noted. • Takes medications as prescribed. • Recognizes adverse effects of medications and calls physician.

SAMPLE MASTER CARE PLAN FOR HOME CARE—

Nursing Diagnoses	Assessment	Planning
b. Ineffective airway clearance of retained secretions.	• Auscultate lung for crackles, wheezes. • Check sputum: amount, color, consistency. • Assess for s/s infection: chills, fever, malaise, discolored sputum (gray, yellow, green) increased shortness of breath, sore throat.	*Short-term and long-term goals* • Decreased to absent adventitious sounds. • Client will be able to state signs of infection and proper action to take. • Client will recognize and be able to control factors in environment that may precipitate infection.
c. Ineffective cough	See airway clearance	• Client will be able to demonstrate cascade (controlled) cough. • Client will be able to state name of ordered medications; contraindications to over the counter cough medications.

CHRONIC LUNG DISEASE (continued)

Intervention: Nursing Orders	Intervention: Resources and Support Systems	Evaluation: Expected Outcomes

• Teach and monitor compliance with medical regimen.
• Prevention and recognition of lung infection.
• Medications: Bronchodilators, Antibiotics
• Hydration—8-10 glasses fluid/day
• Bronchial hygiene as ordered.
  Bronchodilator (inhaled)
  Aersosol therapy
  Chest physical therapy
  Cough technique
		• Observe sputum: should be clean, white, easily expectorated.
		• Calls physician if signs or symptoms of infection present.
		• Demonstrates proper disposal of sputum.
		• Plans and consumes fluid intake in compliance with regimen. Increases fluid intake when sputum thickens.
		• Reports sudden weight gain or edema accumulation.
		• Client/significant other demonstrate proper operation of equipment and performance of bronchial hygiene routine.

• Teach cough technique. • Teach and assess adherence to medication regimen.	• Possible referral to physical therapy. • Respiratory therapist—medical supply company to assist in patient education.	• Cough is productive.

SAMPLE MASTER CARE PLAN FOR HOME CARE—

Nursing Diagnoses	Assessment	Planning
d. Ineffective breathing pattern (obstructive, air trapping)	• Observe use of accessory muscles. • May observe rapid, shallow, uncoordinated pattern. • Observe whether breathing is abdominal or costal.	• Client able to correctly demonstrate: (a) Pursed lip breathing. (b) Abdominal diaphragmatic breathing • Client will utilize pursed lip abdominal breathing when in distress or walking or with other activities.
2. Dyspnea–Anxiety–Dyspnea Cycle	• Observe client for anxiety related to breathing. • Observe for restlessness, increased muscle tension, inability to concentrate. ·	*Short-term goals* • Client will be able to utilize breathing control and relaxation techniques to control anxiety. • Client will state belief that he/she can control breathing and anxiety. • Client report of improved sleep and appetite and decreased muscular tension.
3. Decreased exercise tolerance	• Assess client activity level (See Table 12.3).	*Long-term goals* • Client will be able to increase activity and walking. • Decreased dyspnea when ambulating. • Client will perform abdominal strengthening, chest mobility and upper extremity strengthening exercises daily.

CHRONIC LUNG DISEASE (continued)

Intervention: Nursing Orders	Intervention: Resources and Support Systems	Evaluation: Expected Outcomes

• Teach and evaluate progress:
  1 Pursed lip breathing
  2 Abdominal diaphragmatic breathing
		• Decreased use of accessory muscles.
		• Respiratory rate slowed.
		• Utilizes correct breathing techniques without reminder.

• Teach client relaxation techniques. Assist client to recognize anxiety–provoking situations and how to handle. • Develop supportive relationship with client and family to assist client to cope with anxiety and understand client's reaction to illness.	• Possible referral to biofeedback center • Possible referral to hypnotherapist	*Client's statements reflect:* • no dyspnea • decreased anxiety • belief that he or she controls breathing • utilization of relaxation techniques when in increased anxiety situations Family neither rejects nor overprotects.

• Teach breathing control with activity.
• Activity–exercise program
  (1) Abdominal strengthening exercises
  (2) Chest mobility exercises
  (3) Upper extremity strengthening exercises.
	• See Moser, Kenneth M. et al *Better Living and Breathing*, (St. Louis, C.V. Mosby) pp. 53-61
	• Referral to physical therapy/occupational therapy
		• Client walks each day.
		• Client performs exercises without reminder.

SAMPLE MASTER CARE PLAN FOR HOME CARE—

Nursing Diagnoses	Assessment	Planning
4. Impaired ability to perform independent activities of daily living related to difficulty breathing, weakness, fatigue.	• Assess client for ability to feed, dress, and toilet self, cook, perform light housework. • Assess degree of dyspnea during these activities. (See Table 12.3).	*Short-term goals* *Client will be able to:* • perform ADL: Personal hygiene, dress self, feed self, prepare light meals, light housework • describe and utilize work simplification and energy conservation techniques during ADL.
5. Knowledge deficit related to technical procedures. Respiratory therapy equipment (I.P.P.B., unassisted bronchodilator) oxygen	• Observe client during use and cleaning of equipment. • Observe as client draws up medication. • Inspect equipment. Check for cleanliness and proper operation. • Check liter flow being used.	*Long-term goals* *Client will be able to:* • demonstrate proper assembly, operation, and cleaning of equipment • demonstrate correct medication administration • state precautions related to oxygen therapy • state correct prescribed flow of oxygen • state guidelines for ordering new oxygen supply.

CHRONIC LUNG DISEASE (continued)

Intervention: Nursing Orders	Intervention: Resources and Support Systems	Evaluation: Expected Outcomes
• Teach energy conservation and work simplification techniques. • Teach breathing control.	• Refer to occupational therapist. • Home health aide to assist with personal hygiene and light housework until self sufficient.	• Client utilizes principles of energy conservation and breathing control during Activities of Daily Living (ADL).
• Teach proper assembly, cleaning and operation of equipment. • Teach correct administration of inhalers. • Teach and monitor compliance with medical regimen related to oxygen. • Teach precautions related to oxygen therapy.	• Medical supply company with respiratory therapist to assist in client education and maintain equipment in optimum condition.	• Client demonstrates proper assembly, operation and cleaning of equipment. • Equipment clean and operational. • Precautions related to oxygen observed. • Medication administered correctly. • Uses equipment as prescribed; does not skip or overuse treatments.

SAMPLE MASTER CARE PLAN FOR HOME CARE—

Nursing Diagnoses	Assessment	Planning
6. Altered nutrition related to a. nausea, b. flatus c. shortness of breath and d. financial difficulties.	• Assess weight/height. • Assess for weight loss–weight 20% below ideal body weight. • Diet history–decreased intake. • Poor muscle tone, sore mouth, pale mucous membranes, loss of hair, dry skin. • Assess for diarrhea. • Complains of abdominal discomfort, bloating, gas.	*Short-term goals* *Client will:* • be able to describe and plan proper diet. • consume adequate diet at home. • gain, lose or maintain weight as appropriate.
7. Depression (grief) related to role changes, loss of independence, diagnosis and prognosis leading to social isolation.	• Client verbalizes anger, sadness, sense of loss. • Crying at intervals. • Withdrawal from family, friends • Changes in sleep, activity, appetite.	*Short-term goals* • Client's statements will reflect realistic outlook toward future and acceptance of physical disability. • Client will continue to maintain contact with family/others. *Long-term goals* • Decrease frequency and number of hospitalizations. • Improve quality of life and assist the client to experience greater satisfaction with daily living.

CHRONIC LUNG DISEASE (continued)

Intervention: Nursing Orders	Intervention: Resources and Support Systems	Evaluation: Expected Outcomes
• Instruct client in balanced diet. • Small, frequent meals (5-6) day. • Avoid known gas-forming foods. • Dietary supplements such as Ensure, Instant Breakfast as appropriate. • Weigh client every week. Positive reinforcement for gain, loss or maintenance as appropriate.	• Possible referral to nutritionist. • Possible referral to Meals-on-Wheels.	• Client consumes adequate nutritious diet.
• Observe client/family interaction. • Encourage open communication among family members. • Active listening and an attitude of positive regard toward the patient by health caregivers.	• Church group—volunteers, minister. • Better Breathing Club. • Adult Day Care Center. • Senior Center.	• Client's statements realistic regarding present status and future. • Client verbalizes loss realistically and without undue anger. • Client/family/others continue to have open dialogue regarding future.

CHAPTER 13

SENSORY DEFICITS

Mildred O. Hogstel

One perceives, experiences and enjoys the external environment through the senses. When one of the senses is lost or decreased due to disease, injury or natural changes which occur during the aging process, the individual loses, at least to some degree, his or her contact with the environment. For the older adult, who also experiences many other losses such as job, income, spouse, and/or friends, sensory losses add to feelings of loneliness and depression. Most people, young or old, do not realize how important the senses are to everyday living until one or more is diminished or lost.

Visual Deficits

The most common visual problems that occur as one ages are presbyopia, cataracts, glaucoma, senile macular degeneration, and blindness. Eye problems associated with diabetes are discussed in Chapter 11.

Presbyopia

Presbyopia, or farsightedness, is a normal aging change in which reduced elasticity and translucency of the lenses occur. The "reduced elasticity interferes with accommodation so that, though distance vision remains intact, close vision becomes blurred" (Hall, MacLennon, and Lye, 1978, p. 59). In addition, "the ciliary muscles that help to hold the lens in place may become weaker and lose tone . . . , and fast accommodation from near to far (or vice versa) decreases" (Saxon and Etten, 1978, p. 59). As accommodation decreases, older individuals have difficulty shifting their vision from distant objects to close objects and thus are at risk of falling and having accidents while driving.

Presbyopia requires glasses to see and read close objects. This change usually begins in the early 40s and requires no special care except reading glasses with concave lenses. Clients should be encouraged to have a thorough eye examination about every three to five years, with change in glasses if needed (Caird and Judge, 1977, p. 56), not only to increase reading acuity, but also to detect more serious eye problems. Sometimes the elderly have had the same eyeglasses for 10 to 15 years, usually indicating that they have not had regular eye examinations. Because Medicare does not assist with the purchase of eyeglasses, except after cataract surgery, older people may be hesitant to have a routine eye examination for fear that they will need to purchase new glasses. There are many good resources for health care in the community for older adults at reduced costs, but financial assistance with the purchase of glasses is usually not available unless the client is on Medicaid.

Cataracts

One of the major questions about the aging process is the differentiation between normal aging changes and changes brought on by the disease process. Which aging changes are normal and which ones are caused by disease? One of the major biological theories of aging proposes that tissues lose their elasticity because collagen, a protein substance existing in the various tissues of the body, stiffens with age (Atchley, 1977, p. 35). According to Rockstein, Chesky, and Sussman (1977, p. 12), "one of the most consistent and perhaps universal manifestations of aging in mammals is the series of changes that take place in the composition of the lens of the eye with advancing age." The development of cataracts, therefore, is probably one of the few normal age changes and will occur in everyone sooner or later, perhaps not until the 90s in some individuals (Cataract, 1980). The word cataract is derived from the Latin word "cataracta," which means waterfall, so when the lens of the eye becomes cloudy or opaque, it is like looking through a waterfall and vision is decreased (Cataracts, 1982, p. 1). "Cataract is a leading cause of blindness among adults in the United States, accounting for one out of every seven cases of blindness among persons 45 years of age or over" (Cataract, 1980). There is no way to prevent the development of cataracts or to slow their growth at the present time. Future research may determine the exact cause of cataracts and thus means for prevention or treatment without surgery.

Types of cataracts

Hall, MacLennon, and Lye (1978, p. 60) illustrated three types of cataracts that occur in old age: 1) nuclear (round in shape), 2) cortical (small pie shape), and 3) posterior subcapsular cortical (marquise in shape). Nuclear cataracts start in the center or nucleus of the lens and cortical cataracts form in the outer zone or cortex of the lens (Cataracts, 1982, p. 1). Some cataracts develop rapidly over a period of months and others develop slowly over a period of years.

Assessment

The nurse who has elderly clients in the home setting should determine when the client last had a complete eye examination by an ophthalmologist. Part of the initial history and review of systems will include specific questions about vision. Questions related to the symptoms of cataracts should be asked such as:

- Do you have any difficulty seeing details or reading print?
- Do you have to hold things close to you to read?
- Do you have difficulty distinguishing between colors?
- Do you ever have blurred or cloudy vision?
- Do you ever have double vision?
- Do you ever see spots or ghost images?
- Do you have difficulty seeing at night?
- Do you ever see wagon wheels around lights while driving at night?
- Do you need extra light to see well?
- Does very bright or intense light in your eyes bother you?
- Have you changed your eyeglasses frequently (more often than every three years) in the last few years?

Even if a complete physical examination is not performed initially, positive responses to these questions indicate the need for further assessment of the eyes. The nurse in the home setting, suspecting the presence of cataracts, will assess the eyes for pupil constriction and accommodation. Reactions to light are maintained, but pupil size is frequently smaller than in younger people (Caird and Judge, 1977, p. 56). To check for accommodation, the client is asked to focus on a distant object and then a close object while the nurse observes for both pupil constriction and convergence. Close vision acuity and color can be assessed using the Rosenbaum Pocket Vision Screener. If such a device is not available, the nurse can ask the client to read the headlines of the newspaper for lower visual acuities and the smallest print for higher levels. Finger counting can be used for those with severe visual impairment (Caird and Judge, 1977, p. 57).

Cataracts may be clearly visible as a white, yellow, or milky appearing spot over the dark pupil if the cataract is very advanced, but more than likely fundoscopy with the ophthalmoscope will be necessary to visualize the presence of cataracts. If the pupils are constricted because of medication, for example, in the treatment of glaucoma, the client should be referred to an ophthalmologist because medication will be necessary to dilate the pupils for ophthalmoscopy. If any abnormality of the lens is noted, that is, increased opacity and/or white or yellow color, the client should be referred to an ophthalmologist for diagnosis and treatment.

Treatment

Surgery for cataracts is the only effective treatment and restores "vision in more than 95 out of 100 cases" (Cataract, 1980). If the client is in good health, alert, and cooperative, the surgery can be performed with local anesthesia on an outpatient basis with the artificial lens implanted at the time of surgery. The surgeon and the client, together with the family, will decide if, when, and where the surgery is to be performed, based on the progression of the cataracts and the client's age and current health status. Age should be no deterrent if the client is in relatively good health and will be cooperative. Clients in their 90s tolerate the surgery well. If the client becomes confused easily, general anesthesia may be necessary. In this instance, management of the client before and after surgery is probably of more concern than the surgery itself. If the client can be managed through the pre- and post-operative periods, however, confusion may ultimately decrease when the person is able to see more and move about more freely in his or her environment.

Nursing Care

The client who has cataract surgery will be hospitalized only a few days, if at all. Due to recent developments in microscopic eye surgery, specific precautions following cataract surgery are not as necessary as they once were. The physician may instruct the client to wear an eye patch at night after going home, and an opthalmic antibiotic ointment may be ordered. Some physicians will caution the client not to lift more than ten pounds of weight, not to bend the head or comb the hair for a few days, and to prevent nausea and vomiting. Some anxiety, tenseness and intermittent pain in the operated eye may occur for several days or weeks after surgery for which medication will be ordered by the physician. Symptoms of complications are severe pain, blurring of vision, and/or loss of vision. If any of these symptoms occur, the client should notify the physician immediately. The major concern after surgery, however, is becoming adjusted to a new type of vision. The lens that has been removed may be replaced inside the eye at the time of surgery (intraocular lens), by the use of contact lens (external lens), or special cataract eyeglasses will be prescribed. "Contact lenses or intraocular lenses do provide less distortion than cataract eyeglasses and more complete side vision" (Cataract, 1980). If the elderly client is able to drive a car, peripheral vision, especially at night, may be impaired, so the client should take special care driving. The client usually has to turn his or her head to see clearly to the side. Although Medicare does not pay for eyeglasses in general, it will pay for glasses required after cataract surgery. With the new eyeglasses, the client "will notice that his new vision is different: Objects are larger, colors are altered, the feel for distances must be adjusted" (Cataract, 1980). Usually one eye is operated on at a time, so the client will use the unoperated eye to see until the surgery on both eyes has been completed. Because the operated and unoperated eyes see in different and confusing ways, the operated eye is covered so confusion is lessened.

When caring for the client who has not had or does not intend to have cataract surgery for one reason or another after definite diagnosis, the nurse can assist the person to utilize the vision remaining in the most effective way possible.

Suggestions to clients and families should include the following:

- Increase the wattage of the light bulbs used and place lights above or behind the client.
- Prevent glare from bright lights or direct sun from hitting the client's eyes.
- Keep a light on in the client's bedroom, the hall, and the nearest bathroom during the night and on dark and cloudy days.

- Purchase a magnifying glass, lighted if desired, for use in reading the newspaper and other reading materials with small print.
- Ask the pharmacist to use a large type, or print in large letters the information on medication bottles (especially if the client is responsible for taking his or her own medications).
- Purchase or check out from the local city or church library magazines and other reading materials in large print.
- Use bright reds, yellows and oranges (instead of blues, greens and purples) for clothing, to mark door entries, and steps. Because of the thickening and yellowing of the lens, pastel colors are not seen as clearly as reds, yellows and oranges.
- Add a small round white plastic covering with large black numbers to the telephone so that the numbers can be seen and dialed more easily. A lighted dial is also helpful.
- Post a list of the emergency and most commonly used telephone numbers in large black numbers above or near the telephone. A wide felt-tip pen is excellent for this purpose. Numbers of the fire department, police, ambulance, physician, nearest family member, and neighbor or close friend should be readily and clearly available.
- If the person lives alone and does his or her own cooking, large letters for *ON* and *OFF* on the stove and large printed labels for some foods, such as spices, should be added for easier reading.
- Clients should be reminded not to let a stranger in the home unless a service agency or business has previously telephoned informing them of their visit. Even though some servicemen are required to wear a uniform and/or badge identifying them, the person with decreased vision may not be able to read the name of the person or the agency because of the small print.

The nurse should also review with the client and family a check list for home safety, suggesting revisions in the environment where needed. Falls in the home are very common for the elderly and the person with reduced vision has a greater chance of having such an accident which can be very serious. Reflective red and white or yellow and white tape can be purchased at a local hardware store to be placed on the edge of steps, a safety procedure which helps the visually impaired see the edges of steps as they walk up and down.

Glaucoma

Glaucoma is the second leading cause of blindness in the elderly (Saxon and Etten, 1978, p. 61) and "affects 1 to 2% of the population over 40" (Horowitz, 1982, p. 15). Because there are relatively few, if any, symptoms, the disease often progresses without the client being aware of the presence of the disease. Glaucoma is most likely to develop "somewhere between the ages of 40 and 65 years" (Kart, Metress, and Metress, 1978, p. 63). Glaucoma is caused by an increase in the amount of aqueous humor within the anterior chamber of the eye. When the amount of fluid increases and/or the drainage canal for ocular fluid (canal of Schlemm) is blocked, the excess fluid builds up and causes pressure interfering with the blood supply, particularly to nerve cells and fibers, which eventually damages the optic nerve and causes blindness (Kart, Metress, and Metress, 1978, p. 68; Saxon and Etten, 1978, p. 61).

Types of Glaucoma

There are two major types of glaucoma: 1) chronic simple glaucoma (open-angle glaucoma) and 2) acute glaucoma (angle closure or narrow-angle glaucoma). Open-angle glaucoma is by far the most common, especially in the elderly. It "occurs when, because of degenerative changes, aqueous outflow is impeded" (Soll, 1975, p. 9). "Secondary open-angle glaucoma may be caused by tumors, neovascularization of the angle structures, inflammatory disease, hemorrhage, trauma or drugs such as corticosteroids" (Soll, 1975, p. 11). Narrow-angle glaucoma "often occurs in hyperopic eyes with shallow anterior chambers" (Soll, 1975, p. 9). For this reason, care must be taken in dilating the pupil of an individual with severe hyperopia because it may cause an acute attack of glaucoma (Soll, 1975, p. 9).

Open-angle glaucoma occurs gradually without symptoms, while narrow-angle glaucoma occurs suddenly with symptoms of severe pain, blurred vision, the appearance of halos around lights, and vomiting.

Assessment

While performing the assessment in the home setting, the nurse will include specific questions and observations to detect the possibility of glaucoma. Types of questions which could indicate the presence of glaucoma should, therefore, be included in the health assessment of the elderly such as:

- Have you had any recent blurring of vision?
- Do you have cloudy or foggy vision?
- Have you had any recent headaches or pain in the eyes?
- Do you ever see rainbow-colored halos or rings around lights?
- Have you changed glasses frequently without improvement?
- Has anyone in your immediate family had glaucoma?

Physical assessment should include evaluation of cranial nerve #II (optic), particularly visual acuity and peripheral vision. The experienced practitioner may be able to feel increased pressure by light palpation of the eye over the upper lid which feels "rock hard" when glaucoma is present. However "finger palpation is notoriously inaccurate" (Weinstock, 1973, p. 139). If the history and physical signs are positive for glaucoma, the client should be referred to an ophthalmologist for diagnosis and treatment. The ophthalmologist diagnoses glaucoma by the use of a tonometer, which measures the pressure in the eye by placing the base of the tonometer lightly over the center of the cornea. Only the physician may perform this procedure in some states because medication to anesthetize the surface of the eye is used prior to placing the tonometer on the cornea. Pressure readings over 21 to 22 mm.Hg. are considered suspicious, but glaucoma is not diagnosed on the basis of one elevated pressure reading (Weinstock, 1973, p. 139–140). The procedure is very simple, quick and painless.

If the client in the home is able to be mobile, the nurse can recommend that he or she participate in an annual glaucoma screening program at no cost. In most large communities these screenings are usually available at health fairs and other similar screening programs sponsored by such organizations as the local medical society, medical school, local branch of the National Society to Prevent Blindness, Lions Club, and university sororities. Physicians usually donate their time and expertise in checking pressure for glaucoma. Eyes should be checked for glaucoma at least once every two years after the age of 35 to 40, especially if there is a history of glaucoma in the family (Glaucoma, 1980; Saul, 1975, p. 12). The National Society to Prevent Blindness "recommends yearly screening for all people over 35" (Horowitz, 1982, p. 15).

Treatment

Glaucoma can be treated successfully in most instances, but it cannot be cured. Narrow-angle glaucoma is usually treated with surgery. An iridectomy is performed to remove a small portion of the iris so that the aqueous humor will drain adequately. The surgery is usually not dangerous and only requires a short hospitalization.

Open-angle glaucoma is usually treated with drugs. Miotics are used to decrease the size of the pupil so that the aqueous humor will drain more freely. Drugs used most frequently are direct parasympathomimetic drugs (such as pilocarpine), indirect parasympathomimetic drugs (such as physostigmine-eserine), and medications which decrease the aqueous production rate such as the sympathomimetic agents (Epinephrine) and carbonic anhydrase inhibitors (acetazolamide Diamox) (Soll, 1975, p. 12). The physician will determine the exact drug to be used based upon the type of glaucoma and the client's ability to use the medication.

Common side effects of the eye medications "include dimming of vision, accommodative spasm, ocular pain and headaches. Iris cysts, iritis, conjunctival irritation, lens opacification and even retinal detachment may occur" (Soll, 1975, p. 11). Burning and blurring are probably the two most common complaints clients mention.

Nursing Care

Once open-angle glaucoma has been diagnosed and the treatment started, the most important role of the nurse is to stress the necessity of using the eye medication as ordered by the physician. Clients in the home, especially if they live alone, sometimes do not fully realize the importance of using the eye medication as directed by the physician. They do not use the drops as often as ordered because they forget, because of the uncomfortable side effects of the drugs, or because they have difficulty using the drops themselves.

The client and/or the family should be observed to determine if they understand exactly how to instill the eye medication. Perhaps the ophthalmologist or nurse taught them in the office, but it is important for the nurse in the home to determine if the instructions were understood and are being carried out correctly. The client should be instructed to instill the eye drops if at all possible to encourage independence, although another family member should also be taught so that he or she can give the medication when the client cannot, perhaps because of deformities of the hands and fingers due to arthritis, or will not because of fatigue or fear. It should be stressed to the client and family that eye medication must remain sterile. The hands should be washed and not touch the tip of the medication bottle. Most eye medicines should be kept out of direct sunlight and at room temperature. The family should be instructed that medicine which is not clear or has particles in it should not be used and that they should check the expiration date when new medicines are purchased. The exact procedure for instilling eye drops should be explained in detail and demonstrated. The client should tip the head back slightly and the lower eyelid should be pulled down slightly with one finger tip. The client should be told to look up while instilling only one drop into the lower rim of the eye from the medicine container at least one inch away. It should be stressed that the medicine should not be dropped directly over the middle of the eye (on the cornea) because of the sensitivity of the cornea. The client should be told to close the eye gently and press gently on the inner canthus of the eye for a minute or two to prevent loss of the medication or absorption through the tear duct (Todd, 1983, p. 53).

The nurse should continue to emphasize the importance of taking the medication as ordered, because it is often difficult for the client to realize that blindness will eventually occur without it. An older person may stop using the medication after receiving a negative pressure reading at a community glaucoma screening program. The nurse will need to stress that the medication must be taken for the rest of the client's life.

Senile Macular Degeneration

Another cause of eye problems in the elderly is senile macular degeneration, a condition thought to occur from lack of blood supply to the macula of the eye. The macula is the part of the retina that provides fine or distinct vision. While glaucoma affects peripheral vision first and can result in blindness if not treated, macular degeneration affects the central vision and is less likely to cause blindness.

Assessment

A thorough assessment of the eyes, particularly evaluating the ability to read fine print, watch television, use a needle or thread, or identify people at a distance is important (Kornzweig and Klapper, 1977, p. 27). Diagnosis will be made by the ophthalmologist through fundoscopy.

Treatment

In most older people who have senile macular degeneration, the condition has probably been present for some time, and there is no effective medical or surgical treatment. If discovered early, however, (for example in the 50s) treatment with photocoagulation of local offending retinal blood vessels may be beneficial (The Aging Eye, 1978; Hall, MacLennon and Lye, 1978, p. 61).

Nursing Care

Nursing care will focus on attempts to provide vision assistance, especially for fine or distinct vision such as reading through methods previously discussed (increased light and magnifying glasses). Peripheral vision is not affected, so the person is not totally disabled. However, "threading a needle, reading a newspaper, telling time, or reading directions on a medicine vial may be impossible tasks without use of these devices" (Kart, Metress, and Metress, 1978, p. 64).

Blindness

When cataracts or glaucoma without treatment have progressed to the point of severe visual deficit or blindness, although the quality of life may be decreased, there are multiple programs and services available to aid the client in living life as fully as possible. When the nurse in the home discovers an elderly client who is blind, he or she can ask the client and/or family if they would like to benefit from the services of a rehabilitation counselor with the local society to prevent blindness, usually at no cost. The counselor, or the nurse if preferred, can teach the client and family how to keep the client as independent as possible. It is extremely important that the blind elderly adult not be isolated physically or socially. Physical isolation often leads to physical immobility and the possibility of other multiple problems such as pneumonia, contractures and decubiti.

Nursing Care

The nurse should instruct the family to keep the environment around the client as stable as possible; that is, leaving all of the furniture in the same positions so that the blind person can walk in the house freely, knowing where chairs and tables are located. A cane or walking stick in one hand will help the client feel his or her way around the house. The client should be instructed to hold the other arm bent at the elbow out in front of him or her to keep from running into door frames or tall furniture. Loose rugs or toys should not be left on the floor.

Family members should be taught how to lead a blind person by walking one small step ahead of the person and having him or her hold on to the bent elbow. In this way, the blind person will detect when the other person steps up or down. The person who is guiding should also tell the blind person of impending steps. While walking on a straight surface, the guide can initially count ONE-TWO-THREE-FOUR to help the client take full firm steps. The older newly blind person tends to take small hesitant steps and stand behind the other person for fear of running into some object or stumbling over a hump or hole in the ground. The nurse should demonstrate all of these maneuvers to the family members and observe them as they try them out with the client. It is important that the client have clothing with pockets or a table close to where he or she usually sits so that items used frequently, such as water, kleenex and clock, can be easily reached. Nurses should remind family members to speak before touching the blind person so that he or she will not be unnecessarily startled. Touch is an important source of support and comfort for the blind person. When entering the room of the blind client, the nurse and family member should tell the person their names and who they are. The older blind client who is left alone in a room for periods of time may become severely depressed and experience hallucinations and delusions. Other means of sensory stimulation, therefore, such as music, news and voices are extremely important.

There are numerous services available to the blind through various organizations which assist the blind. Most of these services are free. Examples of these services are:

- talking books, tapes or records available from local libraries (postage for return mailing is free);
- special electronic devices that provide music and news 24 hours a day;
- information about where to purchase talking watches or clocks; or watches with Braille numbers on the dial (Braille was invented in 1829 by a Frenchman, Louis Braille);
- books and magazines in Braille;
- a small "Signature Guide" card that helps the blind person sign his or her name in the correct space on a check or other document.

Family members who transport the blind in their car will qualify for a disabled car sticker and/or license. Certification of visual loss by a physician is required, and there is usually a minimal fee. This license allows the family member to park free at parking meters and in special parking areas designated for the handicapped so that the blind person will have easier access to shopping centers and recreation areas.

The nurse should encourage independence of the client as much as possible. Independence in eating is one important goal. The nurse should teach the family to tell the client what food is on the plate and to always place the food on the client's plate like a clock; for example, the meat will always be at 3, the vegetable at 6, the fruit at 9, and the bread at 12. In this way the client will know where the food is on the plate so that he or she does not have to guess what and where the foods are. Plastic food bumpers can also be purchased very inexpensively at medical supply stores, department stores, or children's toy stores. This bumper fits on the plate on one side and keeps the food from sliding off the plate. The blind person should not be fed unless absolutely necessary. The family should not be concerned about spilled food on the table or floor, as long as the client is getting an adequate amount of nutritious food at each meal. The blind person can be taught to feel with a finger in a cup or glass to determine how hot or full the container is and thus prevent possible burning and spilling.

Additional information, including free pamphlets on cataracts, glaucoma, and other eye conditions for clients as well as professional personnel, may be obtained by writing to any of the organizations listed at the end of this chapter.

Hearing Deficits

Some loss in hearing is also thought to be a normal aging change, although not all older people experience this loss. Many older people in their 90s have little, if any, hearing deficit. Others begin to experience some degree of hearing loss in their 50s. Deafness accompanying aging "is partly due to the natural death of irreplaceable neurones in the acoustic nerve" (Hall, MacLennon, and Lye, 1978, p. 58). Other hearing losses are due to the effects of middle ear infections early in life when antibiotics were not available, environmental factors (such as working in an occupation where there was excessive noise), or simply a buildup of dry, hard wax in the ears which can cause deafness, dizziness, and buzzing (Hall, MacLennon, and Lye, 1978, pp. 58-59). It has been reported that "men tend to show hearing loss earlier than women" probably due to their greater exposure "to high level occupational noise" (Saxon and Etten, 1978, p. 64). "The very aged frequently show collapsed canals which can interfere with sound transmission through the canal to the drumhead" which, together with collection of cerumen, caused a "conductive-type of hearing loss" (Glorig, 1977, p. 44).

Hearing losses can be categorized as conductive, perceptive or mixed. Conductive hearing loss is due "to any disturbance in the conduction of sound impulse as it passes through the ear canal, tympanic membrane, middle ear, and ossicular chain to the footplate of the stapes, which is situated in the oval window" (Judge and Zuidema, 1968, p. 125). Perceptive hearing loss is caused by "a disturbance anywhere from the cochlea, auditory nerve, and on to the hearing center in the cerebral cortex" (Judge and Zuidema, 1968, p. 125). A mixed hearing loss involves both conductive and perceptive factors. Perceptive hearing loss is more common in the elderly.

Presbycusis

Although there are other causes of hearing loss in the elderly, the most common problem is presbycusis. Saxon and Etten (1978, p. 64) have reported four different types of presbycusis: 1) sensory (due to atrophy of hair cells at the base of the basilar membrane); 2) neural (because of loss of neurons in the auditory nerve); 3) metabolic (loss of cells in the cochlea due to insufficient blood supply; and 4) mechanical (due to degenerative changes in the ossicles and basilar membrane). Kart, Metress, and Metress (1978, p. 67) proposed "that the loss of these hair cells in the organ of Corti is the most common cause of presbycusis."

The basic cause of presbycusis is degenerative in nature, therefore, with the loss of higher sound frequencies the first most common sign. "Consonant sounds (such as *c, ch, f, s, h,* and *z*) are typically those in the higher frequencies, and vowel sounds (*a, e, i, o,* and *u*) are those in the lower sound frequencies" (Kart, Metress, and Metress, 1978, p. 67).

Assessment

As part of the initial assessment of the client in the home, the nurse will assess for degree of hearing deficit, if any. Because some elderly people do not like to admit to a hearing deficit (probably because they view this problem as a sure sign of aging), the nurse will probably obtain more information about hearing loss from the physical examination and observation than from the nursing history. The nurse will need to observe closely during the history, however, to determine if the client hears and understands the nurse's questions and comments. One good question to ask is whether the client can hear male voices (lower frequency) better than female voices (higher frequency). The nurse should note if the client asks the nurse to repeat questions or has a blank or questioning look on the face.

Assessment of hearing loss of the client in the home may be performed by several methods. Some of these methods, which evaluate cranial nerve #VIII (acoustic), are described below. All of these tests should be performed in a quiet environment.

The whisper test. In the whisper test, the nurse covers one ear with one hand and stands on the opposite side of the ear being tested, whispering one foot away from the client on his or her side so that the lips cannot be read. Different words or sentences should be used for each ear. Another method is to have the client stand about one or two feet away from the nurse so that the ear to be examined faces the nurse. The client is asked to plug the opposite ear with a fingertip. The nurse then whispers a few words or numbers softly and slowly toward the ear to be tested and asks the client to repeat the words or numbers. Two-syllable words are suggested, "such as 'baseball', 'forty-six', 'hot dog', 'textbook', etc." (Sherman and Fields, 1978, p. 123) "or numbers that include two equally accented syllables, e.g. 14, 25" (Bates, 1979, p.77)

The watch test. In this test, the nurse uses a watch that ticks loudly enough to be heard. The nurse holds the watch several inches (depending on the loudness of the ticks) from the ear and moves the watch toward the ear and asks the client to state when the ticking can be heard. The nurse can estimate how far away to hold the watch based on his or her own ability to hear it, assuming the nurse's hearing is normal. The nurse estimates the distance when the client states that the ticking can be heard. Each ear should be tested separately.

The tuning fork. The tuning fork can also be used to test hearing. The fork should be set to vibrate gently "by stroking it between thumb and index finger or by tapping it on your knuckles" (Bates, 1979, p. 78) and then be held at an equal distance between the client's and the nurse's ears. The client should be asked to let the nurse know when he or she can no longer hear the humming sound of the fork. If the client cannot hear it as long as the nurse, the client has a hearing deficit, assuming that the nurse knows that his or her hearing is normal (Sherman and Fields, 1978, p. 123).

The Weber test. The Weber test also requires the use of the tuning fork. The nurse strikes the tuning fork, holds it by its stem and presses the stem against the midline of the skull or forehead. If hearing is normal, the sound should be heard equally well in both ears. If there is a perceptive hearing loss (for example, nerve damage), there is lateralization of the sound or vibrations to the good ear. If there is a conductive loss (mechanical loss due to otosclerosis or excessive thickened ear wax), the sound lateralizes to the diseased ear (Judge and Zuidema, 1968, pp. 127–128). Excessive or thickened ear wax can be seen with the use of an otoscope.

Whichever test for hearing loss is used in the home by the nurse, any major deficit which interferes with the client's activities of daily living should be referred to the physician for further evaluation.

Treatment

The client may have a condition for which surgery will be helpful (for example, otosclerosis), or the client may only need to have a large amount of dry, hard ear wax removed by an ear specialist. Neither the client, the family, nor the nurse should attempt to remove impacted ear wax without specific instructions from the physician.

It is very important for the nurse in the home to stress to the client and the family that they not purchase a hearing aid without first being examined by an ear specialist. Many elderly people spend money needlessly on hearing aids that do not help their particular type of hearing deficit. Because high-pitched sounds are the most difficult to hear in presbycusis, a hearing aid may only magnify the sound and not help with the high-pitched sounds.

Nursing Care

The nurse in the home must first be sure that he or she is communicating with the client, utilizing a number of simple suggestions which help when talking with the hearing-impaired individual. These techniques should also be taught to family members and friends who are with the client frequently.

It is most important that the nurse assess the client's hearing ability early and use that information in communicating with the client. The nurse should never assume that the older person is hard of hearing and speak in a loud voice to all older

TABLE 13.1
Suggestions For Communicating With Hearing-Impaired Elderly Persons

1. Stand or sit at the same level with the client so that there is direct eye contact.
2. Enunciate words well so that the client can read the lips but do not exaggerate pronunciation.
3. Speak clearly, distinctly and slightly slower and louder, using a low pitch to the voice.
4. Do not ask long, complicated questions or double-barrelled questions (asking two or more questions before waiting for a response).
5. Reduce other environmental noise if possible (such as a television, radio or other people talking).
6. Observe the client's facial expression for understanding or lack of understanding. If there is no response or what seems to be an inappropriate response, repeat the comment or question in a slightly different way.
7. Make a temporary megaphone from a cardboard or plain piece of paper and speak into it after it is placed over the client's ear.
8. Place a stethoscope in the client's ears and speak in a low soothing voice directly into the bell or diaphragm of the stethoscope.
9. Observe which ear the client points to, cups with his or her hand, or tilts toward the speaker and speak directly into that ear.
10. Use the hands to point to various parts of the body, for example, during the history taking.
11. Use sign language, if possible, when both the client and the nurse are familiar with this method.

people. A loud voice often sounds artificial and makes the development of rapport with the client more difficult, especially if the older person has no hearing deficit. Even if there is a hearing problem, if the voice is loud and high-pitched, which is often true for women, the voice will not only not be heard, but it may also cause severe discomfort for the client. "In the cochlea the receptors for soft sounds are more severely degenerated than those for loud ones, which may account for a normal voice being inaudible, but shouting being painful" (Hall, MacLennon, and Lye, 1978, p. 58).

Suggestions for communicating with hearing-impaired elderly persons are listed in Table 13.1. The nurse can also provide a number of other suggestions to the hearing-impaired client and his or her family. The local telephone company can provide information on amplifiers which can be added to the telephone so that the person can better hear conversations. For a minimal fee per month a volume control will be added to the ear piece which can be adjusted by each member of the family when using the telephone. A telephone with an extra loud ring can be obtained, and an attachment with a light that comes on when the telephone rings can be used.

Smoke alarms with a bright blinking light as well as a loud noise can be purchased and should be placed in the bedroom of the deaf person. High pitch and low pitch smoke detectors can also be obtained for the hearing impaired, the selection based on the client's type of deficit. These are important safety features essential in the home environment. Door bells which blink as well as chime can also be purchased.

If the client understands sign language, the nurse can suggest television programs that provide a sign language interpreter. Some television stations also provide a sign language interpreter for their news broadcasts. National television stations now have closed captions for the hearing impaired for a limited number of programs and news broadcasts.

Taste Deficits

Controversy exists about the degree to which taste buds are affected by the normal aging process, but most authors state that there is some change in the perception of taste as one ages. In an early study, Hinchcliffe (1962, p. 50) reported that "all sensory threshold sensitivities seem to show an exponential decrement with age." Saxon and Etten (1978, p. 67) stated that the number of taste buds decrease due to the atrophy and death of some receptors and that the remaining taste buds "require a stronger stimulus to activate them." These changes, they continue, may begin as early as the 40s but are not very obvious until the 70s and 80s. Other reports (Engen, 1977, pp. 64–65; Grzegorczyk, Jones, and Mistretta, 1979, p. 839) have concluded that changes in taste bud perception in the elderly are not as general as previously thought.

The most obvious effects of possible changes in the taste buds are a loss of appetite and less enjoyment of food.

Assessment

While doing the nutrition assessment in the home, the nurse will want to ask the client if he or she has noticed obvious changes in the taste of foods. Usually changes in taste buds are very gradual, if they occur, so the client may not be aware of such changes except in a very general way. The client may simply say that food does not taste as good as it used to or that he or she does not enjoy food as much as in previous years. The nurse, however, should try to obtain more specific information by asking such questions as:

- Can you distinguish between salt, sweet, bitter and sour taste?
- Do you use more sugar to sweeten tea or coffee than in earlier years?
- Do you find yourself craving sweets more than when you were younger?
- Do you put more salt on your food now than in the past in order to have it taste better?

Physical assessment of taste bud perception is not routinely performed except during a thorough neurological examination, but because of the controversy about changes in taste buds in the elderly, the nurse interested in research may wish to pursue a project of this type with older clients in the home. Engen (1977, p. 66) has suggested that any study of perception of taste or odor be performed as part of a general physical examination because changes in these perceptions may be clues to primary health problems. If such an assessment is conducted, the nurse will need samples of four foods to test the four different tastes. Samples of foods which can be used are: 1) sweet (for example, sugar), 2) sour (for example, vinegar), 3) bitter (for example, baker's chocolate) and 4) salt (for example, salt). The food should be dissolved in water and a cotton tip applicator used to place a small amount on the specific section of the tongue being tested. It should be remembered that the taste receptors for sweet and salt are at the tip of the tongue; receptors for sour are along the sides of the tongue; and bitter substances are tasted best at the back of the tongue. For this reason, the client should be asked to rinse his or her mouth between the assessment of each type of taste because saliva will carry the particular food being tested to all parts of the tongue.

Nursing Care

Because there is no effective treatment to increase the function of the taste buds, nursing care will focus on teaching the client and/or family how to prevent changes in taste perception from affecting the diet negatively and ultimately harming the health. Good oral hygiene and review of medications that may affect the taste or perception of foods are also important.

If the client should restrict his or her salt intake because of hypertension, for example, it is important that salt not be added to food at the table. If the client states that the food does not taste good without extra salt, it may be that he or she cannot taste the salt already in the food and therefore tries to add more and more salt to taste. The nurse should suggest seasonings such as lemon juice, vinegar, celery, cinnamon, mustard, paprika, and other spices, if allowed. Salt substitutes may also be suggested. However, it is important to stress that these should also not be used in excess because many of them contain potassium. The salt shaker should be removed from the table so that it will not be easily accessible if the client is on a low–salt diet.

Many older people develop a craving for sweets, especially candy, perhaps because of the theory that the perception for sweet and sour remains while perception for salt and bitter decrease. Or, it may simply be that eating candy is a pleasurable pastime for the older adult not active in other activities.

Nutritious meals based on the four food groups should be prepared and served in an attractive manner to help increase the appetite if the client has lost the desire to eat because food does not taste as good as it once did. Environmental factors are probably as important as taste buds in enhancing appetite. If the older person lives and eats alone, he or she is much less likely to prepare and eat three nutritious meals a day than if the client eats with someone else. Eating is a social event for many people. If the client lives alone, the nurse could suggest that he or she share meals with friends or neighbors who also live alone. Perhaps they could take turns preparing lunch or dinner each day for others in the neighborhood, or they could take their own food to a different neighbor's home each day and eat together. If finances and ability to purchase and prepare food are problems, the nurse should suggest and, if the client agrees, arrange for the client to participate in one of the community nutrition programs such as Meals-on-Wheels.

Olfaction Deficits

Closely related to the decreased perception of taste is the decreased ability to smell. Some neurologists believe that this is one of the first senses to decrease in perception as one ages. Although often not aware of the loss, many older people state that they cannot smell as well as they used to when asked about it.

Research studies on olfaction and aging, however, are few and inconclusive (Saxon and Etten, 1978, p. 68; Engen, 1977, p. 64). Studies on changes in olfaction, as well as taste perception in aging, are confounded by many variables such as individual preference, sex, health, use of drugs, and education (Engen, 1977, p. 66).

Assessment

The nurse will assess possible losses in olfaction during the history and physical assessment. The nurse can ask questions related to smell such as:

- Have you noted any change in your ability to smell?
- Can you smell foods with strong odors such as onions, garlic or cabbage?
- Do you cook or heat your home with natural gas or propane?
- Can you smell the odor of gas when the pilot light on the stove is out?

Physical assessment will reveal more information than the history. Testing for cranial nerve #I, olfactory, the nurse will ask the client to close both eyes while the nurse holds a small container containing an odor-producing substance under the nose. Each nostril should be assessed separately while compressing the nostril on the other side. At least two different substances should be used for each nostril. Examples of substances which can be used are garlic salt, lemon juice, coffee, tea and vanilla.

Nursing Care

If there is a deficit in olfaction, this loss affects the client in several ways. Pleasant odors from foods usually increase the appetite and stimulate the salivary glands which aids in mastication, swallowing, and digestion, an important factor for the client who wears dentures. Other odors the client with an olfaction deficit will miss are fresh flowers, perfume, and dew on fresh mowed grass or hay.

If the client can see well, food should be prepared in a colorful and attractive way, thus relying on sight rather than odors to increase appetite and encourage eating. A fresh flower on the table or tray, a cloth napkin, and colorful dishes as well as food will help the older person look forward to each meal.

One of the dangers of decreased olfaction is the older clients' inability to detect leaking gas or smoke from a fire and spoiled food. The client who lives alone and cooks should be taught to always check the dials on the stove, if gas is used for cooking, after each meal, and before going to bed to be sure they are all turned off. Open gas heaters should not be left on overnight because the flame could go out and gas will escape into the house. An adequate number of smoke detectors should be installed. Pets in the home, such as a dog, may also alert the client to leaking gas or smoke.

Clients should be taught to store left-over foods in clear glass containers in the refrigerator. Containers should also be dated. Foods in glass containers can be seen better than in plastic containers and will more likely be used or discarded, while foods in the plastic containers may be overlooked for days. Then, if there is no date and a bad odor not detected, the older person may become ill from eating spoiled food. Most left-over foods, meats, vegetables and salads should either be eaten or discarded after three or four days in the refrigerator. The nurse in the home should open and assess the contents of the refrigerator of the elderly client who lives alone. Because of limited financial resources, all left-over food is often saved because the individual does not feel that he or she can afford to throw away any food.

Another possible problem which occurs as a result of decreased olfaction is the older client's inability to be aware of personal body odors and/or bad breath. Combined with a visual deficit and periodic urinary or fecal incontinence, the older person may need assistance with personal hygiene to assure that the body and clothes are clean. The older person who has been meticulous in dress and grooming throughout his or her life will appreciate the nurse assisting with and/or supervising general hygiene measures.

If proper care and precautions are taken, any decrease in the sense of smell should not interfere in any major way with quality living for the elderly in the home.

Deficit of Touch

Research on deficit of skin perception as an age-related change is sparse; however, there are probably some changes in the perception of sensory touch, pressure, heat, cold, and pain which occur with age (Saxon and Etten, 1978, p. 69). It is generally believed that the older person experiences less cutaneous pain than younger people. However, there is a lack of convincing evidence that this is the case because of the numerous studies which show conflicting results and the number of variables which affect pain such as ethnic background, socioeconomic status, previous educational experiences, and personality, for example (Kenshalo, 1977, pp. 571–572).

There does seem to be a decreased ability of the elderly to tolerate extreme hot or cold temperatures, but this is probably due to the total temperature regulating system which affects the core body temperature, rather than sensory skin perception alone (Kenshalo, 1977, pp. 568–569).

Research on the changes of touch sensitivity with advancing age is also limited. Kenshalo (1977, p. 575) reported that "Loss in touch sensitivity (appreciation of cotton wool applied to the hairy skin) has been reported to occur in a small percent (25 percent) of an aged population." As is true with other changes observed in the aging process, it is difficult to determine whether the change is due to normal aging or to a pathological condition.

Assessment

The assessment of touch, pain and temperature will be conducted by the nurse during the physical examination. Light touch can be assessed by "using a wisp of cotton . . . on the forehead, cheeks, arms, forearms, hands, chest, thighs and legs" (Sherman and Fields, 1978, p. 261). The client should be asked to compare the difference in sensation from one side of the body to the other while the eyes are closed. Assessment of superficial pain can be performed by pricking lightly with a safety pin in the same manner on the same areas previously mentioned, alternating sharp and dull sides and having the client indicate if it feels "sharp" or "dull". Slight differences from one side to the other are usually not significant (Sherman and Fields, 1978, p. 261). A more extensive examination and referral to a physician should be made if there are definite differences from one side to the other.

Assessment of perception of heat and cold may be performed by filling two test tubes, one with warm water and one with cool water, and holding each one separately against the client's skin of each cheek or inner arm.

Nursing Care

Deficits in the sense of touch, temperature, pressure and pain involve esthetic as well as safety factors. Most individuals receive pleasure from touching the soft smooth skin of an infant, or cannot resist stroking clothing made of velvet, velour or silk.

Because of decreased sensory perception, some older people cease to receive the same pleasure from feeling objects than in past years. This does not mean that they receive less pleasure from being touched. In fact, it is possible that the need to be touched increases in the elderly, perhaps because they cease to receive as much pleasure from touching others.

Although the perception for extreme heat and cold probably remains (even a 90-year-old man will not drink extremely hot coffee), some decrease in reaction of superficial nerve endings may occur. It is for this reason that the family and/or nurse must take special precautions in preparing a bath or hot water bottle or applying a heating pad to the elderly client. A temperature comfortable for the family member or nurse may be too hot for the elderly person. The older individual does not perceive the heat as too hot because of decreased perception of nerve endings, thus increasing the chance of causing a severe burn.

Summary

Sensory perception helps one to fully enjoy the total environment as well as give clues to potential hazards in the environment. The decrease or loss of one or more of these senses affects the older person's quality of life.

Decreased sight, most often caused by cataracts or glaucoma in the elderly, is probably the sensory loss which most adversely affects the ability to remain completely independent, a major goal of most elderly people. Fortunately, however, blindness caused by these conditions can be prevented if they are diagnosed and treated early. Cataracts can be readily and easily removed by surgery, and glaucoma can be controlled by the use of medication. The nurse in the home has a major responsibility to encourage early diagnosis and treatment so that blindness from these conditions will not occur.

Hearing deficits are not universal in the elderly, but when hearing is decreased, communication with others often becomes a major problem. Hearing aids do not always help with presbycusis which begins with a decreased ability to hear high pitches. There are many techniques which can be used to facilitate communication with the hearing impaired older adult. The nurse in the home can help the family increase their communication skills with the older family member who does not hear well.

While deficits in taste, olfaction and touch are less apparent and generally cause fewer problems than deficits in sight and hearing, there are certain esthetic and safety factors which should be considered. Appearance of foods, as well as nutritious content, should be enhanced to increase appetite if needed to counteract decreases in taste and smell. The nurse should teach the client and family about hazards in the environment (particularly gas leaks and extremes of temperature) which can occur as a result of deficits in olfaction and touch.

The nurse in the home can use his or her knowledge, experience and skills to help the client and family provide a healthy and safe environment where the older adult can live a quality life, despite sensory deficits which may occur as a result of the aging process.

A sample master care plan that can be adapted in planning for elderly clients with sensory deficits in the home may be found at the end of this chapter.

REFERENCES

Atchley R C: *The Social Forces in Later Life.* Wadsworth Publishing Co., Inc., Belmont, California, 1977, p 77
Bates B: *Physical Examination.* 2nd ed. J. B. Lippincott Co., Philadelphia, 1979, p 77
Caird F I, Judge T G: *Assessment of the Elderly Patient.* Pitman Medical Publishing Co. Ltd., Tunbridge Wells, Kent, 1977, p 56

"Cataracts." Preprint, Office of Scientific Reporting, National Eye Institute, Bethesda, Maryland 20205, September 1982, pp 1–18

"Cataract—What It Is and How It Is Treated." National Society to Prevent Blindness and Its Affiliates, New York, Pub. No. G–4, March 1980

Engen T: "Does perception of tastes and odors change with age?" in *Sensory Processes and Aging.* Proceedings of A Conference at the Dallas Geriatric Research Institute. University Center for Community Services, Center for Studies in Aging, School of Community Service, North Texas State University, Denton, Texas, 1977, pp 61–67

"Glaucoma . . . Sneak Thief of Sight." National Society to Prevent Blindness and Its Affiliates, New York, Pub. No. G–1, October 1980

Glorig A: "Auditory processing and age," in *Sensory Processes and Aging.* Proceedings of A Conference at the Dallas Geriatric Research Institute. University Center for Community Services, Center for Studies in Aging, School of Community Service, North Texas State University, Denton, Texas, 1977, p 44

Grzegorszyk P B, Jones S W, Mistretta C M: "Age-related differences in salt taste acuity." *J Geront,* Vol 34, No 6, November 1979, pp 834–40

Hall M R P, MacLennon W J, Lye M D W: *Medical Care of the Elderly.* Springer Publishing Company, Inc., New York, 1978, p 59

Hinchcliffe R: "Aging and sensory thresholds." *J Geront,* Vol 17, No 1–4, 1962, pp 45–50

Horowitz J: "A tonometer at Tiffany's." *Sight-Saving,* Vol 51, No 1, 1982, pp 15–18

Judge R D, Zuidema G D: *Physical Diagnosis: A Physiologic Approach to the Clinical Examination.* 2nd ed. Little, Brown and Co., Boston, 1968, pp 124–125

Kart C S, Metress E S: *Aging and Health: Biologic and Social Perspectives.* Addison-Wesley Publishing Co., Menlo Park, California, 1978, pp 63–64

Kenshalo D R: "Age changes in touch, vibration, temperature, kinesthesis, and pain sensitivity," in Birren J E, Schaie K W: *Handbook of the Psychology of Aging.* Van Nostrand Reinhold Co., New York, 1977, pp 562–79

Kornzweig A L, Klapper R M: "Visual processes and aging," in *Sensory Processes and Aging.* Proceedings of A Conference at the Dallas Geriatric Research Institute. University Center of Community Services, Center for Studies in Aging, School of Community Service, North Texas State University, 1977, p 27

Rockstein M, Chesky J A, Sussman M L: "Comparative biology and evaluation of aging," in Finch C E, Hayflick L (eds.): *Handbook of the Biology of Aging.* Van Nostrand Reinhold Co., New York, 1977, p 12

Saxon S V, Etten M J: *Physical Change and Aging.* The Tiresias Press, New York, 1978, pp 53–73

Sherman J L, Fields S K: *Guide to Patient Evaluation.* 3rd ed. Medical Examination Publishing Co., Inc., Garden City, New York, 1978, pp 122–24

Soll D B: "Glaucoma." *Nurs Digest,* Vol; 3, No 2, March-April 1975, pp 9–12

"The Aging Eye." National Society to Prevent Blindness and Its Affiliates, New York, Publ No. G–3, January 1978

Todd B: "Using eye drops and ointments safely." *Geriat Nurs,* Vol 4, No 1, 1983, pp 53–57

Weinstock F J: "Glaucoma detection: A three-step technique." *Am Fam Phys,* Vol 4, No 1, September 1973, pp 136–41

BIBLIOGRAPHY

Hanawalt A, Troutman K: "If your patient has a hearing aid." *Am J Nurs,* Vol 84, No 7, July 1984, pp 900–901

Here's Help! The Five Senses and the Aging Process, American Health Care Association, N.D.

Resler M M, Tumulty G: "Glaucoma update." *Am J Nurs*, Vol 83, No 5, May 1983, pp 752–56

Sensory Processes and Aging. Proceedings of A Conference at the Dallas Geriatric Research Institute. University Center for Community Services, Center for Studies in Aging, School of Community Service, North Texas State University, 1977

Shore H: "Designing a training program for understanding sensory losses in aging." *The Gerontol*, Vol 16, No 2, April 1976, pp 157–65

Resources for Additional Information About Sensory Deficits

Visual Deficits

American Association of Ophthalmology
1100 17th Street, N.W.
Washington, D.C. 20036

American Council of the Blind
1211 Connecticut Ave., N.W.
Suite 506
Washington, D.C. 20036

American Foundation for the Blind
15 West 16th Street
New York, New York 10011

American Speech and Hearing Association
9030 Old Georgetown Road
Washington, D.C. 20014

Library of Congress
Division for the Blind and Physically
    Handicapped
1219 Taylor Street, N.W.
Washington, D.C. 20542

National Eye Institute
National Institutes of Health
Building 31, Room 6A25
9000 Rockville Pike
Bethesda, Maryland 20014

National Federation of the Blind
1346 Connecticut Ave., N.W.
Washington, D.C. 20036

National Society to Prevent Blindness
79 Madison Avenue
New York, New York 10016
(Check the yellow pages in the telephone directory of most major cities for the address of state and local branches.)

Recording for the Blind, Inc.
215 East 58th Street
New York, New York 10022

State Commission for the Blind
(In each state with local offices)

The Public Affairs Committee
Public Affairs Pamphlets
381 Park Ave. South
New York, New York 10016

Hearing Deficits

Better Hearing Institute
1430 K Street, N.W.
Suite 600
Washington, D.C. 20005

Hearing
Box 1840
Washington, D.C. 20013

National Association of the Deaf
814 Thayer Avenue
Silver Spring, Maryland 20910

Registry of Interpreters for the Deaf
P.O. Box 1339
Washington, D.C. 20013

Teletypewriters for the Deaf
P.O. Box 28332
Washington, D.C. 20005

SAMPLE MASTER CARE PLAN FOR HOME CARE—

Nursing Diagnosis	Assessment	Planning
Alterations in visual perception as a result of cataracts, glaucoma or senile macula degeneration.	• Determine whether the client can read, watch television, walk safely in the home environment. • Observe for broken steps, loose rugs, or toys in the yard or house which could cause the client to fall. • Observe for bruises on the arms or legs caused by the client running into walls or furniture because of decreased vision. • Observe for confusion, paranoia, hallucinations which may occur as a result of sensory deprivation.	*Short-term goal* • Client will seek diagnosis and treatment if visual deficits interfere with Activities of Daily Living and make the home environment hazardous. *Long-term goals* *Client will become adjusted to:* • new eyeglasses (presbyopia) • a new type of lens (cataract) • eye medication (glaucoma) • increasing degrees of visual loss (blindness).

SENSORY DEFICITS—SIGHT

Intervention: Nursing Orders	Intervention: Resources and Support Systems	Evaluation: Expected Outcomes
• Suggest that physical environment of home remain as stable as possible (cataracts, blindness). • Teach family how to help the client move about freely in the environment despite visual losses. • Teach client and family importance of eye examinations every 1-2 years. • Teach client and family how to use eye drops (glaucoma).	• Local chapter of the National Society to Prevent Blindness —Large print books —Talking books —24-hour news and weather electronic device —Glaucoma screening • Local Telephone Company —Large numbered dial —Lighted dial —Cordless telephone • Local Lions Club–Assistance with purchase of eye glasses • Local offices of the State Commission for the Blind —Eye medical care —Counseling • Local hospital–Lifeline system to alert support system if emergency occurs • Medicare–Financial assistance with cataract surgery and lens replacement, walking cane for blind • Local YMCA–For transportation to opthalmologist or for glaucoma screening program	*Client:* • adjusts to new glasses following cataract surgery • uses eye medication for glaucoma regularly as ordered by the physician • has and uses a number of assistive devices which add to feelings of security • has a home enviroment which is stable, safe, secure • remains in home as independent as possible for as long as possible.

SAMPLE MASTER CARE PLAN FOR HOME CARE—

Nursing Diagnoses	Assessment	Planning
Decreased hearing as a result of presbycusis accompanying the aging process	• Assess the client's ability to hear the door bell, telephone, and voices of the nurse and family members. • Determine if the client is able to hear male voices (↓frequency) better than female voices (↑frequency). • Note if a hearing aid has been purchased and is being used and works well.	*Short-terms goals* • Increased use of lip reading and sign language by client. • Increased communication skills of family members and friends. *Long-term goal* Ability to function in the home environment safely despite hearing losses.

SAMPLE MASTER CARE PLAN FOR HOME CARE—

Nursing Diagnoses	Assessment	Planning
Decreased taste perception due to possible changes in taste buds because of aging, the use of dentures, and poor oral hygiene resulting in inadequate nutrition.	• Assess possible loss of taste perception through testing each of the taste buds by mixing each substance in water and touching the particular area of the tongue sensitive to that specific taste. —sweet–sugar (tip of tongue) —salty–salt (tip of tongue) —sour–vinegar (sides of tongue) —bitter–baker's chocolate (back of tongue) • Assess number and types of spices and/or flavorings available in the home.	*Short-term goal* Appetite will remain unchanged or increase if additional nutrition is needed. *Long-term goal* Client will reach a desirable weight.

SENSORY DEFICITS—HEARING

Intervention: Nursing Orders	Intervention: Resources and Support Systems	Evaluation: Expected Outcomes
• Utilize effective communication skills while talking with the client such as: —face-to-face contact so that the client can lip read —speak slower, lower and clear —observe for clues to determine if verbal communication is understood. • Teach family members and friends how to communicate with a hearing-impaired person. • Teach use and mis-use of hearing aides.	• Local telephone company —extra loud ring on telephone —light on telephone which comes on when it rings —amplifier for earpiece to facilitate hearing • Local fire department–Information about smoke detectors which light as well as sound, or have low frequency or high frequency sounds as needed. • Electrical companies–Have door bells which light up as well as sound when rung. • Local organizations for the hearing impaired and deaf which provide counseling, educational materials.	*Client:* • has a hearing aid (if prescribed) and uses it effectively • is able to read lips and use some sign language • has family and friends who communicate effectively with the client • feels safe and secure in the home environment.

SENSORY DEFICITS—TASTE

Intervention: Nursing Orders	Intervention: Resources and Support Systems	Evaluation: Expected Outcomes
• Suggest that spices and/or flavorings allowed be added to foods (e.g., lemon juice, vinegar). • Discourage the excess use of salt, sugar, honey. • Teach the client and family about the four basic food groups and essential nutrients required daily. • Weigh the client at each visit. • Encourage daily oral hygiene and proper care of dentures, if used.	• Meals-on-Wheels–For assistance with hot meals daily which help provide an essential quantity and quality of required nutrients. • Local markets and/or stores–For a variety of spices and flavorings which will enhance the taste of foods. • Family and/or neighbors–Suggest they prepare nutritious individual frozen dinners from family leftovers for the older individual who lives alone. • American Dairy Council–For colorful educational literature on the four food groups.	• Client and family use the four food groups and essential nutrients daily in planning and preparing meals. • Client remains at the desired weight.

SAMPLE MASTER CARE PLAN FOR HOME CARE—

Nursing Diagnoses	Assessment	Planning
Decreased perception of odors as a result of normal aging changes	• Note any unusual odors in the home environment such as urine, feces, disinfectants. • Observe any unusual odors about the client which may be caused by incontinence and/or poor personal hygiene. • Observe the type of heating used in the home. • Examine the stove used for cooking to determine if ON and OFF knobs are clearly marked and functioning properly. • Observe the contents of the refrigerator for odors of spoiled foods. • Assess ability of the client to detect several odors.	*Short-terms goals* • The client and his or her environment are clean. • Environmental hazards which could interfere with the safety of the client are eliminated. *Long-term goal* Client has a safe, secure and clean environment.

SAMPLE MASTER CARE PLAN FOR HOME CARE—

Nursing Diagnosis	Assessment	Planning
Altered sensitivity to touch and decreased perception of pain as a result of normal aging changes	• Assess the client's sensitivity to touch and pain. • Look for signs and symptoms of disease and/or illnesses which normally produce pain but which are absent in the client (for example, sudden confusion rather than pain may be the only outward sign of a myocardial infarction). • Note if hot water bottles or heating pads are used by the client.	*Short-term goal* Client and/or family will become aware of decreased sensitivity to touch and/or pain in the client. *Long-term goal* Client and/or family will have the knowledge and ability to seek medical assistance when unusual signs and symptoms occur.

SENSORY DEFICITS—OLFACTION

Intervention: Nursing Orders	Intervention: Resources and Support Systems	Evaluation: Expected Outcomes
• Assist with personal hygiene measures if needed (bath, oral hygiene, clean clothes). • Teach the client and family about safety factors. —check to be sure that all space heaters and gas cooking stoves are turned off before going to sleep —encourage the use of clear glass containers for left-over foods in the refrigerator so that spoiled foods can be seen better and discarded.	• Home Health Care Agency—To provide for a home health aide to assist with personal care and a homemaker to help with household tasks such as cleaning out the refrigerator and doing the laundry • Local Chapter of the American Red Cross—A family member may wish to take a home nursing course so that he or she can provide the client daily assistance with hygiene measures as needed • Local Fire Department—To check for suspected gas leaks. • Neighbors—Who will be alert to odors and/or fire	• Client and/or family begin to observe for hazards in the environment and take action to prevent those hazards from occurring. • A family member, neighbor or friend are regularly available to help with personal hygiene measures.

SENSORY DEFICITS—TOUCH

Intervention: Nursing Orders	Intervention: Resources and Support Systems	Evaluation: Expected Outcomes
• Teach the client and family that special care is needed in the use of hot water bottles, heating pads, and baths. • Ask a family member to decrease the temperature maintained in the hot water heater to prevent accidental burns during bathing.	Local Mental Health Association—A family member may want to participate in a special course that deals with concerns and health problems of the elderly so that he or she will be more alert to the client's problems and needs.	• Client and family are knowledgeable regarding the concerns associated with decreased sensitivity to touch and pain. • The client has a safe home environment.

SECTION IV
THE FUTURE OF HOME HEALTH CARE

CHAPTER 14

TRENDS AND NEEDS IN HOME HEALTH CARE

Lazelle Emminizer Benefield

In this final chapter it seems appropriate to look at the future of home health care.

The Present Health Care Delivery System

Several components of the health care delivery system in the United States are especially relevant to a discussion of home health care services. These include the aging of our population and subsequent increase in the need for chronic care, increased public interest in self-care, distribution of federal expenditures for health care, the restrictive federal reimbursement of home care services, and the changes occurring in health care financing.

Needs of the Elderly Population

The incidence of chronic disease and functional impairment increases in the elderly population. Because "few services are designed to care for clients on a long-term basis or to provide flexibility in service delivery" (Mayer and Engler, 1982), many have suggested the need for comprehensive services for this growing segment of the population (Lane, 1982).

Reimbursement for Home Health Care

Home health care, under the current Medicare reimbursement guidelines, is defined as illness care. Reimbursement is for home care of acute conditions and chronic conditions during acute phases. Although data indicate that caregivers in the home provide both illness care and maintenance care (Mundinger, 1983), regulations governing Medicare home care restricts payment to illness care where a skilled need and homebound status is demonstrated.

Medicare reimbursement is presently not available for basic services essential to *maintenance* of the frail elderly in their homes. Neither is reimbursement available for long-term chronic disease management in the home. From a holistic perspective, the current system of home care services is fragmented in scope and delivery methods (Mayer and Engler, 1982).

Federal Health Care Expenditures

The United States spends the majority of its health care dollars financing illness care rather than prevention of illness or maintenance of health. Total health expenditures in 1977 equalled $162.6 billion or 8.8 percent of the Gross National Product (GNP) or $737 per person. "Of this amount, $721 per capita was spent for treatment of illness, while only $16 per capita was spent for prevention or health promotion" (Gibson and Fisher, 1977). Three years later, 1980 data indicated that health care costs totalled 9.4% of the Gross National Product (GNP) (US Bureau of the Census, 1981).

Health Care Payment System

Health care financing is changing. Previously, whatever the cost of the care, third party payors reimbursed the provider that dollar amount. The leader in health care financing, the federal government, has shifted the method of Medicare payment for in-hospital care from cost-based to prospective payment (Schaeffer, 1983). This means that for each patient the hospital will be paid a set rate, based on the Diagnostic Related Group (DRG) that the patient's illness or condition matches. Additionally, most private insurance companies have initiated some form of cost containment, perhaps through higher deductibles for certain services or preferred provider organizations (PPOs). "PPOs involve health care organizations who receive a guaranteed volume of patients in trade for discounted fees and other cost saving benefits . . . A hospital, physician group, or third party administrator organizes a PPO by brokering selected provider services at negotiated rates" (Kodner, 1982, p. 60).

The subsequent search for efficiency in a now competitive marketplace will force hospitals to monitor all parameters of patient care, specifically patient length of stay. This may result in premature discharge and patients discharged in more acute stages of illness (Livengood, Smith, and Hallstead, 1983).

High technology ("high tech") care for these patients is being performed at home, rather than in a hospital. Home health agencies provide intermittent visits by registered nurse staff to provide technical skill and teach clients and families to care for these conditions. Medicare reimbursement for these home care services is presently based on the cost of services provided; however, prospective payment for home health care services is a strong possibility in the near future.

Consumers and Health

Finally, consumers of all ages have shown an interest in self care and decision making regarding their personal health and their medical care. Consumers have begun to take a more active role in the maintenance of their health. Self-help groups abound and the general knowledge level regarding health behaviors has improved. The elderly are beginning to seek and utilize free or low–cost health care services in the community, such as hypertension and glaucoma screening and health education programs which emphasize self help and wellness.

The population of the United States is aging, and large numbers of consumers are in need of services to meet their illness and health care needs. The method for payment of services is changing and cost containment is essential for all health institutions and agencies that plan to stay in business. Current federal reimbursement for home health services focuses on illness care. Many believe in a more comprehensive model of service delivery; providing such care in a marketplace of limited resources is a continuing challenge. Consumers are becoming aware of the limited resources available for comprehensive health care. They are also becoming more aware of health maintenance and are beginning to take a more active role in individual maintenance of a healthy state.

The Future of Home Health Care

Health care costs have skyrocketed in the last few years. The Health Care Financing Administration (HCFA) is attempting to curb the continuing increase by using the DRG system of reimbursement for hospital care. The DRG system has introduced competition into the marketplace. Cost containment is now the norm, and how policymakers divide up the dollars available for health care (illness and wellness) has taken on new significance. Assuming the need for cost containment, home health care services will expand and diversify; competition will increase; qualified staff and managers will be in short supply; and creative management of human, capital and fiscal resources will be the norm.

Illness and Wellness for Home Care?

The scope and purpose of home health care services will expand and grow as the need arises and when and if reimbursement for services expands. Service expansion will occur because: 1) there is a population in need of assistance to maintain stability at home and/or recuperate from illness after hospitalization and 2) home health care in many cases is less costly than hospitalization. Whether the expansion in home services will be primarily in illness care or chronic maintenance care and health maintenance depends on the allocation of dollars by federal and state governments and/or private insurance companies.

Many groups suggest expansion to a more comprehensive health care model that would include prevention as well as health maintenance and promotion. The ideal home care model would provide illness care, health maintenance, chronic care, and disease prevention. This model would interface with community–supported programs that assist clients in maintaining their independence. However, the ideal home care model may not prevail because of the narrow reimbursement focus which does not provide for comprehensive services. The illness model may continue to shape home care for some time. In the future, there may be a more active response by Congress in implementing chronic health care funding. Over the last four years, several bills have been introduced into Congress that would provide for such funding (Palley and Oktay, 1983).

For any comprehensive model to receive congressional support and funding, society will need to indicate its willingness to accept the model and finance its cost. The United States has struggled to finance care for the poor and the less fortunate. Comprehensive care would require much more financial support and planning. There is also an attempt "to strike a better balance between promoting wellness and treating illness" (Nelson and Simmons, 1983).

Diversification in Services

Home health agencies have begun to diversify, both in health services and in other non-health related ventures. Services will include care throughout the life span such as maternity, pediatric, and hospice care, and private pay homemaker/companion services. Mothers and newborns can be discharged from hospitals to home care within 24 hours of delivery; pediatric oncology care is being provided in the home; and hospice services have proven their worth in improving the quality of life.

Expansion of home health services will occur for three major reasons: (1) the need for services has been created through increasing public awareness and strong home health care marketing to potential clients; (2) home care services may be a less costly alternative to hospitalization; and (3) agencies will attempt to increase the non-Medicare population (to decrease the percentage of potentially "prospective pay" clients) by increasing the percentage of charge-based payors.

Diversification is occurring in high technology areas such as intravenous (IV) therapy, 24-hour assisted ventilation, total parenteral nutrition (TPN), and chemotherapy. The change in hospital reimbursement, with the potential for earlier hospital discharge and the need for services that provide care for sicker individuals, promote this expansion of services.

High technology skills will be needed to provide these expanded services. Agencies will not survive without providing staff coverage 24-hours a day, seven days a week.

Expansion is also occurring in areas not traditionally seen as home care such as transportation services, the supplying of durable medical equipment, offering supplemental nursing and aide services to hospitals, and subcontracting with nursing homes for use of agency therapists. Agency diversification will be viewed as expanded business ventures. The economic climate mandates fiscal accountability; thus, agencies will expand to other reimbursable services to maintain their viability so that the primary mission of providing a range of home services to consumers can be maintained.

Consumer Interest will Increase

As public awareness of home health services increases, so will the utilization of these services by consumers. At the present time home care may have less than its rightful share of consumer support, probably due to lack of knowledge about available services. However, the public has begun to focus on the advantages of home care, such as recuperation in a familiar environment, maintenance of independence, and a less costly alternative to institutionalization. Many private insurance companies also are encouraging home care. This public awareness is increasing among those consumers under age 65.

Expansion in Number of Agencies

The number of home care providers is rapidly increasing. From 1977 to 1982 there was a 62% increase in Medicare-certified agencies. In 1977 there were 2,589 certified agencies and as of November, 1983 their number had jumped to 4,204. Hospitals, physicians, nursing homes, private corporations and individuals have started home health agencies. For example, most hospitals are evaluating their need for a home care program as a means to: (1) move patients quickly from the hospital so as to maximize income from DRG prospective payment; (2) keep patients within the hospital corporate structure; and (3) provide continuity of care to patients who may have acute needs upon discharge.

Competition Will Continue

Competition for patients will continue to be strong since all providers want to protect their marketshare. In the past, physically adjacent hospitals and home health agencies may have operated with separate boards and mission; now formal coordination of service is beginning to occur. Home health agencies have begun to discuss coordination of services and joint business ventures with hospitals, with industry health coalitions, and with health maintenance organizations (HMOs). As a result of the competition, mergers may occur between agencies or groups of home health agencies.

Shortage of Qualified Practitioners and Managers

The expansion in number of agencies and the diversification into high technology services will cause an acute need for qualified nursing staff. Knowledge of public health principles, family and individual counseling, health education and strategies of adult learning, as well as mastery of advanced technical care (such as intravenous therapy and total parenteral nutrition) are prerequisites to providing care in the home setting. Home health care is not hospital care in the home setting. More independent judgment is necessary to function in home care than within the structure of a hospital where immediate assistance and supervision is usually available. Also, the traditional public health or community health nurse may not have had preparation or experience in some of the newer "high tech" skills being performed in the home. Unfortunately, many currently practicing nurses have little experience in home care nursing. Also, most nursing education programs provide their students with only limited education or supervised experience in home care nursing. Therefore, the pool of *qualified* nurse candidates for employment in home health care is limited. The need for and training of practitioners in other disciplines should also be stressed.

The complexities of managing an agency require individuals with knowledge of home health care administration, clinical care, fiscal planning, marketing, and long-range planning as well as skill in personnel management. Managers are needed who can creatively manage human, capital and fiscal resources. In this time of fiscal restraint, the major question all agencies must ask is how to provide quality service with limited resources. As hospitals are presently doing, all home health agencies have and will continue looking for methods to cut expenses. The largest percentage of the budget is usually direct salary expenses. The future will bring increased emphasis on productivity standards, staffing schedules, and the use of contract and part-time staff.

Computerization of data (although not identified as a separate topic) is certainly essential to efficient and effective home care management in the future. Administrators can manage only when internal and external agency data can be quickly condensed to provide reports that accurately monitor the functions of an agency. Most agencies will use some form of in-house computer/management information system for a range of services such as: (1) billing, (2) cashflow, (3) statistics, (4) productivity standards, (5) demographics of referral patterns, (6) strategic planning, (7) staff recruitment, and (8) staff availability 24 hours a day, seven days a week.

Home Health Care Advocacy

What can nurses do to impact the delivery of home health care services? How can nurses educate others about the complex needs that clients and families have when caring for themselves or a family member at home? What strategies will promote a more comprehensive model of home health care delivery?

Involvement in Health Care Planning and Policymaking

Nurses must increase their involvement in health care planning and policymaking. If nurse experts in home health care do not determine priorities for home care, policymakers at the national and state level will do so without suggestions from providers. The 1982 merger between the National Association of Home Health

Agencies and the NLN Council of Home Health Agencies/Community Health Services (Wortley, 1982) is an example of two organizations merging to develop a more unified voice representing home care.

Research in Resource Allocation

Nurses must also determine the human and capital resources needed to provide comprehensive care and must develop creative ways to deliver and evaluate quality care. Research is certainly needed in these areas. Further investigation is needed in how "different configurations of service, different mixes of service, and different providers of service are suited for different communities . . . . We need to learn more about different kinds of organizational models, and the cost effectiveness of a variety of combinations of services for different mixes of patient characteristics" (Vladeck, 1983). It cannot be assumed that our current models of home health care delivery are the most cost efficient.

Clinicians, researchers and administrators must work quickly to evaluate current methods of home care delivery and to investigate creative alternatives. For example, it could be said that patient satisfaction must be present for quality care, yet policymakers respond that limited data are present to validate that assertion.

What specifically contributes to patient satisfaction? Can it be observed and measured? Does patient satisfaction equal quality care? Can patient outcomes and well-being be measured? Does it cost more to provide quality nursing care? Is the Congress (and the general public) willing to increase health care spending or reallocate dollars to achieve quality care?

Education for the Future

Nurses in home health care agencies must educate their colleagues in hospitals about home health care services and discharge planning. The patient assessment that a professional nurse performs when a patient is admitted to a hospital provides clues to the need for later home care services. For example, is there a family support system? Was the patient admitted because he or she could not cope with the chronic disease medication regimen? Are there multiple medical and/or nursing diagnoses? The hospital nurse should assess and determine early in the patient's hospitalization if the individual and/or family will need home care.

Home health care nurses must maintain a strong clinical base. McCormick (1983) reviewed and documented the technologic future. Home health nurses are needed who are knowledgeable, thorough and understand how to provide nursing care in this increasingly complex society. Besides the need for technical skills and maturity of judgment, comfort with independent functioning is critical to satisfactory performance. Efficiency is also expected when caring for clients in their homes. In addition, the nurse in home health care needs a high degree of sophistication in dealing with families in all stages of wellness and illness. The nurse will provide the "high touch" needed in this "high tech" environment

(Naisbitt, 1984). Kelly (1984) stated that it is the "highly qualified nurse who attends to the human factor—the patient as an individual. It is the nurse who can identify and sometimes prevent potential problems, teach, counsel, reassure and provide the continuity of care necessary beyond hospital walls—the high touch that all the high tech available cannot replace."

Educators have the responsibility of providing students with these experiences in public health science and home care nursing. Presentation of content in geron-tological nursing care is particularly important in preparing future practitioners to care for an aging society. In addition, more agency administrators will need to open their agencies for student learning experiences as well as provide sites for re-search.

Finally, caregivers must understand the health care delivery system and the complexities and inequities of financing health care. Students and practitioners should be aware that, in reality, access to health care may not be a right of every individual. Lest nurses become discouraged that a two-tiered system of health care is evolving, one for those with "good insurance" or self payment and the other for those with no ability to pay, nurses need to recognize that health care policy is changing. For example, in recent years resource growth "in Medicaid and the private sector has been diverted from institutions to community-based services" (Vladeck, 1983). However, the process is slow. The challenge is to work with the current system and attempt to change components that are undesirable while promoting those that are vital to quality care in the future.

Summary

The aging population, changes in health care financing, and the need for more comprehensive services will all affect the need for expansion in home health care. In the future agencies will continue to increase in number, diversify to meet consumer need, and market their diversification as business ventures in a com-petitive marketplace. Qualified staff and managers will be in short supply to meet the demands of an increasingly complex technological and humanistic field of home health care services delivery.

Nurses can affect change in the home health care system by increasing their involvement in health care planning and policymaking by documenting the com-plex needs of clients and families in home care and by developing cost–effective means to provide quality services. Nurses need to understand the complexities of home health care delivery and coordinate the education of student practitioners in the areas of community health, home care, and gerontology. Research is needed to validate and develop new strategies for health care delivery and management of resources.

Health policy that increases the scope and funding of home health care will occur when public policy and documented research influence congressional decision making.

REFERENCES

Gibson R, Fisher C: National Health Expenditures: Fiscal year 1977. *Social Security Bulletin*, July 1978, 41, 3–20

Kelly L: "High tech/high touch—now more than ever." Editorial. *Nurs Outlook*, Vol 32, No 1, January 1984, p 15

Kodner K: "Competition, getting a fix on PPOs." *Hospitals*, Vol 56, No 22, 1982, pp 59–66

Lane L: "Long term care: The challenge from the 1981 White House Conference on Aging." *Pride Institute Journal of Long Term Home Health Care*, Vol 1, No 1, 1982, p 29

Livengood W, Smith C, Hallstead S: "The impact of DRGs on home health care." *Home Health Care Nurse*, Vol 1, No 1, 1983, pp 29–34

Mayer M, Engler M: "Demographic change and the elderly population: Its implications for long term care." *Pride Institute Journal of Long Term Home Health Care* Vol 1, No 1, 1982, pp 21–28

McCormick K: "Preparing nurses for the technologic future." *Nursing and Health Care*, Vol 4, No 7, 1983, pp 379–382

Mundinger M: *Home Care Controversy–Too Little, Too Late, Too Costly*. Aspen Systems Corporation, Rockville, Maryland, 1983, pp 104–105

Naisbitt J: *Megatrends*. Warner Books, New York, 1982

Nelson E, Simmons J: "Health promotion—the second public health revolution: Promise or threat?" *Family and Community Health*, Vol 5, No 4, 1983, pp 1–15

Palley H, Oktay J: "In-home and other community-based long-term care: A critical review of some legislative proposals and recent national legislation." *Home Health Care Services Quarterly*, Vol 4, No 7, 1983, pp 379–382

Shaffer F: "DRGs: History and overview.: *Nursing and Health Care*, Vol 4, No 7, 1983, pp 388–396

U.S. Bureau of the Census. Statistical Abstracts of the United States, 1981. 102 Ed. Washington, D.C., U.S. Government Printing Office, 1981, pp 99

Vladeck B: "Two steps forward, one back: The changing agenda of long term care reform." *Pride Institute Journal of Long Term Health Care*, Vol 2, No 3, 1983, pp 3–9

Wortley D: Chairman's Editorial. *Caring*, October, 1982, p 1

BIBLIOGRAPHY

Moore F, Layzer E: "Supporting the homemaker-home health aide as a valuable player on the home care team." *Pride Institute Journal of Long Term Home Health Care*, Vol 2, No 3, 1983, pp 19–23

APPENDIX: Organizations of Home Health Care Agencies

Name (Abbreviation)	Address	Goal/Purpose	Membership
National Association for Home Care (NAHC)	519 C Street, N.E. Stanton Park Washington, D.C. 20002	To provide an organized and unified voice for home care industry	*Voting Members:* Home Health Agencies Hospices Homemaker/Home Health Aide Organizations Corporations or groups interested in home care *Non-Voting Members:* Individuals interested in home care State associations representing home care providers
American Federation of Home Health Agencies, Inc. (AFHHA)	429 N Street, S.W. Suite S-605 Washington, D.C. 20024	To influence public policy regarding home health care	Medicare certified home health agencies
National HomeCaring Council	235 Park Avenue South New York, N.Y. 10003	To promote high quality homemaker-home health aide services	Agencies providing homemaker-home health aide services Individuals concerned with quality home-maker-home health aide services State associations interested in develop-ing and expanding quality homemaker home health aide services
National League for Nurs-ing Council of Community Health Services	10 Columbus Circle New York, N.Y. 10019	To promote NLN's com-mitment to nursing and quality health care	Agencies providing community health services
Home Health Services and Staffing Association (HHSSA)	815 Connecticut Ave., N.W. Suite 206 Washington, D.C. 20006	To advance the views of the home health care in-dustry before Congress, federal regulatory bodies, and state legislatures	Free standing, investor owned, taxpaying home health agencies
American Affiliated Visit-ing Nurse Associations/ Services	21 Maryland Plaza Suite 300 St. Louis, MO. 63108	Promotes voluntary, non-profit VNA/S as the pro-vider of choice in home health services delivery	Open to VNAs/Ss

INDEX